Anesthesia
Pearls

Anesthesia Pearls

JAMES DUKE, MD
Associate Director of Anesthesiology
Denver Health Medical Center
Associate Professor of Anesthesiology
University of Colorado Health Sciences Center
Denver, Colorado

DUKE

WO 215   H0802636

HANLEY & BELFUS, INC. / Philadelphia

Publisher: HANLEY & BELFUS, INC.
                 Medical Publishers
                 210 S. 13th Street
                 Philadelphia, PA 19107
                 (215) 546-7293, 800-962-1892
                 FAX (215) 790-9330
                 Website: http://www.hanleyandbelfus.com

Library of Congress Control Number: 2002107107

ANESTHESIA PEARLS   ISBN 1-56053-495-8

Last digit is the print number: 9 8 7 6 5 4 3 2 1

CONTENTS

Patient   **Page**

CONTRIBUTORS

Rita Agarwal, MD
Associate Professor, Fellowship Director, Department of Anesthesiology, The Children's Hospital, University of Colorado Health Sciences Center, Denver, Colorado

Craig A. Andersen, CRNA, MA
Staff Nurse Anesthetist, Denver Health Medical, Denver, Colorado

Rodger E. Barnette, MD
Professor, Departments of Anesthesiology and Internal Medicine, Temple University School of Medicine, Temple Hospital, Philadelphia, Pennsylvania

Elaine F. Broad, MD
Department of Anesthesiology, University of Colorado Health Sciences Center, Denver, Colorado

Alexander A. Carrillo, MD
Resident, Department of Anesthesiology, University of Colorado Health Sciences Center, Denver, Colorado

Mark H. Chandler, MD
Department of Anesthesiology, University of Colorado Health Sciences Center, Denver, Colorado

Shawn Dufford, MD
Resident, Department of Anesthesiology, University of Colorado Health Sciences Center, Denver, Colorado

James C. Duke, MD
Associate Director of Anesthesiology, Denver Health Medical Center, Associate Professor, Department of Anesthesiology, University of Colorado Health Sciences Center, Denver, Colorado

Brian J. Hopkins, MD
Resident, Department of Anesthesiology, University of Colorado Health Sciences Center, Denver, Colorado

Kathryn P. King, MD
Assistant Clinical Professor, Department of Anesthesiology, Duke University Medical Center, Durham, North Carolina

Jason P. Krutsch, MD
Resident, Department of Anesthesiology, University of Colorado Health Sciences Center, Denver, Colorado

Sunil Kumar, MD
Assistant Professor, Department of Anesthesiology, University of Colorado Health Sciences Center, Denver Health Medical Center, Denver, Colorado

Anthony Lee, MD
Resident, Department of Anesthesiology, University of Colorado Health Sciences Center, Denver, Colorado

John D. Lockrem, MD
Director of Anesthesiology, Denver Health Medical Center, Associate Professor, Department of Anesthesiology, University of Colorado Health Sciences Center, Denver, Colorado

Howard J. Miller, MD
Assistant Professor, Department of Anesthesiology, University of Colorado Health Sciences Center, Denver Health Medical Center, Denver, Colorado

Cyrus Mirshab, MD
Resident, Department of Anesthesiology, University of Colorado Health Sciences Center, Denver, Colorado

Gordon H. Morewood, MD
Assistant Professor, Director of Perioperative Echocardiography, Department of Anesthesiology, Temple University School of Medicine, Philadelphia, Pennsylvania

William Nel, MD
Assistant Professor, Department of Anesthesiology, University of Colorado Health Sciences Center, Denver, Colorado

David M. Polaner, MD
Associate Professor, Department of Anesthesiology, University of Colorado Health Sciences Center, Attending Pediatric Anesthesiologist, The Children's Hospital, Denver, Colorado

Marc A. Rozner, MD, PhD
Associate Professor of Anesthesiology, Associate Professor of Cardiology, Director of Perioperative Program, Division of Anesthesiology and Critical Care, University of Texas, MD Anderson Cancer Center, Houston, Texas

Scott A. Schartel, DO
Associate Professor and Director of Resident Education, Department of Anesthesiology, Temple University School of Medicine, Temple Hospital, Philadelphia, Pennsylvania

Kenneth M. Swank, MD
Assistant Professor, Department of Anesthesiology, University of Colorado Health Sciences Center, Denver Health Medical Center, Denver, Colorado

Ronald Valdivieso, MD
Assistant Professor, Department of Anesthesiology, University of Colorado Health Sciences Center, Denver Health Medical Center, Denver, Colorado

Philip M. Vercio, MD
Private Practice, Great Falls, Montana

Kristin T. Woodward, MD
Resident, Department of Anesthesiology, University of Colorado Health Sciences Center, Denver, Colorado

Eric Zeeb, MD
Resident, Department of Anesthesiology, University of Colorado Health Sciences Center, Denver, Colorado

DEDICATION

For my mom and dad, Lorraine and Dave, with love.

PREFACE

Anesthesia Pearls was written to complement *Anesthesia Secrets,* a popular text currently in its second edition. Both texts were edited by me and created with the assistance of my peers at Denver Health Medical Center and across the country, and also with contributions from anesthesia residents of the University of Colorado Department of Anesthesiology. While the format of *Anesthesia Secrets* was topical, *Anesthesia Pearls* uses a patient scenario format. This text differs somewhat from other volumes of the Pearls Series® as the practice of anesthesia tends to be less diagnosis-driven, and therefore you will find fewer "guess the diagnosis" chapters than in other Pearls books. So what is emphasized? One might think of them as "issues," perhaps a phenomenon receiving increasing scrutiny, such as postoperative visual loss, saline infusion-related metabolic acidosis, or the response under anesthesia to medications that blunt the renin-angiotensin system. Many of the cases review therapy or address treatment dilemmas. As anesthesia is a procedure-intensive specialty, some chapters are devoted to procedural difficulties that have proven troublesome. Finally, I challenged myself and encouraged my contributors to address their topics from an evidence-based perspective, balancing brevity with "the whole story." I appreciate that readers have a life beyond their profession, other interests and obligations, and significant time limitations. **All chapters conclude with take-home messages called Clinical Pearls.**

Anesthesia Pearls consists of 50 chapters, but, as this is written, I'm thinking of more chapters for the second edition! And I can always use some help. If you have an interesting case or a favorite topic you'd like to review, I'd be happy to consider your contribution. Thank you for your interest in *Anesthesia Pearls.*

James Duke, MD
Department of Anesthesiology
Denver Health Medical Center
MC 0218 777 Bannock Street
Denver, CO 80204
james.duke@dhha.org

Alexander A. Carrillo, MD

PATIENT 1

A 47-year-old woman with post–spinal anesthetic pain and dysesthesias

A 47-year-old woman is scheduled for a diagnostic dilation and curettage for dysmenorrhea. She has a 20-year history of hypertension that has been treated with β-blockers. She has no history of neurologia disease or back pain and is otherwise healthy. She consents to subarachnoid block. The anesthesia is performed in a standard fashion and is technically unremarkable. The position of the 24G pencil-point Sprotte needle was confirmed by free flow of cerebrospinal fluid. After aspiration of cerebrospinal fluid, 75 mg of hyperbaric lidocaine (5% in 7.5% dextrose) is injected. No pain or paresthesias are elicited during placement of the needle or drug injection. The patient is returned to the supine position until an anesthetic level of T8 is achieved, then is placed in the lithotomy position. No episodes of hypotension or hypoxemia occur during the procedure, which is uneventful and lasts 15 minutes. The patient has full return of sensorimotor function within 45 minutes, is able to void, and soon thereafter is discharged home in good condition.

The following day, the patient calls complaining of a burning, aching pain that has developed in the buttocks and radiates down bilaterally through her posterior thighs and calves. The pain is worse at night and improves with ambulation. She denies headache, fever, numbness, or weakness, and there has been no difficulty with bowel or bladder function. She returns for evaluation.

Physical Examination: Vital signs normal. Neurologic: normal. No nuchal rigidity.

Questions: What is the diagnosis?
What are the common findings in patients with this disorder?
What recommendations do you have for the patient?
Form a differential diagnosis for a patient with lower extremity neurologic complaints after subarachnoid block.

What is the diagnosis? Transient neurologic syndrome (TNS).

What are the common findings in patients with TNS? Common findings in patients with TNS include pain or dysesthesias in the buttocks radiating to the dorsolateral aspect of the thighs and calves. The pain has been described alternately as sharp and lancinating or dull, aching, cramping, or burning. Usually, symptoms improve with moving about, are worse at night, and respond to non-steroidal antiinflammatory drugs (NSAIDs). The pain is moderate to severe in at least 70% of patients with TNS and diminishes over time, resolving spontaneously within approximately 1 week in about 90%. It is extremely rare for pain to continue beyond 2 weeks. Significantly, no objective neurologic findings are encountered.

Schneider et al[3] first described TNS in 1993. They reported four cases of significant buttock and lower extremity radicular pain occurring after resolution of hyperbaric lidocaine spinal anesthesia in women undergoing procedures in the lithotomy position. Pain was the principal complaint, and the patients had no sensorimotor deficits or bowel and bladder dysfunction. The pain symptoms resolved spontaneously within days. Schneider et al[3] proposed positional stretching of the cauda equina while exposed to the local anesthetic solution may have played a role in these transient syndromes and that a direct neurotoxic effect of lidocaine itself should be considered.

A prospective, blind, nonrandomized study followed from the same institution in 1995. The patients underwent gynecologic or obstetric procedures using spinal anesthesia with either 5% hyperbaric lidocaine or 0.5% hyperbaric bupivacaine. Hampl et al[4] found that 44 patients (37%) receiving lidocaine developed transient neurologic symptoms compared with only 1 patient administered bupivacaine. All patients receiving lidocaine were placed in the lithotomy position, whereas 62% of the bupivacaine group were placed in the lithotomy position. The one patient who developed a neurologic finding after receiving bupivacaine had transient numbness along the lateral aspect of the right foot after having had a 200-minute procedure with her feet in ankle straps; a pressure effect from the strap was considered to be the cause in this case. The procedures performed using bupivacaine lasted significantly longer (51 minutes) than the procedures using lidocaine (16 minutes), suggesting the duration of exposure in the lithotomy procedure was not a contributing feature.

Subsequently, Pollock et al[5] performed a randomized, double-blinded, prospective study to identify further factors associated with TNS. They found 16% of their patients receiving lidocaine experienced TNS compared with no patients receiving bupivacaine. Developing TNS was independent of the presence of dextrose or concentration of lidocaine used (5% hyperbaric versus 2% isobaric lidocaine). They found no association with gender, weight, age, needle type, difficulty with block placement, or paresthesias during block placement. Positioning may have been a factor.

Despite several years of lidocaine use, this syndrome has been described and investigated systematically only more recently. Although recognition may have been delayed because of the mild and self-limited nature of the symptoms, greater consideration given to postanesthetic complaints followed the occurrence of cauda equina syndrome associated with use of 28G microcatheters for continuous spinal anesthesia. Patients developing cauda equina syndrome experienced long-standing or permanent perineal and lower extremity sensorimotor deficits and bowel, bladder, and sexual dysfunction. It seemed in these cases that satisfactory levels of anesthesia were not achieved reliably because of nonuniform distribution of the local anesthetic. Practitioners redosed these catheters repeatedly, exposing the patient to large concentrations of local anesthetic (doses of > 200 mg of hyperbaric lidocaine were reported). Laboratory models later determined that a lack of turbulence associated with injection of these microcatheters led to pooling of the local anesthetic distal to the lordotic curve of the lumbar vertebrae. Microcatheters subsequently were removed from the market.

Neither the presence of dextrose, opioids, or epinephrine nor the baricity or osmolarity of the solution seems to be a factor in producing TNS. Chemical contaminants, such as detergents used for cleaning, and reusing supplies have been implicated in the past in producing arachnoiditis, but spinal kits are now disposable and nonreusable. Stretching of the spinal cord nerves or roots (as might occur in the lithotomy position), potentially producing nerve root ischemia, has been considered a potential factor, although in Hampl's study patients in the litothomy position who received bupivacaine did not develop TNS. Freedman et al[6] described factors that did not apparently increase the risk of developing TNS, including age, gender, preexisting neurologic disorder or back pain, needle type or size, or bevel direction during injection. Lithotomy position after receiving lidocaine and outpatient procedures did increase risk of TNS. Experimental studies in animals have provided ample evidence that some local anesthetics in clinically relevant concentrations can injure nerve tissue, and lidocaine is more neurotoxic than bupivacaine. Pollock et al[5] found that the concentration of lidocaine administered (2% versus 5%) did not affect the incidence of TNS. Significant objective manifestations of local anesthetic neurotoxicity when administered spinally in single doses have not been evident in large-scale studies, however. The cause of TNS has yet to be elucidated fully.

What recommendations can be made to a patient who is found to have lower extremity pain after a spinal anesthetic? The patient's prior medical history and medications and the anesthetic record should be reviewed. Did the patient receive a lidocaine spinal anesthetic? Were pain or paresthesias elicited during needle insertion or drug injection? Was the patient hypoxemic or hypotensive intraoperatively or postoperatively? Systemic signs and symptoms (e.g., fever, headache) should be sought and queries made for objective neurologic findings (weak or numb extremities, bowel and bladder dysfunction). If any such abnormalities are detected or if pain is incapacitating, a return to the hospital for evaluation is warranted. If the interview reveals nothing remarkable except for the complaints of pain in the buttocks and legs, it is reasonable to reassure the patient that the symptoms likely will resolve in a matter of days and might respond favorably to NSAIDs and ambulation. Patients should be advised to contact the physician or return to the hospital should symptoms worsen. It is advisable to continue follow-up until the patient's complaints resolve.

Should the use of lidocaine as a spinal anesthetic be discontinued? Authorities disagree on this issue. As has been mentioned, lidocaine has a long history of effective and safe use. If lidocaine spinal anesthesia caused functional impairment, it would have been recognized some time ago. It also seems that the morbidity is relatively minor and of brief duration. It seems that the higher end of lidocaine neurotoxicity was observed when continuous spinal microcatheters were used; we may be observing the lower end of lidocaine neurotoxicity in patients developing TNS. The decision to discontinue use of lidocaine would be an easy one if an alternative nontoxic local anesthetic of short duration were available, but no such compound currently is available. Until that time, practitioners must decide for themselves whether to continue using lidocaine when considering spinal anesthesia.

Form a differential diagnosis for a patient with lower extremity neurologic complaints after subarachnoid block. The differential diagnosis for the patient's symptoms includes cauda equina syndrome, nerve root injury, herniated intervertebral disk, meningitis, ischemic neurologic injury, and epidural abscess or hematoma. Because the patient lacks bowel or bladder dysfunction and objective sensorimotor defects, cauda equina syndrome is unlikely. Nerve root injury would be associated with pain during performance of the spinal anesthetic, either during placement of the needle or during injection of local anesthetic. The patient's history is not what usually is associated with a herniated disk, and although it is conceivable that the spinal needle could encounter a disk, it is rare, and the patient probably would have objective neurologic findings with disk herniation. Meningitis would be associated with systemic signs and symptoms, headache, and nuchal rigidity. Hypotensive episodes or hypoxemia would accompany an ischemic neurologic injury. Epidural abscess likely would be associated with fever, pronounced back pain, and objective neurologic findings. Although not invariable, patients with epidural hematoma usually are on anticoagulants, have stigmata of a bleeding disorder, or have a prior history of bleeding events. Additionally, objective neurologic findings would be evident. With the exception of pain in her buttocks and lower extremities, the patient had absolutely no neurologic findings, which led to the diagnosis of TNS associated with spinal anesthesia with 5% lidocaine.

Clinical Pearls

1. TNS should be suspected in a patient who has received a lidocaine spinal anesthetic and has postanesthetic complaints of pain in the buttocks and dorsal lower extremities. There are no objective neurologic findings with this syndrome.

2. The incidence of TNS is not inconsequential (16% to 37%), and patients who are being considered for lidocaine spinal anesthesia should be apprised of symptoms they may experience as part of the consent process.

3. After careful questioning to rule out serious causes for the patient's symptoms, NSAIDs and ambulation can be recommended for patients experiencing TNS. Severe pain and objective symptoms warrant evaluation by a medical provider.

4. TNS has not been associated with bupivacaine. Some practitioners may decide to use this drug as an alternative for lidocaine at the expense of a prolonged postoperative recovery.

REFERENCES

1. Lambert DH, Hurley RJ: Cauda equina syndrome and continuous spinal anesthesia. Anesth Analg 72:817–819, 1991.
2. Rigler ML, Drasner K, Krejcie TC, et al: Cauda equina syndrome after continuous spinal anesthesia. Anesth Analg 72:275–281, 1991.
3. Schneider M, Ettllin T, Kaufmann M, et al: Transient neurologic toxicity after hyperbaric subarachnoid anesthesia with 5% lidocaine. Anesth Analg 76:1154–1157, 1993.
4. Hampl KF, Schneider MC, Ummenhofer W, et al: Transient neurologic symptoms after spinal anesthesia. Anesth Analg 81:1148–1153, 1995.
5. Pollock JE, Neal JM, Stephenson CA, et al: Prospective study of the incidence of transient radicular irritation in patients undergoing spinal anesthesia. Anesthesiology 84:1361–1367, 1996.
6. Freedman JM, De-Kun L, Drasner K, et al: Transient neurologic symptoms after spinal anesthesia. Anesthesiology 89:633–641, 1998.
7. Hodgson PS, Neal JM, Pollock JE, et al: The neurotoxicity of drugs given intrathecally. Anesth Analg 88:797–809, 1999.

Jason Krutsch, MD

PATIENT 2

A 60-year-old man with postoperative visual loss

A 60-year-old man was scheduled for a three-level lumbosacral laminectomy and diskectomy. He had a history of type 2 diabetes mellitus, hypertension, and a 50-pack-year smoking history. Previous anesthetics were without complication. Medications included glyburide and captopril. He had no known drug allergies.

Physical Examination: Afebrile, pulse 77, respirations 14, blood pressure 152/92, oxygen saturation 94%. General appearance: Moderately obese man in no apparent distress. HEENT: unremarkable without gross visual deficits. Neck: carotids 2+ bilaterally with normal upstroke and no bruits. Chest, heart, abdomen, and extremities examinations were unremarkable. Neurologic: bilateral lower extremity stocking-distribution sensory loss; otherwise unremarkable.

Laboratory Findings: Hct 40%, blood glucose 178 mg/dL. Remaining hematology, coagulation profiles, and chemistries: normal. ECG: normal sinus rhythm. Chest radiograph: normal.

Hospital Course: The patient underwent induction and intubation. He was turned prone, he was well padded, and ventilation and hemodynamics were satisfactory. The procedure lasted for 6 hours, and during a period of vigorous blood loss, the patient had a period of relative hypotension lasting roughly 30 minutes. His blood pressure averaged 90/40 mmHg for about 30 minutes and for 5 minutes was 60/30 mmHg. Fluid resuscitation totaled 4 L of crystalloid and 1 Liter of colloid. Estimated blood loss was approximately 2,500 mL with a postoperative hematocrit of 24%. On awakening, the patient immediately complained of bilateral loss of vision without ocular pain. Neurologic examination was otherwise normal.

Postoperatively, ophthalmologists examining the patient find markedly decreased visual acuity (counting fingers at 10 feet). The pupils are minimally reactive to light bilaterally but react briskly to convergence. Anterior segment and funduscopic examinations are unremarkable. A CT scan is performed 24 hours later and reveals only enlargement of the intraorbital optic nerve.

Questions: What is the diagnosis?
What are the possible causes of postoperative visual loss?
Describe the vascular supply of the retina and optic nerve.
What patient factors and intraoperative factors may predispose one to postoperative visual loss?

What is the diagnosis? Ischemic optic neuropathy (ION).

What are the possible causes of postoperative visual loss? Postoperative visual loss (POVL) is a devastating postoperative complication. It has been reported after cardiopulmonary bypass, prone spine surgery, hip arthroplasty, general surgical abdominal procedures, craniotomies, and procedures on the head and neck. Overall, POVL is relatively infrequent. A retrospective review found only 1 case of visual loss in 60,965 nonocular surgical procedures. Visual loss associated with cardiopulmonary bypass is more frequent, however, and may be 1%. There is a perception that POVL has increased; this may be due to increased reporting, or surgeries may be more frequent in patients at risk. The American Society of Anesthesiologists (ASA) Committee on Professional Liability has established a POVL database to understand this problem better.

The differential diagnosis of POVL includes ION, cortical blindness, retinal artery occlusion, and ophthalmic venous obstruction. ION is of greatest interest to the anesthesiologist. The reader is referred to the excellent review by Williams et al[2] for a broader discussion.

Describe the vascular supply of the retina and optic nerve. A review of the blood supply of the retina and optic nerve is pertinent (see Figure below). The anterior portion of the optic nerve, including the optic disk and the part of the nerve within the scleral canal, is supplied by short posterior ciliary arteries, branches of the ophthalmic artery. These ciliary arteries subdivide within the choroid layer of the optic disk into the choriocapillaris. The choriocapillaris has repetitive lobular divisions consisting of a feeding capillary in the center and draining venules at the periphery. This is an end-arterial circulation with little cross-circulation and, under the proper circumstances, may be prone to ischemia. The posterior optic nerve (anterior to the optic chiasm) is served by branches of the ophthalmic artery and the central retinal artery; blood flow to the posterior optic nerve is significantly less than the anterior optic nerve.

What patient factors and intraoperative factors may predispose one to POVL? ION is the most common cause of POVL and may be designated anterior (AION) or posterior (PION), depending on the location of the optic nerve lesion (see Figure on next page). Visual loss of AION is due to infarction at watershed zones of the choriocapillaris but may not be *all or none*. The most common visual field defect in AION is painless vision loss, often within the lower hemifield (altitudinal hemianopsia) with central vision spared; it

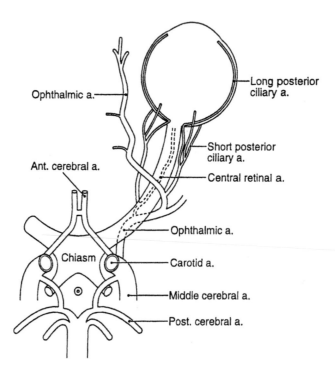

Vascular supply to the retina and optic nerve. (From Williams EL, Hart WM, Tempelhoff R: Postoperative ischemic optic neuropathy. Anesth Analg 80:1018–1029, 1995.)

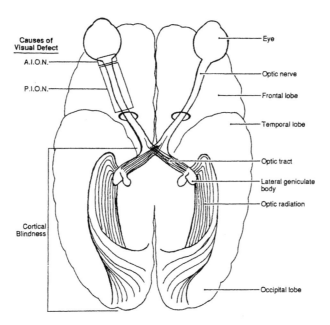

Causes of blindness according to the anatomic source of the visual disturbance. AION, anterior ischemic optic neuropathy; PION, posterior ischemic optic neuropathy. (From Williams EL, Hart WM, Tempelhoff R: Postoperative ischemic optic neuropathy. Anesth Analg 80:1018–1029, 1995.)

often is unilateral. The degree of impairment may vary from a slight decrease in visual acuity to no light perception at all. AION associated with hemorrhagic hypotension usually presents bilaterally, however, with a fixed visual defect. AION is most commonly nonarteritic.

The rare arteritic form is inflammatory in nature, diagnosed by temporal artery biopsy, and responds to steroids. Nonarteritic AION is usually the result of a transient decrease in oxygen delivery in the choriocapillaris and may be secondary to hypoperfusion or increased resistance to flow. Patient-dependent factors associated with nonarteritic AION include diabetes, hypertension, atherosclerosis and other vasculitides, obesity, smoking, and age >50 years. The ASA POVL database found procedure-related risk factors to include cardiopulmonary bypass, prone procedures, surgical durations >5.5 hours, blood loss > 2 L and Hct <25%, and hypotension (mean arterial pressure 40% below baseline). Increases in intraocular pressure (IOP) also may contribute to ocular hypoperfusion. IOP increases during cardiopulmonary bypass. Also, eyes with AION have been shown to exhibit greater increases in IOP with changes in position; venous outflow may be impaired, and this may result in crucial reductions in perfusion pressure. This may partially explain POVL after head and neck surgery.

Many treatments have been attempted to reverse POVL, including anticoagulation, antiplatelet therapy, retrobulbar steroid injections, norepinephrine infusions (to improve perfusion pressure), phenytoin, osmotic diuretics, blood replacement, carbonic anhydrase inhibitors, steroids, and optic nerve decompression. No modality has met with great success, and optic nerve decompression has resulted in deterioration in visual acuity in some cases. The most common prognosis is little return of visual function.

PION occurs less frequently than AION and is less well understood but probably is caused by decreased oxygen delivery to the most vulnerable portion of the optic nerve, that part between the optic foramen at the orbital apex and the central retinal artery's point of entry. PION is associated strongly with hemorrhagic hypotension and presents as acute loss of vision with visual field defects similar to nonarteritic AION. Anatomic abnormalities noted in some patients sustaining PION include congenital absence of the central retinal artery or venous obstruction. There also may be a greater delay in visual deterioration when compared with AION. The prognosis and treatment of PION are similar to those of nonarteritic AION. With the exception of occlusive vascular disease, risk factors for developing PION are similar to those for nonarteritic AION.

ION should be suspected if a patient complains of painless visual loss during the first postoperative week and may be noticed first on awakening from sleep, when IOP is highest. Urgent ophthalmologic consultation should be sought to examine the patient comprehensively, establish the diagnosis, and recommend further evaluation and therapy. Although the prognosis tends to be poor, prompt treatment may be the patient's only chance at recovering vision.

Describe some strategies for preventing ION. Strategies to avoid ION include avoiding external pressure on the eye. However, POVL has been noted in patients when supine and when prone but in Mayfield pins. Compression on the eyes is a rare intraoperative event. Perhaps more beneficial is maintaining acceptable blood pressure and Hct, particularly in patients with multiple risk factors. More than half the patients already entered in the ASA POVL database were positioned prone and often were noted to have significant facial swelling. Perhaps we can infer that there were significant in-creases in IOP or decreases in venous drainage in these cases. When associated with systemic hy-potension, ocular perfusion pressure certainly would be diminished. The trend toward ever-decreasing Hct transfusion triggers may not be as prudent as previously supposed because a low Hct in the presence of other factors seems to put surgi-cal patients at risk for visual loss. Induced hy-potension and hemodilution during prone spine procedures ought to be considered carefully when patients have risk factors for POVL.

It would be difficult at this time to recommend discussion during informed consent of potential POVL to most patients. Patients refusing to con-sent for transfusion when large blood losses are anticipated may be a subgroup, in which this dis-cussion seems more pertinent.

Clinical Pearls

1. POVL is a devastating occurrence. ION is the most common diagnosis. Although patient-related and procedure-related risk factors have been identified, it is still a rare event.

2. AION is diagnosed most commonly in supine cases in patients with atherosclero-sis. POVL after cardiopulmonary bypass is most often AION.

3. PION is diagnosed most commonly after prone operations or when venous con-gestion of the head and neck are encountered.

4. Recommendations to prevent ION include maintenance of acceptable blood pres-sure and Hct in patients at risk and avoidance of external ocular pressure.

5. Early detection of POVL and ophthalmologic consultation are essential because although the prognosis usually is grim, any improvement likely depends on urgent treat-ment.

REFERENCES

1. Brown RH, Schauble JF, Miller NR: Anemia and hypotension as contributors to perioperative loss of vision. Anesth Analg 80:222–226, 1994.
2. Williams EL, Hart WM, Tempelhoff R: Postoperative ischemic optic neuropathy. Anesth Analg 80:1018–1029, 1995.
3. Roth S, Thisted R, Erickson P, et al: Eye injuries after nonocular surgery. Anesthesiology 85:1020–1027, 1996.
4. Myers MA, Hamilton SR, Bogosian AJ: Visual loss as a complication of spine surgery: Review of 37 cases. Spine 22:1325–1329, 1997.
5. Lee LA: Postoperative visual loss data gathered and analyzed. American Society of Anesthesiologists Newsletter 64:25–27, 2000.
6. Remigio D, Wertenbaker C: Post-operative bilateral vision loss. Surv Ophthalmol 44:426–432, 2000.

Kenneth M. Swank, M.D.

PATIENT 3

A 36-year-old woman with multiple sclerosis presents for repair of left anterior cruciate ligament

A 36-year-old woman with multiple sclerosis (MS) presents for repair of the left anterior cruciate ligament, which she tore during a fall while jogging 2 weeks previously. Her MS was diagnosed 4 years ago after two episodes of optic neuritis that caused permanent but mild visual impairment. She reports one exacerbation since that time, approximately 3 years ago involving another episode of optic neuritis and bilateral upper extremity paresthesias, which remitted without lasting impairment after therapy with steroids and interferon. She reports no other medical problems and takes no medication other than oral contraceptives. She relates having had a cesarean section 2 years ago under lumbar epidural anesthesia, which worked well and was without complication. Because of this experience, she requests to have another epidural anesthetic if possible.

Physical Examination: No pertinent findings.

Laboratory Findings: β-Human chorionic gonadotropin negative.

Questions: What is the etiology and natural history of multiple sclerosis?
What are the potential advantages and disadvantages of performing regional anesthesia in a patient with MS?
Is spinal anesthesia preferable to epidural anesthesia?

What is the etiology and natural history of multiple sclerosis? MS is a chronic, relapsing-remitting disease of the central nervous system characterized by multifocal demyelination. This demyelination slows nerve conduction, resulting in motor and sensory impairment. Because MS is associated with multiple, varied neurologic disturbances that occur seemingly at random, diagnosis and evaluation of disease progression are difficult.

The incidence of MS varies with latitude, being rare in equatorial regions but occurring with an incidence of 30:100,000 to 80:100,000 in the northern United States. The incidence is greater in urban, upper socioeconomic groups. There is a genetic component with first-degree relatives having a 6- to 14-fold higher incidence than the general population. The cause is unknown; viral infection leading to immunologically mediated destruction of myelin is one hypothesis. Onset is usually between 20 and 40 years of age.

Common symptoms include motor weakness, sensory impairment, gait and coordination disturbance, bowel and bladder dysfunction, optic neuritis leading to visual loss, and spasticity. The disease course is variable; some patients experience few exacerbations over long periods with little or no cumulative impairment, whereas others experience more frequent exacerbations and accumulate greater amounts of impairment.

MS has no cure. Steroids decrease the duration of exacerbations but do not affect the long-term course of the disease. Other therapies, such as immunosuppressive drugs, interferon, and plasmapheresis, are often of benefit.

Exacerbations occur seemingly at random, but certain factors, such as stress, fatigue, trauma, surgery, hyperthermia, and infection, can trigger an exacerbation. Pregnancy seems to have a protective effect, but a *rebound* occurs, with exacerbations being more common in the postpartum period. During a typical exacerbation, symptoms usually progress over several days, last several weeks, and resolve to varying degrees over weeks.

What are the potential advantages and disadvantages of performing regional anesthesia in a patient with MS? Because many potential exacerbating factors exist in the perioperative period and because of the seemingly random nature of the disease itself, it is difficult to determine the role of anesthesia as a trigger for MS. The literature regarding MS and anesthesia is not extensive and is limited mostly to case reports and small case series. No clear relationship exists between the type of anesthesia administered and the subsequent incidence of postoperative MS exacerbation. General anesthesia does not seem to increase the risk of MS exacerbation, and most of the commonly used agents seem to be safe. Early (1940s to 1960s) case reports implicated barbiturates and nitrous oxide as potential exacerbating factors, but these agents have been exonerated by subsequent reports. Controlling the known factors associated with MS exacerbation is more important than the choice of medications for general anesthesia.

Regional anesthesia may be beneficial in the patient with MS because of decreased stress response to surgery. Local anesthesia has been used extensively in patients with MS and has been shown to be safe. The safety of neuraxial anesthesia in patients with MS is not as well known, with controversy over the subject dating back to the 1940s. Above threshold concentrations, local anesthetics are neurotoxic. This potential may be amplified in the setting of MS because of the loss of the protective effect of the myelin resulting in the spinal cord and nerves being exposed to higher local anesthetic concentrations. This theoretical increase in sensitivity to local anesthetics is not apparent clinically, however, because patients with MS respond appropriately to typical neuraxial dosages. Neuraxial local anesthetics have the potential to exacerbate MS, but whether they actually exacerbate MS is unclear.

Is spinal anesthesia preferable to epidural anesthesia? Epidural block may be safer than spinal block because the local anesthetic concentration at the spinal cord is lower than after spinal block. Early (1940s to 1960s) case reports of MS exacerbation after spinal anesthesia implicated spinal anesthesia as a trigger and led to recommendations against neuraxial blockade in patients with MS. More recent reports and series involving obstetric patients failed to show any correlation, however, between anesthetic type (general versus epidural) and MS exacerbation. On the basis of this information, epidural anesthesia seems to be an acceptable technique for patients with MS.

Since the early case reports implicating spinal block as an exacerbation trigger, other case reports and series have shown that spinal blockade does not cause any complications. There are several reports of the use of intrathecal opioids in the setting of MS without complication. Because of these conflicting reports and a lack of other information, it is unclear whether spinal block is a safe choice in the setting of MS. Spinal block should be used with caution and only in situations in which the benefits of spinal anesthesia are clear.

The major perioperative concerns regardless of type of surgery or anesthetic involve minimizing the known risk factors for MS exacerbation. Patient temperature should be monitored closely, and any degree of hyperthermia should be treated aggressively. Throughout the perioperative course, physiologic stress should be minimized. There is no evidence that prophylactic treatment with steroids or other agents preoperatively is of any benefit.

Other considerations for the patient with MS include neuromuscular blockade and choice of relaxants. Because these patients (particularly patients with severe disease) can have significant motor impairment with associated muscle wasting, succinylcholine may be best avoided owing to potential hyperkalemic response. Lower dosages of nondepolarizing relaxants should be used in patients with baseline motor weakness. Also, shorter duration nondepolarizing relaxants may be advantageous in this situation. MS is not a risk factor for malignant hyperthermia. Severe disease often is accompanied by varying degrees of dementia. Demented patients likely have an increased sensitivity to the sedative effects of anesthetic agents; short-acting agents are recommended.

The Present Patient

After a discussion with the present patient regarding the controversies about epidural and general anesthesia in patients with MS, she chose to have another epidural anesthetic. Continuous lumbar anesthesia was administered without difficulty using 0.5% bupivacaine and 100 μg of fentanyl. Midazolam, 5 mg, was used intraoperatively for sedation. The patient's axillary temperature was monitored throughout the surgery and was at no time above 36.1°C. The block worked well for the 2-hour surgery and resolved normally. The patient was discharged to home 4 hours after arrival to the postanesthesia care unit with return of baseline lower extremity neurologic function. The patient reported no change in her baseline neurologic status during telephone follow-ups on postoperative days 1 and 7.

Clinical Pearls

1. Neuraxial blockade is not contraindicated for patients with MS. Anesthetic choice depends on individual circumstances and discussion with the patient. Based on the limited literature available, epidural anesthesia may be safer than spinal anesthesia for patients with MS.

2. Care should be exercised in the choice and dosing of neuromuscular relaxants because patients with MS may exhibit an increased sensitivity to these drugs secondary to muscle weakness or wasting.

3. Prophylactic steroids are not beneficial preoperatively. The best perioperative prophylaxis is the avoidance of known MS exacerbation triggers, such as hyperthermia, infection, and stress.

REFERENCES

1. Bamford C, Sibley W, Laguna J: Anesthesia and multiple sclerosis. Can J Neurol Sci 5:41–44, 1978.
2. Jones RM: Anaesthesia and demyelinating disease. Anaesthesia 35:879–884, 1980.
3. Crawford JS, James FM, Nolte H, et al: Regional anaesthesia for patients with chronic neurological disease and similar conditions. Anaesthesia 36:821–828, 1981.
4. Warren TM, Datta S, Ostheimer GW: Lumbar epidural anesthesia in a patient with multiple sclerosis. Anesth Analg 61:1022–1023, 1982.

PATIENT 4

A 54-year-old man with cyanosis and deteriorating pulse oximetry

A 54-year-old man was scheduled for a radical neck dissection secondary to carcinoma of the larynx. He had a long history of alcohol abuse and an 80-pack-year smoking history. Previous anesthetics for inguinal hernia repairs were well tolerated. He was not under the regular care of a physician. He denied medications and known allergies.

Physical Examination: Vital signs normal. General appearance: thin, disheveled man without respiratory distress. Vital sounds normal. Throat: direct laryngoscopy: a fungating mass enveloping the right vocal cord and anterior third of the glottic aperture. Chest: distant breath sounds, slightly barrel-shaped thorax, no retractions. Cardiac auscultation: normal.

Laboratory Findings: Hct 51%; WBC 8,700/μL. Electrolytes normal. ABG (room air): pH 7.43, PCO_2 47 mmHg, PO_2 68 mmHg, HCO_3 28 mmHg. Chest radiograph: decreased lung markings with hyperlucent lung fields, no masses, normal cardiac silhouette. ECG: normal sinus rhythm with occasional premature atrial contractions.

Hospital Course: The patient underwent awake, sedate flexible fiberoptic intubation in preparation for surgery. After standard monitors were placed and supplemental oxygen was administered, the patient was sedated slowly with intermittent doses of fentanyl and midazolam. Intermittent sprays of Cetacaine (active ingredients, 14% benzocaine and 2% tetracaine) provided topical anesthesia. Vocal cords and trachea were visualized by direct fiberoptic bronchoscopy and anesthetized with sprays of 4% lidocaine, total dose approximately 200 mg. Awake intubation proceeded without incident, correct placement of the endotracheal tube was verified, and general anesthesia was induced in a routine intravenous fashion.

Over the next few hours, the pulse oximetry readings progressively declined, from 98% to the mid-80s. The surgeon comments that the blood is unusually dark, yet ABG analysis while breathing 100% oxygen showed partial pressures of oxygen of 180 mmHg and calculated oxygen saturation of 98%. All gas monitors appeared in order, and bilateral chest auscultation is unchanged.

Questions: What is the likely cause of the patient's decline in pulse oximetry oxygen saturations?
Describe how blood gas and pulse oximetry values clarify the diagnosis.
What is the treatment for this clinical condition?

What is the likely cause of the patient's decline in pulse oximetry oxygen saturations? Acquired methemoglobinemia secondary to benzocaine.

Methemoglobin (MetHb) is formed continuously in the body when the ferrous (Fe^{2+}) iron moiety of hemoglobin (Hb) is oxidized to the ferric (Fe^{3+}) state. The enzyme MetHb nicotinamide-adenine dinucleotide (reduced form) reductase is responsible for reducing 95% of the ferric iron back to the ferrous state, reestablishing normal Hb. Normal MetHb levels are about 1% to 1.5% of total Hb. Not only is MetHb incapable of carrying oxygen, but also it increases the affinity of normal oxygenated hemoglobin (HbO_2) for oxygen; preventing off-loading at the cellular level.

Methemoglobinemia may be congenital or acquired. Congenital forms may be associated with enzymatic deficiencies or abnormal Hb species. Hemoglobin M favors iron in the ferric state. By far, the most likely cause of elevated MetHb levels are medications, in particular, those that possess highly electrophilic nitrogen atoms. Commonly encountered medications that may result in elevated MetHb levels include local anesthetics (prilocaine, benzocaine, lidocaine, and procaine), nitroglycerin, amyl nitrate and sodium nitrite (used to produce MetHb in the management of cyanide poisoning), and sulfonamides. Other medications and chemicals known to produce methemoglobinemia include phenacetin, phenazopyridine, flutamide, acetanilid, aminobenzenes, nitrobenzenes, and aniline dyes. Methemoglobinemia is rarely symptomatic at a level less than 20%, although cyanosis may be evident at levels between 5% and 15%. Patients may be lethargic or dizzy or complain of headaches at levels of about 30% to 40%, and levels greater than 70% may be fatal.

Describe how blood gas and pulse oximetry values clarify the diagnosis. Methemoglobinemia should be suspected when cyanosis is present and a disparity exists between normal blood gas analysis and pulse oximetry values. Clarifying the situation requires knowledge of how blood gas and pulse oximetry values are derived.

Although many hospitals now routinely use actual saturation measurements, Hb saturation may be calculated from nomograms based on the measured partial pressure of oxygen, taking into account temperature, pH, and partial pressure of carbon dioxide and assuming all Hb is the normal species. Pulse oximetry measures pulsatile light absorbance at two wavelengths (660 and 940 nm), calculates an absorbance ratio, and compares this value with an algorithm derived from measurements taken from volunteers breathing hypoxic gas mixtures. A given absorbance ratio corresponds to a given pulse oximeter–derived oxygen saturation (SpO_2). Because only two wavelengths are used, the concentrations of only two unknowns, oxygenated and reduced hemoglobin (RHb), can be determined. The limitations of both these measurement methods in detecting dyshemoglobinemias should become clear. Hb saturation is not measured directly during routine ABG analysis, and accurate measurement of an aberrant Hb species by pulse oximetry would require measuring light absorbance of more than two wavelengths of light.

Co-oximetry measures light absorbance at four wavelengths. Four unknowns can be determined (HbO_2, RHb, MetHb, and carboxyhemoglobin [COHb]). Oxyhemoglobin saturation is the percentage of HbO_2 of all species of hemoglobin present.

Pulse oximetry and co-oximetry are based on the spectrophotometric principle, the Beer-Lambert law, which is stated:

$$I_{trans} = I_{inc}\, e^{-CL\alpha}$$

where I_{trans} is the light transmitted through the species; I_{inc} is the light shown on the species; C is the concentration of the species under investigation (and it is usually C we are determining); L is the width of the cuvette holding the solution; and α is the extinction coefficient, a constant for the solution dependent only on the wavelength of light used for the measurements. The extinction coefficients for the different hemoglobin species over a spectrum of wavelengths are shown in the Figure. At the wavelengths measured by pulse oximetry, the extinction coefficients for MetHb are nearly equal. Consequently the absorbance ratios determined by pulse oximetry as MetHb concentrations rise tend toward unity. By the previously mentioned algorithm, the pulse oximeter reads the sample as having a saturation of approximately 85%, despite the fact that true HbO_2 saturation is much lower. For this reason, as MetHb concentrations rise, the pulse oximetry readings trend down but level off at a spurious reading of 85%.

What is the treatment for methemoglobinemia? Treatment involves administration of methylene blue, given intravenously at 1 to 2 mg/kg, which acts as a cofactor in an enzymatic reaction and reduces MetHb. If methemoglobinemia has not resolved in 1 hour, the dose may be repeated. Doses of methylene blue should not exceed 7 mg/kg because this paradoxically would lead to oxidation of hemoglobin, increasing MetHb. Methylene blue should be avoided in patients with glucose-6-phosphate dehydrogenase deficiency because a hemolytic anemia may be precipitated. Discontinuing likely offending agents and increasing inspired oxy-

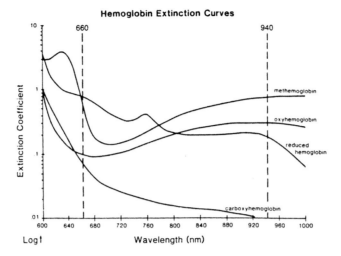

Hemoglobin Extinction Curves

Extinction coefficient versus wavelength for the four hemoglobin species: RHb, HbO$_2$, MetHb, COHb. Pulse oximeters use two wavelengths 660 nm and 940 nm. (From Barker SJ, Tremper KK, Hyatt J: Effects of methemoglobinemia on pulse oximetry and mixed venous oximetry. Anesthesiology 70:112–117, 1989.)

gen concentration to 100% are important management strategies. Ischemic ECG changes should be treated and hemodynamics supported as necessary if these prove a concern.

The Present Patient

The patient had cyanosis, progressively deteriorating pulse oximetry values, and confusing routine blood gas analysis. Methemoglobinemia secondary to the use of benzocaine for awake intubation was diagnosed only after ABGs were analyzed by co-oximetry and treated effectively with methylene blue administered intravenously. This diagnosis is likely to be missed without understanding the technical limitations of routine oxygen analysis and monitoring.

Clinical Pearls

1. Methemoglobinemia should be suspected if cyanosis is present despite normal oxygen tension and high calculated oxygen saturation by routine blood gas analysis.

2. Pulse oximetry values are misleading because commonly used technology measures pulsatile light absorbance at only two wavelengths and assumes the presence of only two hemoglobin species, oxygenated and reduced hemoglobin.

3. The diagnosis can be confirmed by ABG analysis by co-oximetry, in which measurement of light absorbance at four wavelengths can determine accurately concentrations of oxygenated and reduced hemoglobin, methemoglobin, and carboxyhemoglobin.

4. Treatment includes administration of methylene blue 1 to 2 mg/kg, discontinuing offending agents (likely to possess nitrogen atoms), increasing oxygen administration, and supportive care as needed.

REFERENCES

1. Anderson ST, Hajduczek J, Barker SJ: Benzocaine-induced methemoglobinemia in an adult: Accuracy of pulse oximetry with methemoglobinemia. Anesth Analg 67:1099–1101, 1988.
2. Barker SJ, Tremper KK, Hyatt J: Effects of methemoglobinemia on pulse oximetry and mixed venous oximetry. Anesthesiology 70:112–117, 1989.
3. Tremper KK, Barker SJ: Pulse oximetry. Anesthesiology 70:98–108, 1989.
4. Jackson SH, Barker SJ: Methemoglobinemia in a patient receiving flutamide. Anesthesiology 82:1065–1067, 1995.

PATIENT 5

A 9-year-old girl with posttonsillectomy bleeding

A 9-year-old girl underwent tonsillectomy for chronic tonsillitis 4 days before presentation. At the time of her original surgery, she had no significant personal or family medical history. No one in her family had a prior surgery; her mother recalled no significant problems surrounding delivery of her children. Two days postoperatively, the girl experienced a posttonsillectomy bleed. As in the first surgery, she underwent general endotracheal anesthesia, and bleeding sites in the tonsillar bed were cauterized. She was sent home in the care of her parents late that day. Two days later, she again presents with similar oropharyngeal bleeding. Her parents note she has been vomiting undigested blood.

Physical Examination: Temperature normal, heart rate 123, respirations 21; blood pressure 110/78. General appearance: Pale, mildly distressed 9-year-old girl appropriate in physical development. No petechiae, hematomas, or other stigmata noted. HEENT: venous oozing and no pulsatile bleeding from tonsillar beds bilaterally. Remainder of physical examination unremarkable.

Laboratory Findings: Hct 31%, WBC 7,300/μL, platelet count 135 × 103/cm², prothrombin time 13 seconds, partial thromboplastin time 28 seconds, template bleeding time 14 minutes.

Questions: What diagnosis is the cause of the child's bleeding?
Review the functional defect.
Discuss the classification system.
What is the importance of accurate characterization for treatment?
Describe the treatment options.

What diagnosis is the cause of the child's bleeding? von Willebrand's Disease (vWD).

The most common inherited coagulopathy, vWD affects approximately 1% of the population. von Willebrand first recognized this disorder in 1926 and astutely characterized it as having combined functional platelet and vessel wall defects. The most common forms are inherited as autosomal dominant, although recessive forms also are known and tend to be more severe. Heterozygotes vary remarkably in the severity of their disease. The usual presentation is bleeding from mucosal surfaces, including epistaxis, post–dental extraction, bleeding, gastrointestinal or female genital tract bleeding, or trivial wound bleeding. Women may experience profound menorrhagia or severe abdominal pain secondary to rupture of hemorrhagic ovarian cysts. Often vWD manifests postoperatively, as in ear, nose, and throat surgery. Severe forms are noted early in life and may manifest with hemarthrosis; muscular hematomas; or intracranial, retroperitoneal, or intraabdominal bleeding. Acquired forms of vWD are known and may be found associated with myeloproliferative or autoimmune disease, hypothyroidism, glycogen storage disease, uremia, and connective tissue disease or secondary to medications, including hydroxyethyl starch, dextran, heparin, and thrombolytic medications.

Review the functional defect. The primary defect is a quantitative or qualitative deficiency of the glycoprotein known as *von Willebrand factor* (vWF). Manufactured within platelets or endothelium and found circulating in plasma, vWF mediates adhesion of platelets to exposed subendothelium, promoting thrombus formation. vWF also forms noncovalent, dissociable complexes with factor VIII, preventing its rapid removal from the circulation. Production and release of factor VIII are stimulated by vWF, and for these reasons, when vWF is deficient, factor VIII levels and activity are deficient as well. Another characteristic of the vWF glycoprotein is its ability to link up with other vWF molecules, forming large multimers to which platelets can bind. The largest multimers are products of platelets themselves.

Discuss the classification system. The classification system of vWF is complex but of more than academic interest because treatment strategies depend on accurate identification of vWD subtype. Type I vWD is characterized by a decreased amount (usually 5% to 30% of normal) of normal vWF. Found in about 75% to 80% of all individuals affected with vWF, bleeding tends to be of mild-to-moderate severity. Numerous subtypes have been identified, usually based on platelet vWF content. Notable subtypes are discussed subsequently only as they affect treatment. Factor VIII activity is depressed to the extent that vWF levels are depressed.

Qualitatively abnormal vWF is characteristic of type II vWD, which accounts for 10% to 15% of all vWD patients. Inheritance may be dominant or recessive. Although vWF levels are normal, normal multimeric patterns are absent, and bleeding can be severe at times. Factor VIII levels may be normal or decreased. Severe vWD, or type III, is characterized by virtual absence (usually <1%) of vWF; multimers are absent, and factor VIII activity is about 2% to 10% of normal. Inheritance is recessive, and the prevalence is 0.1 to 5 cases per 1 million. There is a rare platelet type of vWD, which manifests with thrombocytopenia and decreased vWF and factor VII.

What is the importance of accurate characterization for treatment? Adequate characterization of vWD type is complex and requires review of family history, characterization of platelet and plasma vWF levels and activity, factor VIII activity, and multimeric electrophoretic analysis. Although the sine qua non is considered a prolonged bleeding time in association with a normal platelet count, bleeding times may not be particularly sensitive. vWF is an acute-phase reactant whose levels typically increase in response to epinephrine or vasopressin release or surgical stress or in liver disease, cancer, or infection. Levels also increase with age, during pregnancy, and during the follicular phase of the menstrual cycle. Patients with mild disease at times may have normal bleeding times, and repeated testing often is necessary. Template (Ivy) bleeding times are more reliable than Duke bleeding times, which may not be prolonged in mild disease. Normal Ivy bleeding time is <9 minutes.

Of additional value in the characterization of vWD is the platelet response to the antibiotic ristocetin. A sufficient amount of vWF must be available for ristocetin to induce platelet agglutination. Ristocetin cofactor activity (Rcof) is a test system using formalin-fixed normal platelets and the patient's platelet-poor plasma that assesses the capacity of the vWF to interact with platelet glycoprotein Ib. Low Rcof is noted whenever there is abnormal multimeric structure or a decrease or absence of large multimers. A related assessment is ristocetin-induced platelet aggregation (RIPA), in which ristocetin produces platelet aggregation when instilled into the patient's platelet-rich plasma. Partial thromboplastin times may be elevated slightly in type I and type II vWD and may be prolonged in type III vWD.

Describe the treatment options. Therapy may be prophylactic, as when surgery is planned, in response to acute bleeding, as for accidental or spontaneous bleeding, or postoperatively, perhaps in a patient previously unrecognized as having vWD. Many treatment options exist, with the goal being stimulation of vWF release or replacement therapy by transfusion of clotting factors. DDAVP (1-desamino-8-D-arginine vasopressin) or desmopressin is a synthetic analog of vasopressin and the treatment of choice for mild vWD. About 80% of patients respond favorably. When given intravenously in a dose of 0.3 μg/kg (up to 20 μg), an average 3-fold to 4-fold rise in vWF is noted, with a peak effect in 30 to 60 minutes. The effect is realized for several hours as reflected in correction of bleeding times. Bleeding times may be too insensitive to guide therapy, and Duke bleeding times correct more easily than Ivy bleeding times. DDAVP may be readministered every 12 hours, but repeated doses cause tachyphylaxis. Side effects include facial flushing, headaches, nausea, abdominal cramps, tachycardia, hypertension, and hypotension. A rare but concerning complication is water intoxication and hyponatremia. This problem should be suspected in patients who become oliguric or confused, particularly the elderly and very young. Serum sodium should be followed, and hypotonic IV fluids should be avoided. DDAVP also may be administered subcutaneously, and an intranasal preparation (Octostim) is ideal for home treatment of bleeding episodes. DDAVP also is useful in the preoperative preparation of vWD patients because response to this therapy can be assessed. Testing should be undertaken about 1 week before surgery, and if a benefit is observed, DDAVP should be administered preoperatively and at 12 and 24 hours postoperatively.

Although in the past cryoprecipitate has been the blood replacement product of choice, it carries with it the risk of transmission of hepatitis B and C and human immunodeficiency virus (HIV). New clotting factor concentrates that have undergone viral inactivation are now available. In particular, Haemate-P (Behring) is a pasteurized plasma product with normal vWF factor levels and multimeric patterns. For modest bleeding in mildly affected individuals, Haemate-P should be administered in doses of 30 IU/kg (1 U being defined as the clotting factor activity found in 1 mL of fresh plasma); severely affected individuals should receive 40 to 70 IU/kg. Therapy should be guided by correction of bleeding times, and the previous caveats concerning bleeding times hold. If Haemate-

P is unavailable, cryoprecipitate may be administered. A bag of cryoprecipitate possesses 40% to 70% of the original vWF, and a bag should be administered for each 10 kg of body weight. Although infrequently given because it is not an intensive therapy and carries the risk of viral transmission, fresh frozen plasma may be administered at times. Occasionally, adjunctive antifibrinolytic therapy with ε-aminocaproic acid (Amicar) or tranexamic acid (Cyclokapron) is useful to prevent plasminogen activation and clot lysis.

There are important exceptions to general treatment guidelines in the context of vWD type. In type I vWD, in which normal vWF usually is found but in lesser amounts, DDAVP is the treatment of choice, but in patients whose platelet content of vWF is low, as shown by low RIPA, the response may not be substantial. Likewise, in type II vWD, characterized by abnormal vWF multimers, DDAVP is often ineffective and is contraindicated in type IIB vWD because these patients develop thrombocytopenia in response to DDAVP treatment. Type IIB patients have all multimers present in platelets and are hyperresponsive to ristocetin treatment as shown by elevated RIPA. Recommendations are to treat type II patients with normal or decreased RIPA with DDAVP and patients with increased ristocetin cofactor activity with plasma products.

Type III patients do not respond to DDAVP; not only are plasma products indicated (factor VIII and vWF must be replaced) and in repeated doses, but also antithrombolytic therapy and platelet infusions often are needed. Finally, the platelet type vWD has low Rcof but increased RIPA because all platelet multimers are present. Response to DDAVP may be platelet aggregation and worsened thrombocytopenia.

The Present Patient

The patient received two 20 mL/kg fluid boluses of lactated Ringer's solution before anesthesia. She underwent IV induction of anesthesia with ketamine, 1.5 mg/kg. Induction was carried out with cricoid pressure, and intubation was unremarkable. With cautery and soon after treatment with DDAVP, all oozing from the tonsillar bed resolved. Extensive testing postoperatively found vWF factor levels 25% of normal, Rcof decreased, RIPA decreased, and electrophoretic multimeric pattern normal. The patient was discharged with desmopressin nasal spray and advised to have DDAVP therapy before any future surgical procedure. Her mother and two siblings were found to have type I vWD as well.

Clinical Pearls

1. Because it is the most common inherited coagulopathy, vWD should be considered in any situation in which unexpected bleeding is encountered. Because most bleeding is mild, postoperative bleeding may be the initial presentation of vWD.

2. vWD is a surprisingly heterogeneous disorder, and although 80% respond to DDAVP, in some situations it is contraindicated. If possible, a complete coagulation assessment should be performed before instituting treatment.

3. Where possible and appropriate, preoperative testing with DDAVP should be performed to assess efficacy. Antiplatelet medications should be avoided as well.

4. Severely affected individuals are likely to need non–virally inactivated blood products and should be immunized for hepatitis A and B. Health care providers should be fastidious in using universal precautions.

5. In the patient with posttonsillectomy bleeding, the likelihood of a full stomach and hypovolemia should be entertained and appropriate decisions made for preanesthetic fluid therapy, aspiration prophylaxis, choice of induction agents, and induction and intubation technique (rapid sequence with cricoid pressure).

REFERENCES

1. Ruggeri ZM: Structure and function of von Willebrand factor: Relationship to von Willebrand's disease. Mayo Clin Proc 66:847–861, 1991.
2. Holmberg L, Nilsson IM: von Willebrand's disease. Eur J Haematol 48:127–141, 1992.
3. Hathaway WE, Goodnight SH Jr: Disorders of Hemostasis and Thrombosis. New York, McGraw-Hill, 1993.
4. Association of Hemophilia Clinic Directors of Canada: Hemophilia and von Willebrand's disease: 2. Management. Can Med Assoc J 3:205–214, 1995.

James Duke, MD

PATIENT 6

A 20-year-old woman with long bone fractures and pulmonary and hemodynamic instability

A 20-year-old woman was involved in a major mechanism motor vehicle accident. She is alert and complaining of severe leg pain. IV fluid administration before arrival is 3L of crystalloid.

Physical Examination: Pulse 134, respirations 24, blood pressure 138/88, oxygen saturation 96% on 40% oxygen. General appearance: Pale, agitated, but responds appropriately to questions. Head, neck, chest, heart, and abdomen examinations are unremarkable. Lower extremities are swollen and deformed with intact peripheral pulses on neurologic examination.

Laboratory Findings: Hct 41%, platelets 154,000/μL. Clotting functions and electrolytes: normal. Recumbent chest radiograph and CT scan of the chest: no pulmonary injuries. CT scans of the abdomen and pelvis: negative. Radiographs: closed left and open right femoral fractures and bilateral closed tibial fractures.

Hospital Course: Intramedullary rodding of the femoral and tibial fractures is undertaken under general endotracheal anesthesia. Rodding of the open femoral fracture proceeds without incident. During the second femoral rodding, on essentially no anesthesia, the patient's arterial blood pressure decreases to 100/55 mmHg. Peak inspiratory ventilatory pressures have increased gradually to the mid-40s (cm H_2O) on controlled minute ventilation of 11 L/min. Oxygenation saturation decreases into the high 80s. PEEP, 5 cm H_2O, is added. Tachycardia develops and reaches 140 beats/min. Fluid resuscitation to this point has included 6 L of crystalloid and 4 U of packed RBCs in response to an estimated blood loss of about 2 L. Dopamine infusion is begun and titrated upward, but blood pressure continues to decrease. A pulmonary artery catheter is inserted; initial pulmonary artery pressures are 58/49 mmHg, pulmonary capillary wedge pressure is 22 mHg, mixed venous oxygen saturation is 65%, and cardiac index is 1.8 L/min/m². As a result of the deterioration in her condition, surgery was interrupted, and the patient was taken to the intensive care unit. A chest radiograph was taken (Figure).

Questions: Interpret the chest radiograph. What is a likely diagnosis?
What are the criteria for making this diagnosis?
What treatment options are available?
Review the important issues regarding timing of fracture fixation.

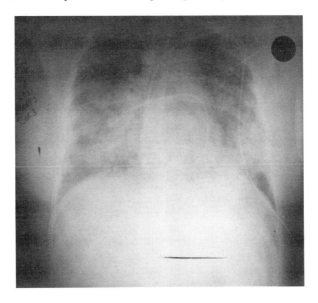

Interpret the chest radiograph. What is a likely diagnosis? Fat embolism syndrome resulting in adult respiratory distress syndrome (ARDS).

Discussion: Although some degree of fat embolism occurs in 90% of patients with long bone fractures, only 3% to 4% of the patients develop fat embolism syndrome (FES). Of patients with multiple fractures, 5% to 10% are at risk for this syndrome. Clinical deterioration can be dramatic, occurring over only a few hours, and 90% of patients show symptoms within 24 hours of injury. In the 1960s and 1970s, mortality was 20%, but improvements in pulmonary therapy likely have reduced this percentage. Coma, severe ARDS, pneumonia, and acute congestive heart failure are particularly grave prognostic signs.

What are the criteria for making this diagnosis? The principal areas affected by FES are pulmonary, central nervous system, and skin. Major and minor criteria have been established to support diagnosis; one major and four minor criteria are needed to make the diagnosis of FES. Major criteria are axillary or subconjunctival petechiae, hypoxemia ($PaO_2 < 60$ mmHg, $FIO_2 \leq 0.4$), central nervous system depression disproportionate to hypoxemia, and pulmonary edema. Minor criteria are tachycardia (>110 beats/min), pyrexia ($> 38.5°C$), emboli observed in the fundi, fat present in urine, sudden unexplainable decrease in Hct or platelet counts, increased sedimentation rate, and fat globules in the sputum. Pulmonary signs are usually the first recognized, and tachypnea, dyspnea, and cyanosis are common. Cerebral findings (found in 80% of patients) include headache, irritability, delerium, stupor, convulsions, hemiparesis, and coma. A nondependent petechial rash over chest, anterior axillary folds, or conjunctiva may be recognized by the second or third day in about 50% of patients.

Mechanical and chemical theories explain the observed effects of FES. Torn marrow veins and disrupted marrow fat allow passage of fat droplets into the circulation, especially when the marrow cavity is exposed to increased pressure, such as during femoral reaming. Fat droplets <8 μ in size can pass through the pulmonary bed, entering the systemic circulation, depositing fat into the brain, kidney, eye, and liver. Pulmonary precapillary shunts and a patent foramen ovale (found in 20% to 35% of patients) may allow systemic fat embolization, especially in the setting of acute cor pulmonale.

The chemical theory of fat embolization maintains that circulating free fatty acids deposit in the lung and are directly toxic to pneumocytes, producing inflammation, inactivating surfactant, and increasing capillary permeability, contributing to the development of ARDS. Cerebral edema may be secondary to a direct toxic effect of free fatty acids.

What treatment options are available? Although many agents have been used to treat FES, including bicarbonate solutions, ethyl alcohol, low-molecular-weight dextran, and heparin, significant benefit has not been shown consistently. Trials of corticosteroids are employed in some centers. Therapy remains supportive and includes ventilatory management and treatment of right heart failure.

Stabilization of fractures is considered by most authorities to be essential in prevention and management of FES. Contemporary management of femoral fractures stresses early operative fixation (EOF), with the belief that numerous complications, including FES, are lessened. Agreement with this concept is not universal, however.

In patients with isolated femoral fractures, there is general agreement that when the patient has received satisfactory resuscitation, early fixation has numerous benefits and is preferred to delayed repair. Traction forces the patient into recumbency, complicating nursing care and rendering the patient prone to numerous complications. Pulmonary secretions are retained, and there is loss of intrathoracic volume, placing the patient at risk for atelectasis, pneumonia, ventilation-perfusion inequalities, and shunting. EOF has been associated with a decreased incidence of ARDS and decreased ventilator and intensive care unit days. Venous stasis and thromboembolism are lessened. Débridement of necrotic tissue limits the systemic inflammatory response. Fracture outcome also is improved. There is improved joint mobility and less muscle wasting and fewer problems with decubitus ulcers. Embolization of marrow material declines when the fracture is stabilized.

Greater concern and controversy surrounds timing of femoral fracture repair in patients with coexisting pulmonary injury. Most American studies favor EOF in these patients. Pape et al[6] believed, however, that EOF increases ARDS and mortality. Comparison of studies is difficult because most studies are retrospective, matching of groups and satisfactory controls may be poor, and scoring systems for severity of injury and definitions of ARDS are inconsistent.

Many factors may predispose the patient to posttraumatic respiratory insufficiency. Shock, number of blood units transfused, advanced age, and long bone injuries are factors, and direct trauma to the chest itself is particularly important as a cause of ARDS.

Review the important issues regarding timing of fracture fixation. Many authorities stress that the degree of pulmonary injury, not the associated fracture, is the significant factor in subsequent pulmonary complications. Clinical judgment regarding timing of operative repair is important, and ensuring adequate resuscitation and treatment of associated injuries is paramount. Modest delays to optimize patient status are likely to be beneficial. There also is some evidence that suggests unreamed femoral nails may produce less fat embolism and ARDS than reamed femoral rodding. An important objective in this instance is to limit intramedullary pressure increases.

Pulmonary embolization of marrow contents has been well shown by transesophageal echocardiography (TEE) during femoral fracture fixation. Smaller quantities of emboli have been noted during EOF when compared with delayed fixation. The magnitude of embolization varies from minimal evidence of embolization to copious showers of small emboli to embolization of large (>10 mm) fragments. Because 90% of fractures are associated with fat embolization and few patients go on to develop the fulminant FES, guidelines for use of TEE have not been forthcoming. TEE monitoring may alert anesthesiologists to portions of the reaming procedure, however, that incite particularly worrisome degrees of embolization.

Anesthetic management my be facilitated as well if the extent of left heart underfilling or right heart distention and failure are known, guiding therapy in these problematic situations.

The Present Patient

After transfer to the surgical intensive care unit, the present patient required increasing vasopressor support. Dobutamine infusion was added to the dopamine infusion; this proved ineffective, and epinephrine infusion was substituted for dobutamine. The chest radiograph showed diffuse alveolar infiltrates and normal cardiac silhouette consistent with ARDS. Transthoracic echocardiography showed normal left ventricular contractility with underfilling of the left ventricle, and right atrial and right ventricular dilation with hypocontractility consistent with acute right ventricular failure. Elevations in pulmonary capillary wedge pressure were thought to be consistent with diffuse pulmonary capillary and arteriolar disease, consistent with fat embolism. Blood pressure and heart rate declined, and the patient experienced full cardiac arrest. She was resuscitated, but subsequently she was found to meet brain death criteria. Postmortem examination revealed fat emboli in lungs, liver, brain, spinal cord, and kidneys. Microscopic examination of the organs revealed cerebral edema and changes consistent with ARDS within the lungs.

Clinical Pearls

1. During internal fixation of long bone fractures, the clinician should be alert for deterioration in pulmonary and hemodynamic function because this may suggest that significant fat embolization is taking place. Although few go on to the fat FES, patients with multiple long bone fractures are at increased risk. When FES is established, management is mainly supportive.

2. Especially in the multiply-injured patient, operative fixation should be delayed to optimize hemodynamic status and to treat associated injuries. Significant blood loss attends these injuries before and during repair. Invasive monitoring, ABGs, serial Hct measurements, and lactic acid determinations are useful to assess oxygen carrying capacity and cellular perfusion.

3. During acute cor pulmonale, increased pulmonary artery and capillary wedge pressures may reflect diffuse embolization and right heart failure despite left ventricular underfilling. TEE may be useful in this instance in guiding fluid therapy. Fat embolization can be detected as well.

REFERENCES

1. Riska EB, Myllynen P: Fat embolism in patients with multiple injuries. J Trauma 22:891–894, 1982.
2. Levy D: The fat embolism syndrome. Clin Orthop 261:281–286, 1990.
3. Pell ACH, Christie J, Keating JF, et al: The detection of fat embolism by transesophageal echocardiography during reamed intramedullary nailing. J Bone Joint Surg Br 75:921–925, 1993.
4. Bone LB, Babikian G, Stegemann PM: Femoral canal reaming in the polytrauma patient with chest injury: A clinical perspective. Clin Orthop 318:91–94, 1995.
5. Reynolds MA, Richardson JD, Spain DA, et al: Is the timing of fracture fixation important for the patient with multiple trauma? Ann Surg 222:470–48, 1995.
6. Pape HC, Regel G, Tscherne H: Controversies regarding fracture management in the patient with multiple trauma. Curr Opin Crit Care 2:295–303, 1996.

James C. Duke, MD

PATIENT 7

A 33-year-old man with oliguria and ventilatory insufficiency

A 33-year-old man was involved in a rollover motor vehicle accident. On arrival to the emergency department, his principal complaint is abdominal pain and difficulty breathing.

An emergency laparotomy reveals stellate lacerations of the liver. The surgeons decide to delay definitive repair and pack the liver for hemostasis, leave the fascia open, and close with towel clips. Interoperatively the patient receives 12 U of packed RBCs, 10 U of platelets, 4 U of fresh frozen plasma, and 6 L of normal saline. In the ICU, mechanical ventilation is initiated with the following settings: FIO_2 100%, rate 16, tidal volume 12 mL/kg, PEEP 5 cm H_2O. Peak and mean airway pressures are 36 cm H_2O and 29 cm H_2O. Static compliance is 36 mL/cm H_2O. ABG values are pH 7.31, PCO_2 31 mmHg, PO_2 95 mmHg.

Over the next 12 hours, urine output decreases to 15 mL/h, and the patient's respiratory status deteriorates with an increasing shunt and progressive hypercapnia. Bladder pressures are measured to be 32 cm H_2O.

Physical Examination: Temperature 36.2°C, pulse 135, respirations 35, blood pressure 90/75. General appearance: alert, agitated, pale and diaphoretic. Neck: immobilized and nontender. Chest: no tenderness, normal breath sounds. Cardiac: normal. Abdomen: distended and tender. Extremities: unremarkable.

Laboratory Findings: Initial findings: Hct 35%. All other laboratory findings within normal limits. Peritoneal lavage: gross blood. Repeat findings: Hct 29%, platelet count 65,000/ μL, prothrombin time 16 seconds, lactate 3.2 mmols/L. Pulmonary artery catheterization revealed pulmonary arterial pressures of 28/16 mmHg, central venous pressure 10 mmHg, and pulmonary artery occlusion pressure 14 mmHg. Cardiac index 2.8 L/min/M², systemic vascular resistance 1300 dyne·sec·cm^{-5}.

Questions: What is the cause of the patient's oliguria?

                Why may pulmonary artery catheter data be misleading in this scenario?

                Describe surgical scenarios where this phenomenon is commonly encountered.

                What effect does this syndrome have upon the pulmonary, cardiovascular, and renal systems?

                What is the treatment?

What is the cause of the patient's oliguria? Abdominal compartment syndrome (ACS). An acute elevation in intraabdominal pressure (IAP) is increasingly recognized as a cause of physiologic compromise in critically ill patients. The principal manifestations are declining cardiac output, hypoxemia, and oliguria in the setting of increasing intraabdominal pressure, increased systemic vascular resistance, increased airway pressures, and decreased pulmonary compliance. Although trauma patients are at highest risk, ACS may occur in any setting characterized by coagulopathy, massive fluid resuscitation, unrelenting intraabdominal or retroperitoneal bleeding, or significant third-space fluid accumulations.

Why may pulmonary artery catheter data be misleading in this scenario? Acute increases in IAP decrease cardiac output by interfering with venous return. In this setting, normal central venous and pulmonary artery occlusion pressures may falsely suggest adequate or even excessive fluid resuscitation. These measurements often are spuriously elevated, however, because IAP is transmitted progressively to the pleural space, especially when IAP rises about baseline values by >20 cm H_2O. A transarterial or *true* pulmonary artery occlusion pressure, which is the difference between the measured pulmonary artery occlusion pressure and pleural pressure, provides a more accurate gauge of intravascular fluid status and more than likely will indicate underresuscitation in this clinical setting.

All intraabdominal organs become underperfused as IAP increases, with the curious and unexplained exception of the adrenal glands. Although renal underperfusion is the principal cause of oliguria in ACS, the kidneys also experience a direct pressure effect that increases renal vascular resistance. Renal blood flow and glomerular filtration rate decrease.

ACS also alters pulmonary functions by raising IAP and decreasing static compliance of the respiratory system. Resulting decreases in tidal volume produce atelectasis with deterioration in oxygenation and ventilation. PEEP may be required to maintain adequate tidal volume and to preserve oxygenation. ACS may affect cerebral perfusion adversely in patients with coexisting head trauma. IAP in this setting raises intrapleural pressure and impairs cerebral venous outflow, raising ICP. The increased ICP combined with ACS-induced depression of cardiac output decreases cerebral perfusion. Some patients with head and abdominal injuries may require abdominal decompression to decrease an abnormally elevated ICP.

Describe surgical scenarios where this phenomenon is commonly encountered. In addition to during abdominal trauma, ACS occurs postpartum and during recovery from hypothermia, cardiac arrest, septic shock, and elective or emergency intraabdominal surgeries, including abdominal aortic procedures and liver transplantation. ACS is observed regularly after abbreviated laparotomy for significant trauma-associated injuries, especially hepatic lacerations and major vascular injuries. Perihepatic packs are suspected to be causative, although intraabdominal fluid collections, bowel clots, and bowel edema likely play contributory roles.

What effect does this syndrome have upon the pulmonary, cardiovascular, and renal systems? ACS should be considered in any patient with severe intraabdominal injuries who experiences declining cardiovascular, renal, or pulmonary function. The presence of ongoing hemorrhage, coagulopathy, or resuscitation with large fluid volumes should raise clinical suspicion further. When suspected, the diagnosis of ACS is established by measuring bladder pressures, which reflect IAP. After instillation of 50 mL of water into the bladder, the Foley catheter is clamped, and pressures are measured at the level of the symphysis pubis via the Foley catheter's sampling port. Pressures >35 cm H_2O indicate a need for immediate laparotomy to prevent permanent organ failure or death from elevated IAP. Pressures between 20 and 35 cm H_2O require interpretation within the clinical context. Pressures <20 cm H_2O rarely require operative intervention.

What is the treatment? A promptly performed abdominal decompression may reverse all deleterious effects of ACS. Ongoing hemorrhage should be controlled, and coagulation disturbances and hypothermia should be reversed. Blood pressure usually is maintained postdecompression if fluid resuscitation was adequate before reexploration. Reclosure is considered on a case-by-case basis. If primary closure is not possible because of persistent bowel edema or retained abdominal packs, temporary closure may be instituted using opened, sterilized 3-L genitourinary irrigation bags.

The Present Patient

The present patient underwent emergent laparotomy. As the towel clamps were removed, a fountain of serosanguineous fluid sprang from the wound. A total of 3 to 4 L of fluid was suctioned from the abdominal cavity. As abdominal packs were teased from the hepatic injuries, some oozing was noted and the packs were left in place. Urine output, cardiac output, and pulmonary function improved, and the patient was closed with a 3-L genitourinary irrigant bag. Abdominal packs were removed 24 hours later, and the patient gradually recovered.

Clinical Pearls

1. ACS should be suspected in any critically ill patient with decreasing cardiac output, progressive respiratory failure, and oliguria, especially in the setting of coagulopathy, significant fluid resuscitation, third-space fluid losses, or continued bleeding.

2. Because intraabdominal pressure is well transmitted to the pleural space, central venous pressure or pulmonary artery occlusion pressure may overestimate cardiac filling and fail to detect underresuscitation.

3. In the presence of systemic hypotension, a trial of fluid therapy is indicated despite *normal* measured central venous pressures in patients with ACS.

4. The diagnosis of ACS is confirmed by measuring elevated bladder pressures. Pressures >35 cm H_2O warrant urgent abdominal decompression; pressures between 20 and 35 cm H_2O are borderline values and require interpretation within the clinical context.

5. Although preload augmentation usually is a satisfactory temporizing measure, the treatment for ACS is abdominal decompression. The clinician should be prepared to treat ongoing hemorrhage and coagulation disturbances.

REFERENCES

1. Meldrum DR, Moore FA, Moore EE, et al: Cardiopulmonary hazards of perihepatic packing for major liver injuries. Am J Surg 170:537–542, 1995.
2. Ridings PC, Bloomfield GL, Blocher CR, et al: Cardiopulmonary effects of raised intra-abdominal pressure before and after intravascular volume expansion. J Trauma 39:1071–1075, 1995.
3. Burch JM, Moore EE, Moore FA, et al: The abdominal compartment syndrome. Surg Clin North Am 76:833–842, 1996.
4. Saggi BH, Sugerman HJ, Ivatury RR, et al: Abdominal compartment syndrome. J Trauma 45:597–609, 1998.
5. Maxwell RA, Fabian TC, Croce MA, et al: Secondary abdominal compartment syndrome: An underappreciated manifestation of hemorrhagic shock. J Trauma 47:995–999, 1999.
6. Ertel W, Oberholzer A, Platz A, et al: Incidence and clinical pattern of the abdominal compartment syndrome after "damage-control" laparotomy in 311 patients with severe abdominal and/or pelvic trauma. Crit Care Med 28:1747–1753, 2000.

James Duke, MD

PATIENT 8

A 47-year-old man with chest pain and imaging abnormalities

A 47-year-old man was a restrained driver in a motor vehicle accident. His automobile was struck on the driver's side, and a prolonged extrication was required. On arrival in the emergency department, he is alert and cooperative, complaining only of chest pain. He was previously healthy and denies medications and allergies.

Physical Examination: Temperature normal, pulse 120, respirations 40, blood pressure 132/93. General appearance: immobilized on a hard board with Philadelphia collar, pale, slightly diaphoretic, alert. Neck: no cervical tenderness, masses, or asymmetry. Chest: left-sided rib cage tenderness, slight bruising, no crepitance, breath sounds clear and equal. Cardiac: regular rate with 1/6 systolic ejection murmur at left sternal border. Abdomen: normal. Extremities: normal, symmetric pulses. Neurologic: Glasgow coma scale 15.

Laboratory Findings: Hematocrit 44%, WBC 7,000/μL, electrolytes normal. ECG: sinus tachycardia. Cervical spine radiographs (cross-table lateral, anteroposterior, and odontoid view): normal. Chest radiograph: see Figure. Arch aortogram: see Figure.

Questions: Interpret the chest radiograph and arch aortogram.
What is the natural history of this malady?
Describe the anesthetic management of this problem, including choice and site of insertion of invasive monitoring.

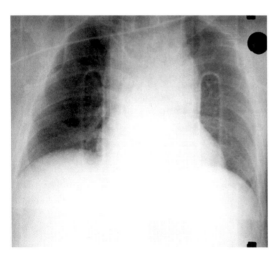
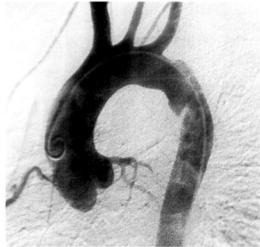

Interpret the chest radiograph and arch aortogram. Widened mediastinum and intimal tear secondary to traumatic dissection of the proximal descending aorta.

What is the natural history? Traumatic dissection of the aorta usually occurs as a result of deceleration injuries (motor vehicle or motorcycle accidents, motor vehicle/pedestrian accidents, and falls) and has an initial mortality of 70% to 90%. Prehospital survival depends on containment of the dissection by an intact aortic adventitium. Although injury is usually at the level of the ligamentum arteriosum just distal to the left subclavian artery (about 90%), dissection also may occur at the ascending aorta, great vessels, or diaphragmatic hiatus.

Coexisting injuries are common and include myocardial contusion (>50%), pulmonary contusion, head and cervical spine injury, long bone fractures, and abdominal visceral injury. Patients who are conscious may complain of ripping or tearing chest or back pain. There may be external signs of chest trauma, such as bruising, rib or sternal fractures, or flail segments. If the dissection has produced arterial occlusion, focal neurologic signs may be evident and confused with spinal cord or head injuries. Pulses may be asymmetric, or there may be disparity in blood pressure readings, either between right and left upper extremities or between upper and lower extremities. The patient may be hypotensive from blood loss or hypertensive and in need of immediate blood pressure control to prevent extension of the dissection. Because 50% of patients have no external signs of injury, a high index of suspicion based on the mechanism of injury is required.

Chest radiographs may reveal a widened superior mediastinum, but only about 17% of trauma patients with a widened mediastinum are proved to have dissection after aortography. Occasionally, initial chest radiographs are normal. Additional valuable radiologic features include blunted aortic contours; depression of the left main stem bronchus; leftward deviation of the endotracheal tube or trachea; rightward deviation of the nasograstric tube; sternal, clavicular, or rib fractures (fractures of the first and second ribs suggest extreme forces were transmitted at injury); hemothorax; and left apical hematoma. CT and MRI are not as informative as arch aortography, which should identify clearly the location and extent of dissection, as evident in the Figure on the previous page.

Describe the anesthetic management of this problem, including choice and site of invasive monitoring. Patients sustaining this injury should undergo standard early resuscitation, but a few points require emphasis. If endotracheal intubation was not secured in the field, this procedure should be undertaken with great care and attention to hemodynamic stability. In addition to possible cervical spine injury, laryngoscopy and intubation may produce hypertension and tachycardia, resulting in extension or rupture of the dissection. If associated injuries and general condition are not a contraindication, β-adrenergic blockade with the short-acting agent esmolol and hypertensive control with sodium nitroprusside may be instituted. This combination has the advantage of not only lowering blood pressure, but also controlling heart rate and contractile force (dP/dt). The likelihood of cardiac contusion must be entertained because this may complicate operative management.

Concomitant visceral injuries requiring exploratory laparotomy are frequent, and such injuries should be ruled out by diagnostic peritoneal lavage, abdominal ultrasound, or CT. Laparotomy to control intraabdominal sources of bleeding usually precedes thoracotomy for aortic repair. Pulmonary artery catheterization is necessary because the aorta proximal and distal to the injury will be cross-clamped, subjecting the heart to increased afterload. Right radial arterial monitoring is preferred because the left subclavian may be involved in the injury or occluded during aortic cross-clamping. Femoral arterial monitoring is indicated to monitor distal perfusion. Urine output should be followed via an indwelling Foley catheter.

Because the repair will be undertaken through a left lateral thoracotomy with the patient placed in the right lateral decubitus position, a double-lumen endotracheal tube (or other device to isolate lungs) should be placed for single-lung ventilation of the right lung. If the patient already is intubated, exchanging a single-lumen tube for a double-lumen tube is challenging because of concerns for aspiration of gastric contents, immobilization of the cervical spine, oxygenation, and tight hemodynamic control.

Surgical alternatives include the *clamp and sew* technique, passive arterial shunts, and active shunts (cardiopulmonary or partial left heart bypass). The clamp and sew technique has the highest associated rates of paraplegia and requires proficiency because cross-clamp times of >30 to 35 minutes are associated with higher rates of paraplegia. Complete cardiopulmonary bypass requires full anticoagulation, and patients often exsanguinate subsequently. Partial left heart bypass has been used successfully with essentially no subsequent paraplegia. Cannulae are inserted proximally into the left atrium or left superior pulmonary vein, with distal cannulation into the femoral artery. Using centrifugal pumps and heparin-bonded tubing, flows of 1.5 to 5 L/min (usually 2 to 3.5 L/min) are generated, and no or minimal heparinization is needed. Perfusion is maintained to the distal spinal cord, renal and splanchnic beds, and skeletal muscle; superior afterload reduction is obtained as well. An additional beneficial effect of afterload reduction is lessening of intracranial and cerebrospinal fluid pressures, maintaining spinal cord perfusion pressure. Declamping phenomena and ischemia-reperfusion injuries are lessened as well.

As mentioned, paraplegia is the principal postoperative complication and has been noted in 15% to 40% of patients undergoing surgical repair. Causes include interruption of intercostal vessels supplying the anterior spinal cord and hypoperfusion. Other postoperative complications include renal failure, adult respiratory distress syndrome, sepsis, and multiple organ failure. The association with myocardial contusion is particularly worrisome because patients with both injuries have a 38% postoperative mortality.

The Present Patient

The present patient was administered esmolol (500 μg/kg load and 50 μg/kg/min infusion) and nitroprusside (10 μg/min). He was brought to the operating room, a right radial arterial catheter was inserted, and other standard monitors were applied. After preoxygenation, a modified rapid sequence induction with in-line cervical stabilization and cricoid pressure was performed, and the trachea was intubated with a 39F, left-sided double-lumen endotracheal tube. Pulmonary arterial and right femoral arterial catheterization was instituted. After placement in the right lateral decubitus position with the hips turned back to the left, right-sided single-lung ventilation, left posterolateral thoracotomy, and isolation of the left femoral artery were performed. Heparin-bonded cannulae were inserted into the left superior pulmonary vein and left femoral artery. Partial left heart bypass was instituted, a descending aortic dissection distal to the left subclavian artery was mobilized and opened between cross-clamps, and an interposition aortic graft was sewn successfully. Distal perfusion pressures of 70 to 80 mmHg were achieved at partial left heart bypass flow rates between 3 and 5 L/min. Except for mild pulmonary dysfunction, which resolved, the patient experienced no postoperative complications and was discharged in 3 weeks from the hospital.

Clinical Pearls

1. Because of the high mortality of traumatic aortic dissection and the need for urgent diagnosis, all patients with blunt chest trauma and a widened mediastinum should undergo aortography.

2. Patients with aortic dissections require careful control of hemodynamic pressures. Esmolol and sodium nitroprusside are particularly beneficial during intubation to prevent a pressor response.

3. Traumatic aortic dissections are associated commonly with other injures that involve the head and cervical spine, intraabdominal organs, and long bones.

4. Partial left heart bypass has the fewest associated postoperative complications, especially paraplegia, in patients undergoing repair of aortic dissections. Afterload reductions may enhance spinal cord perfusion pressure by lowering spinal cord cerebrospinal fluid pressure.

REFERENCES

1. McCroskey BL, Moore EE, Moore FA: A unified approach to the torn thoracic aorta. Am J Surg 162:473–476, 1991.
2. Read RA, Moore EE, Moore FA, Haenel JB: Partial left heart bypass for thoracic aortic repair: Survival without paraplegia. Arch Surg 128:746–752, 1993.
3. Forbes AD, Ashbaugh DG: Mechanical circulatory support during repair of thoracic aortic injuries improves morbidity and prevents spinal cord injury. Arch Surg 129:494–498, 1994.
4. Hunt JP, Baker CC, Lentz CW, et al: Thoracic aorta injuries: Management and outcome of 144 patients. J Trauma 40:547–556, 1996.

PATIENT 9

A 27-year-old health care worker with intraoperative cardiovascular collapse

A 27-year-old female anesthesiology resident developed moderate low abdominal pain and slight vaginal bleeding. She was 3 weeks past due for her menstrual cycle and thought she might be pregnant. Prior medical and surgical histories were unremarkable, she was on no medications, and she denied allergies to medications. Her only complaints were recurring nasal stuffiness and watery eyes, which dated back, as best she could remember, to the end of her internship 6 months prior. She also complained of eczema to her hands, managed with over-the-counter hydrocortisone cream.

The patient was diagnosed with a tubal pregnancy and scheduled for an exploratory laparotomy. Anesthetic induction and endotracheal intubation using propofol, 150 mg; fentanyl, 150 µg; and succinylcholine, 100 mg, was unremarkable. Cefotetan, 2 g, was administered as IV piggyback without difficulty, and at the time of skin incision vitals signs were stable. The abdomen was opened, and a contained right adnexal tubal pregnancy was identified. About 20 minutes into the procedure, while mobilizing the right fallopian tube, the patient's systolic blood pressure falls precipitously to 40 mmHg. Airway pressures rise precipitously to 50 cm H_2O, and the patient becomes difficult to ventilate.

Preoperative Physical Examination: Temperature normal, heart rate 74 supine with no change when sitting, respirations 14, blood pressure 122/78 supine with no change when sitting. General appearance: healthy-looking woman appears well except for minimal low abdominal discomfort. Good skin color. Chest, heart, and abdominal examinations unremarkable except for low abdominal tenderness. Pelvic examination: fullness in right adnexa.

Laboratory Findings: Hematocrit 38%. β-human chorionic gonadotropin positive. Pelvic ultrasound: right adnexal mass and blood in the cul-de-sac.

Questions: What diagnosis can explain the precipitous decrease in blood pressure and increase in airway pressure?
Are there any features of the history or physical to assist in making a diagnosis?
Formulate a treatment plan to address this instability.
What is the key to protection for health care workers?

What diagnosis can explain the precipitous decrease in blood pressure and increase in airway pressure? Latex anaphylaxis secondary to occupational exposure.

Universal precautions have become an everyday practice for health care workers. The benefit of such practice is to protect health care workers from exposure to viral illnesses, such as HIV, hepatitis B and C, and other communicable diseases. **Latex gloves** are an essential feature of universal precautions, but increased use of gloves and other latex products has created allergic reactions in patients and health care workers. Of the general population, 8% may have latex allergy. About 17% of health care workers have latex sensitivity, and about 70% of adverse events related to latex are in health care workers. A few thousand allergic reactions are reported annually to the Food and Drug Administration, with about 1% resulting in death.

There are numerous proteins within latex that may produce allergic reactions. Chemicals introduced during the manufacturing process of commercial latex products also may result in allergic reactions. With the dramatic increase in the need for latex products, quantity has been sacrificed for quality, and latex products differ dramatically in the number of allergens detectable. There are multiple routes by which patients and health care workers can be exposed to the allergens, including contact with intact or abraded skin, contact with mucous membranes, by inhalation, or by exposure to an open vascular tree.

There are three forms of allergic reactions that may result from latex exposure. Potentially the most serious is the **immediate hypersensitivity,** or type I allergic reaction. This allergic reaction requires previous exposure to the latex protein allergen and depends on formation of IgE antibodies. Individuals also may experience the delayed hypersensitivity, or type IV allergic reaction from chemicals introduced in the manufacturing process. Type IV reactions are due to lymphocyte activation. Nonimmunologic skin reactions may result in skin irritation.

Are there any features of the history or physical to assist in making a diagnosis? Patient populations at risk include patients born with meningocele, myelomeningocele, and spina bifida. Patients requiring long-term bladder catheterization, such as those with spinal cord injury or developmental abnormalities of the genitourinary system, also are at risk. Patients having had multiple operations have more frequent allergic reactions, as do patients with allergic histories, known as *atopy*. Individuals who have problems with latex products

such as condoms, diaphragms, gloves, or dental dams may have severe latex-associated allergic reactions. Anyone having had a severe allergic reaction during medical care in the past may have latex hypersensitivity.

Extensive preparation for patients suspected or known to have latex allergy is required for surgery to be performed safely. The cases should be scheduled first in the morning because the amount of airborne latex particles is least at the beginning of the day. Nonlatex surgical and anesthesia supplies and nonlatex gloves are essential. Increasingly, latex-free medical supplies are the standard for all patients, but it is important to be familiar with supplies used in your department because a totally latex-free environment for all cases has yet to be achieved. Ordinarily, latex-containing supplies are labeled as such.

Formulate a treatment plan to address this instability. The typical presentation for a severe reaction is a patient with prior exposure and symptoms developing some 20 to 60 minutes after the current exposure. Respiratory symptoms include edema, especially of mucous membranes and the larynx, bronchospasm, and pulmonary edema. Cardiovascular symptoms include hypotension and tachycardia. Cutaneous manifestations include flushing and hives. These are the manifestations of the most severe, potentially fatal, IgE-mediated reaction, known as *anaphylaxis*. Should a real or likely anaphylactic reaction be recognized, the following actions should be undertaken: (1) Call for help and remove offending stimulus. (2) Limit use of anesthetic agents as much as possible. (3) Complete the procedure as quickly as possible. (4) Administer 100% oxygen. (5) Be aggressive with volume expansion. (6) Administer accelerated doses of epinephrine based on patient response, or norepinephrine in refractory cases, and antihistamines and corticosteroids. (7) Administer aminophylline and albuterol for bronchospasm.

There are basically three types of allergy testing. In the skin-prick test, a dilute latex solution is placed on the skin, the skin below the solution is scraped, and redness and swelling are noted. The risk of this skin test is that a severe, systemic reaction may be produced. Blood may be analyzed for IgE antibodies (radioallergosorbent test). There may be a 30% false-negative rate with these tests, however, and they are expensive. A third alternative is to place a latex glove on one hand and a nonlatex glove on the other and later inspect for a reaction. Despite best efforts, a latex allergy may be missed where one exists, or a severe reaction may be produced during testing. There is no universally accepted standardized serum test to assess type I latex allergy. The best method to identify at-risk patients is to take a careful history. Testing is probably not indicated, **except perhaps in people with occupational exposure**.

What is the key to protection for health care workers? Currently, about 70% of all allergic reactions are reported in health care workers, and it is estimated that 15% of anesthesia personnel have developed some degree of latex sensitivity. Most allergic reactions probably are due to inhalation exposure from latex particles adhering to the powder of powdered gloves. Because signs and symptoms may be nonspecific (puffy eyes, nasal congestion, sneezing, wheezing, coughing, hoarseness), the connection may not be made to an occupational exposure. Health care workers who develop hand dermatitis or have an atopic history may be at increased risk. Although sensitization may occur at work, severe allergic manifestations may occur while health care workers are receiving medical care themselves. The key to the protection of health care workers is to reduce work-related exposure ("Stop the Sensitization!"). The use of nonpowdered latex gloves or latex-free gloves is probably the most important intervention. Maintaining good skin care is important, and health care workers who develop skin rashes might consider visiting an employee health clinic and possible latex sensitivity testing. It is important to not wear scrub suits home because there are reports of family members developing latex sensitivity by this route.

The Present Patient

Suspecting the present patient was experiencing an anaphylactic reaction, epinephrine was administered intravenously, starting with 1 mg and doubling every subsequent dose until the patient's blood pressure improved. The volatile anesthetic was reduced, and 100% oxygen was delivered. Inhaled nebulized albuterol was administered to correct the bronchospasm. Diphenhydramine (Benadryl) and hydrocortisone were administered intravenously. The surgeons switched to latex-free gloves, the latex-containing blood pressure cuff was replaced, and all other latex products were removed from patient contact. No further medications were drawn up through latex stoppers, and a Neoprene ventilating bag was placed on the anesthesia machine. The patient achieved hemodynamic stability, the surgery was completed expeditiously, and the patient was taken to the intensive care unit for further care. No further instability was noted, and she recovered well. Subsequently, radioallergosorbent testing was positive for latex allergy. The resident later returned to training. Powderless gloves for herself and all individuals within her operating room were used to reduce her latex exposure. The nasal stuffiness and watery eyes she previously experienced resolved.

Clinical Pearls

1. To prevent severe latex-related allergic reactions, it is important to identify patients at risk, and taking a good history is key.

2. Proper preparation of the operating room environment is crucial. Patients at risk should be scheduled as first cases. Latex-containing and non–latex-containing supplies should be identified clearly and the former avoided.

3. The proper medications needed to treat a reaction adequately should it occur must be at hand. Allergic reactions should be treated aggressively. Epinephrine doses should be accelerated if needed.

4. Health care workers are at increased risk for latex hypersensitivity. The use of powdered gloves should be avoided wherever possible. Health care workers should be alert for the development of symptoms that might be latex allergy.

5. Health care workers with type I latex allergy should have proper allergy identification and always carry an epinephrine autoinjector device.

REFERENCES

1. Natural Rubber Latex Allergy: Considerations for Anesthesiologists (Handbook). Park Ridge, IL, American Society of Anesthesiologists.
2. Leynadier F, Pecquet C, Dry J: Anaphylaxis to latex during surgery. Anaesthesia 44:547–550, 1989.
3. Yassin MS, Lierl MB, Fisher TJ, et al: Latex allergy in hospital employees. Ann Allergy 72:245–249, 1994.

Websites of Interest

American College of Allergy, Asthma, and Immunology. www.allergy.mcg.edu

American Society of Anesthesiologists. www.asa. org

National Institute for Occupational Safety and Health. www.cdc.gov/niosh

James C. Duke, MD

PATIENT 10

A 70-year-old hypertensive man with postinduction hypotension

A 70-year-old man complains of pain, numbness, and tingling in the right leg. MRI reveals spinal stenosis from lumbar levels 1 to 4, and he is scheduled for a three-level spinal decompression. He has hypertension under good control. His exercise tolerance is limited by his leg symptoms. Prior surgeries include two laminectomies about 10 years ago. Medications include hydrochlorothiazide, 25 mg daily; atenolol, 50 mg daily; and losartan, 50 mg daily.

Physical Examinations: Temperature normal, heart rate 71, respirations 12, blood pressure 111/60. General appearance: obese man (6 feet tall, weighing 109 kg) complaining only of leg discomfort. Cardiac, pulmonary, and abdominal examinations are unremarkable. Decreased right patellar reflex and pain on straight-leg raise.

Laboratory Findings: Sodium 135 mEq/L; potassium 4.4 mEq/L, chloride 98 mEq/L, bicarbonate 25 mEq/L. BUN 31 mg/dL, creatinine 1.4 mg/dL. Hematocrit 53%. Platelet count and coagulation studies unremarkable. ECG: normal sinus rhythm, left anterior fascicular block, and inverted T waves in leads II and III. Dipyridamole (Persantine)-thallium scan: fixed inferior subendocardial defect and no myocardium at ischemic risk. Transthoracic echocardiogram: mild left atrial and ventricular dilation, moderate mitral regurgitation, and mild diastolic dysfunction. Overall left ventricular function mildly depressed.

Anesthetic induction and endotracheal intubation proceeded using sufentanil, 20 μg; propofol, 150 mg; and rocuronium, 70 mg. Before intubation, his blood pressure decreased to 60/35 mmHg, and he was treated with multiple 100-μg boluses of phenylephrine with improvement of blood pressure to 80/50 mmHg. Blood pressure did not improve with the stimulus of laryngoscopy and intubation. He received multiple intravenous fluid boluses. He continued to receive 100-μg phenylephrine and 10-mg ephedrine boluses, but his systolic blood pressure could not be increased beyond 90 mmHg. He developed inferior ST segment depression and was started on dopamine, 10 μg/kg/min, and nitroglycerin, 0.25 μg/kg/min. Radial arterial and pulmonary artery catheters were inserted. Initial pulmonary arterial pressure was 53/22 mmHg, and pulmonary artery occlusion pressure was 21 mmHg. Blood pressure stabilized at 100/50 mmHg. Chest auscultation revealed bilateral moist rales. Plans for surgery are cancelled, and he is transferred to the surgical intensive care unit intubated. Total fluid received is 2.5 L.

Questions: What caused his poor hemodynamic response to anesthetic induction?
Discuss the components of the renin-angiotensin system.
Discuss the management of these hypotensive episodes.

What caused this poor hemodynamic response to anesthetic induction? Refractory hypotension secondary to long-term use of angiotensin receptor antagonists (losartan).

Discuss the components of the renin-angiotensin system. Blood pressure is mediated through sympathetic nervous system stimulation, release of vasopressin, activation of the renin-angiotensin system, and activation of other hormonal systems. The renin-angiotensin system is activated when renin is secreted from juxtaglomerular cells within the kidney in response to decreased renal artery perfusion, decreased sodium delivery to the macula densa, or sympathetic nervous system activation. Renin then cleaves the hepatically produced α_2-globulin angiotensinogen to generate angiotensin I. This decapeptide is cleaved rapidly to the octapeptide angiotensin II by angiotensin-converting enzyme (ACE). The principal site of this conversion is within the pulmonary circulation, and the principal effect of angiotensin II is within the vascular endothelium. Angiotensin II is a potent vasopressor, stimulates the release of aldosterone from the adrenal cortex (increasing sodium retention), promotes fluid retention by stimulating release of vasopressin, metabolizes bradykinins, and decreases the release of renin in a negative feedback fashion.

ACE inhibitors (ACEIs) are effective in the treatment of hypertension, decrease mortality in congestive heart failure and left ventricular dysfunction after myocardial infarction, and delay the progression of diabetic nephropathy. Overall, ACEIs have a favorable side-effect profile compared with other antihypertensives, contributing to their popularity. They have fewer central nervous system effects than centrally acting antihypertensives, avoid the effects of β-blockade (e.g., heart failure, bronchospasm), have fewer metabolic effects than diuretics, and lack rebound when discontinued. However, renal function may deteriorate in the presence of bilateral renal artery stenosis, hyperkalemia may be observed in the renal impaired patient, and hypotension may be observed in volume-depleted individuals. Cough has been noted secondary to increased bradykinins.

Other enzymes besides ACE contribute to the generation of angiotensin II, and the effect of ACEIs on angiotensin II production is incomplete. Recognizing this, angiotensin receptor antagonists (ARAs) were developed; these drugs competitively inhibit the binding of angiotensin II at its receptor. ARAs are approximately equally efficacious with ACEIs in the treatment of hypertension. Similar to ACEIs, ARAs improve left ventricular function in chronic congestive heart failure. Be-cause some of the beneficial effects of ACEIs may be due to bradykinin potentiation, however, the salutary effect of ACEIs on renal insufficiency may not be observed with ARAs. Similarly, because they do not inhibit bradykinin metabolism, they do not have cough as a side effect.

Hypotension on anesthetic induction has been noted in patients taking ACEIs and in patients taking ARAs. The mechanism is believed to be loss of sympathetic tone superimposed on renin-angiotension system blockade. The vasopressin system is the only intact system left to maintain blood pressure. Because vasopressin more effectively improves arterial resistance than systemic vascular capacity, fluid loading should be beneficial during such hypotensive episodes.

The hypotensive effect at anesthetic induction has been noted regardless whether the patients were administered these medications for hypertension or ischemic heart failure, and magnitude of hypotension seems about equal in both groups. Patients on multiple antihypertensives or with left ventricular diastolic dysfunction may be particularly at risk because they are volume-dependent individuals.

Discuss the management of these hypotensive episodes. Investigations from Coriat and Colson[1,2,5] suggest the hypotensive episodes are managed easily with fluids and the vasopressors phenylephrine and ephedrine. Eyraud et al[6] disputed the ease of treatment of such patients because vasopressin analogs were required in 20% of their patients to correct hypotension refractory to other pressors. Hypotension has been noted in 75% of patients on ACEIs and ARAs at anesthetic induction and intraoperatively. Brabant et al[4] found the hypotensive episodes associated with ARAs were more severe and refractory to treatment than episodes associated with ACEIs. Greater amounts of ephedrine or phenylephrine were required, and vasopressin analogs were administered to approximately 30% of patients to improve blood pressure. (The effects of receptor blockade are more profound than enzyme inhibition, because other enzymes are available to convert angiotensin I to angiotensin II.) As noted by Bertrand et al, the incidence and severity of hypotensive episodes associated with ARAs were greater if the drug was not withheld the day of surgery.

The Present Patient

The present patient achieved hemodynamic stability, was weaned from his infusions, and was extubated the same day. A repeat echocardiogram showed no change in ventricular function, although the chambers were dilated slightly secondary to his fluid resuscitation. Pulmonary edema resolved with diuretics, and a myocardial infarction was ruled out. Further cardiac evaluation showed no change from his preoperative evaluation. His precipitous and severe hypotension was attributed to the use of losartan and exacerbated by the multiple antihypertensive regimen and likely volume depletion. Three weeks later, the patient returned for his surgical procedure. Losartan was withheld the day of surgery. He received a cautious anesthetic induction with fentanyl and etomidate, titrated to loss of responsiveness. Hemodynamic stability was noted through induction, and arterial and central venous catheters were inserted. The patient's intraoperative course was unremarkable; he was awakened and extubated immediately postoperatively and had a satisfactory postoperative course.

Clinical Pearls

1. Patients treated with long-term ACEIs or ARAs have a high risk of hypotension on anesthetic induction, particularly if they are on a multiple antihypertensive regimen.

2. Patients on ACEIs and ARAs are volume dependent; preoperative volume depletion places patients particularly at risk for hypotension on induction. Surgical procedures associated with large blood loss or fluid shifts may lead to refractory intraoperative hypotension. Volume infusions are beneficial in both settings.

3. ACEIs and ARAs reduce responsiveness to the usually administered exogenous pressors.

4. Although conventional practice is to administer antihypertensives the day of surgery, ACEIs and ARAs should be held the day of surgery. Withholding angiotensin antagonists when administered for chronic heart failure (rather than hypertension) should be individualized.

5. Vasopressin analogs may improve hypotension when sympathetically mediated agents such as phenylephrine and ephedrine prove ineffective.

REFERENCES

1. Colson P, Saussine M, Sequin JR, et al: Hemodynamic effects of anesthesia in patients chronically treated with angiotensin-converting enzyme inhibitors. Anesth Analg 74:805–808, 1992.
2. Coriat P, Richer C, Douraki T, et al: Influence of chronic angiotensin-converting enzyme inhibition on anesthetic induction. Anesthesiology 81:299–307, 1994.
3. Ryckwaert F, Colson P: Hemodynamic effects of anesthesia in patients with ischemic heart failure chronically treated with angiotensin converting enzyme inhibitors. Anesth Analg 84:945–949, 1997.
4. Brabant SM, Bertrand M, Eyraud D, et al: The hemodynamic effects of anesthetic induction in vascular surgical patients chronically treated with angiotensin II receptor antagonists. Anesth Analg 88:1388–1392, 1999.
5. Colson P, Ryckwaert F, Coriat P: Renin angiotensin system antagonists and anesthesia. Anesth Analg 89:1143–1155, 1999.
6. Eyraud D, Brabant S, Dieudonne N, et al: Treatment of intraoperative refractory hypotension with terlipressin in patients chronically treated with an antagonist of the renin-angiotensin system. Anesth Analg 88:980–984, 1999.
7. Bertrand M, Godet G, Meersschaert K, et al: Should the angiotensin II antagonists be discontinued before surgery? Anesth Analg 92:26–30, 2001.

James C. Duke, MD

PATIENT 11

A 74-year old man with diffuse weakness during critical illness

A 74-year-old man with chronic obstructive pulmonary disease previously had undergone left hemicolectomy for an obstructive carcinoma. He was given a colostomy and mucus fistula and was now scheduled for takedown of the colostomy and enteric reanastomosis. His prior history was remarkable for numerous pneumonias with a significant reactive airway component. He has been on steroids but has taken none in >1 year. He currently is relatively stable from a pulmonary status. He is on home oxygen, 2 L/min, and administers nebulized albuterol treatments to himself at least four times daily. He takes theophylline (Theo-Dur), 300 mg twice daily.

After a preoperative nebulized albuterol treatment, he underwent balanced general anesthesia with endotracheal intubation. His procedure was uneventful, and he was extubated at case conclusion. Blood loss was 300 mL, fluids administered were 2,500 mL, and urine output was 200 mL. After recovery, he was transferred to the floor.

On postoperative day 3, the patient developed a temperature of 39°C. He was dyspneic, and his lips were dusky. Chest auscultation revealed bilateral wheezes and decreased breath sounds at the bases. He was transferred to the intensive care unit (ICU) for close observation, placed on clindamycin and ceftazidime, and received bronchodilator therapy. Despite increasing oxygen concentrations, the patient's blood gases were deteriorating and he was obviously tiring. He was intubated and mechanically ventilated. By the next day, a chest radiograph showed diffuse alveolar infilatrates. Peak airway pressures had increased >50 cm H_2O, and albuterol therapy was not improving the patient's reactive airway disease. Aminophylline and methylprednisolone (Solu-Medrol) were administered by infusion. Ventilatory status did not improve, and the patient was fighting the ventilator. He received intermittent doses of lorazepam (Ativan) and was placed on a doxacurium infusion for 3 days. Over the next 4 days, the patient improved but attempts to wean the patient failed. He is noted to be weak in all four extremities. He responds to questions appropriately, sensation appears intact, reflexes are diffusely depressed, and cranial nerves are intact.

Laboratory Findings: Electrolytes, phosphorus, magnesium, calcium, all normal. Liver and renal profiles normal. Creatine kinase markedly elevated.

Questions: What is the diagnosis?
What historical information and physical findings aid in diagnosis?
What tests are available to confirm a diagnosis?

What is the diagnosis? Critical illness myopathy. Differential includes critical illness polyneuropathy, persistent neuromuscular blockade, catabolism/disuse atrophy, and steroid myopathy. Use of muscle relaxants was popularized in the operating room setting and became commonplace in ICUs. There is a significant difference in the pattern of use between these two environments, however. Patients may be administered relaxant doses in the ICU 100-fold greater than usual operating room use and receive these medications over extended periods. Close monitoring of neuromuscular function does not occur to the extent of hemodynamic or respiratory monitoring. Under these circumstances, and complicated by the severity of these patient's illnesses, it is not surprising that prolonged weakness and paralysis has been noted in this population. Prolonged weakness usually is identified when attempts to wean from mechanical ventilation fail. Prolonged weakness extends ICU stays and hospitalization overall, requires extensive patient rehabilitation and has significant mortality.

What historical information and physical findings aid in diagnosis? Electrolyte abnormalities are easily identifiable and readily treatable causes of weakness. Hypokalemia, hyponatremia, hypocalcemia, hypophosphatemia, and hypermagnesemia result in weakness, as does respiratory acidosis. Hepatic and renal dysfunction regularly occurs in critically ill patients, impairing metabolism of all relaxants except the atracurium compounds. Many steroid-based relaxants have active metabolites. A metabolite of vecuronium, 3-desacetyl vecuronium, has about 50% of the relaxant activity of the parent compound. Relaxants may potentiate the neuromuscular effects of other drugs, such as antibiotics. If these causes of weakness are ruled out, consideration should shift to abnormalities of nerves, muscles, and the neuromuscular junction.

Of patients with sepsis, multiple organ dysfunction, or systemic inflammatory response syndrome, 70% develop generalized weakness associated with sensory loss and other neurologic findings. This syndrome has been termed **critical illness polyneuropathy.** The longer the duration of the underlying illness, the more severe the weakness. Patients with mild or moderate underlying critical illness are likely to improve in strength when their primary condition improves, although death is frequent in patients severely affected (and usually related to the primary illness). The mechanism, although unknown, is thought to be a disturbance of microvasculature, resulting in neuronal ischemia and increased capillary permeability. Under these circumstances, relaxants may

penetrate neuronal and muscle membranes in toxic concentration. Failure to wean is the most common presentation, but coexistent encephalopathy often clouds the clinical picture. Severe cases may present as areflexic quadriparesis. Other clinical characteristics include predominantly distal limb weakness with muscle wasting, decreased or absent deep tendon reflexes, and variable sensory loss, often in a stocking-and-glove distribution. Cranial nerves are intact. Creatine kinase levels are normal or slightly elevated. Cerebrospinal fluid is normal. Biopsy specimens of nerves show fiber loss with axonal degeneration, whereas muscle biopsy specimens show denervation atrophy. Electrophysiologic studies reveal an axonal polyneuropathy.

Numerous myopathies occur in the critically ill. Disuse atrophy is common, and it is estimated there may be 5% loss of strength per week when a patient is bed-ridden; muscle relaxants exacerbate disuse atrophy. Septic and injured patients are catabolic and waste muscle.

A myopathy has been identified that is associated with concurrent use of steroids and relaxants. This myopathy has gone by many names, including acute quadriplegic myopathy, acute necrotizing myopathy, and **critical illness myopathy.** This myopathy and critical illness polyneuropathy account for most cases of severe weakness in the ICU, and they may be difficult to distinguish from one another. In these situations, it is likely that features of both illnesses are present.

Critical illness myopathy is independent of persistent muscle relaxant or metabolite levels. Although most often associated with prolonged relaxant use, extended weakness has been reported after 2 to 3 days of relaxant use. Titrating relaxant use to train-of-four monitoring also has failed to eliminate cases of critical illness myopathy completely. This myopathy has been associated regularly with steroid administration in conjunction with muscle relaxants. Initially, this myopathy was believed a risk for steroidal relaxants such as vecuronium and pancuronium, but cases associated with use of the isoquinolinium relaxants atracurium and doxacurium also have been identified. The mechanism is uncertain. Chemical denervation secondary to relaxant use may render muscle more prone to toxic effects of steroids. Corticosteroid receptors are noted to increase, and as in steroid myopathy, they correlate with increased weakness. It also has been established that, similar to burns or physical denervation, neuromuscular blockade up-regulates acetylcholine receptors and increases the receptor population at extrajunctional sites. Lee[3] theorized that the common pathologic process of all relaxant-associated myopathies, regardless of the underlying critical illness, may be a disorder of the neuromuscular junction and motor membrane.

Diffuse muscular weakness with atrophy is characteristic. Profoundly affected individuals are quadriparetic. Facial, ocular, and respiratory muscles sometimes are involved. Deep tendon reflexes are reduced or absent, and sensation and autonomic function are intact. Creatine kinase levels usually are elevated substantially.

Steroid myopathy independent of the use of relaxants is well described but usually presents gradually. Weakness tends to be proximal. As mentioned, membrane corticosteroid receptors are increased and may play a causative role. Creatine kinase levels are not elevated appreciably.

Other neuromuscular disorders that may manifest during critical illness include myasthenia gravis, motor neuron disease, and Guillain-Barré syndrome. Comprehensive review is beyond the scope of this discussion, and the reader is referred to Raps et al.[1] Patients who have had any anesthetic neuraxial procedures should be evaluated for epidural hematoma or abscess. Incontinence is a feature of spinal cord dysfunction that may not be observed with neuropathies of critical illness. Cranial nerve findings, with the occasional exception of ophthalmoplegia, suggest brainstem injury. Autonomic dysfunction is a neuropathic finding and not a feature of the major illnesses discussed. Of interest to anesthesiologists, exacerbations of acute intermittent porphyria may follow administration of barbiturates and present with neuropathies, psychiatric disturbances, abdominal pain, and autonomic dysfunction.

What tests are available to confirm diagnosis? Electrodiagnostic examinations discriminate between disorders of nerve, muscle, and neuromuscular junction and include nerve conduction studies and electromyography. Performing and interpreting these examinations requires considerable expertise, and appropriate consultation is necessary. These examinations are invaluable when evaluating prolonged weakness. The Table reviews the clinical, electrophysiologic, and biopsy findings and usual creatine kinase levels.

Differential Diagnosis of Weakness in Critical Care Settings

Condition	Clinical Features	Electrophysiologic Studies	Biopsy Results	Creatine Kinase
Critical illness polyneuropathy	Weakness, distal > proximal Respiratory muscle weakness May be quadriparetic Decreased sensation Reflexes decreased or absent	Decreased nerve conduction Normal electromyography	Axonal degeneration	Normal to slightly elevated
Critical illness myopathy	Diffuse weakness Respiratory muscle weakness Reflexes decreased or absent Sensation intact	Relatively normal nerve conduction Abnormal electromyography	Myonecrosis	Markedly increased
Persistent neuromuscular blockade	Diffuse weakness Respiratory muscle weakness Reflexes normal or reduced Sensation intact	Decreased repetitive stimulation	Normal	Normal
Catabolism/ disuse atrophy	Diffuse weakness Respiratory muscle weakness Reflexes intact Sensation intact	Normal	Atrophy	Normal
Steroid myopathy	Gradual weakness Reflexes intact Sensation intact	Normal	Atrophy	Normal

The Present Patient

Electrophysiologic studies confirmed critical illness myopathy. Nerve conduction was normal, whereas motor action potentials were severely reduced. The patient underwent tracheostomy and was weaned from mechanical ventilation in approximately 1 month. Over a 3-month period of rehabilitation, the patient's strength eventually returned to a functional but incomplete level.

Clinical Pearls

1. Use of muscle relaxants in the ICU requires thought in terms of indication, selection of relaxant and dose, duration of paralysis, and, importantly, a consideration of alternatives to neuromuscular blockade. Sedation and analgesia as an alternative suffices in many situations.

2. Common causes of prolonged weakness in critically ill patients include organ dysfunction; electrolyte abnormalities; medications; and disorders of neurons, neuromuscular junction, and muscle. Muscle relaxants may exacerbate weakness resulting from many of these disorders.

3. Administration of relaxants titrated to train-of-four stimulation reduces but does not eliminate the possibility of an ICU neuromuscular syndrome. Monitoring relaxant effect is likely to reduce overall relaxant dose. Relaxant use should be limited to 48 hours if possible.

4. Review of muscle relaxant dosing, physical findings, electrolytes, hepatic and renal panels, creatine kinase, electrophysiologic studies, and nerve and muscle biopsy assists in establishing the cause of prolonged weakness.

REFERENCES

1. Raps EC, Bird SJ, Hansen-Flaschen J: Prolonged muscle weakness after neuromuscular blockade in the intensive care unit. Crit Care Clin 10:799–813, 1994.
2. Lee C: Intensive care unit neuromuscular syndrome? Anesth Analg 83:237–240, 1995.
3. Sigg DC, Hasinof IK, Iaizzo PA: Prolonged paralysis and muscular weakness in critically ill patients: I. Pathophysiology and differential diagnosis. Am J Anesthesiol 27:265–272, 2000.
4. Sigg DC, Hasinoff K, Iaizzo PA: Prolonged paralysis and muscular weakness in critically ill patients: II. Neuromuscular blockers. Am J Anesthesiol 27:321–328, 2000.

James C. Duke, MD

PATIENT 12

A 47-year-old man with cardiovascular collapse under spinal anesthesia

A 47-year-old man was scheduled for right femoral head decompression as treatment for avascular necrosis. He is otherwise healthy, takes no medications, and has no prior surgeries. Because he is an occasional cigarette smoker, he is given the American Society of Anesthesiologists' physical class II.

He was brought into the operating room after having an 18-G IV catheter inserted. Lactated Ringer's solution was running freely. Automated blood pressure device, ECG, and pulse oximeter were attached. All findings were normal except for a sinus bradycardia with P-R interval of 0.22 seconds (first-degree atrioventricular block). An oxygen cannula was placed and oxygen flowed at 3 L/min. Midazolam, 2 mg, and fentanyl, 100 μg, were administered intravenously. The patient was placed in a lateral decubitus position, and 12.5 mg of hyperbaric bupivacaine with fentanyl, 25 μg, was administered intrathecally without difficulty. He was returned supine, and after 10 minutes a T4 level was verified by pinprick. He was turned again to a lateral position and prepared for surgery. Total IV fluids administered by this time was 500 mL.

An additional 2 mg of midazolam is given and a propofol infusion is begun at 50 μg/kg/min. The surgery begins, and all appears well. The patient seemed to go to sleep. Oxygen saturations declined to 90%, so a nonrebreathing mask replaced the nasal cannula and improved oxygen saturation. Soon thereafter, the blood pressure is noted to be 80/45 mmHg. Ephedrine, 10 mg, is administered, and IV fluids are increased; this fails to improve the patient's blood pressure. The anesthesiologist notes that the patient's heart rate has decreased precipitously, and the patient suddenly develops asystole.

Questions: What happened to the patient?
What effect does spinal (or epidural) anesthesia have during intravenous sedation?
What is the effect of neuraxial anesthesia on volatile anesthetics?
Describe the role of afferent spinal cord impulses on consciousness.
Describe the factors that may result in cardiac arrest during spinal (or epidural) anesthesia.
Discuss the treatment of cardiac arrest in the setting of spinal anesthesia.

What happened to the patient? Increased sensitivity to sedatives secondary to deafferentiation. Relative hypovolemia during spinal anesthesia associated with increased vagal tone.

Although long ago it was noted that patients under spinal anesthesia experience increasing drowsiness as the level of blockade rises, a landmark publication discussing predisposing factors for unexpected cardiac arrest during spinal anesthesia has stimulated investigation into causes of this concerning phenomenon. As part of the American Society of Anesthesiologists' study of closed insurance claims for major anesthetic mishaps, Caplan et al[1] identified a concerning subset of 14 patients who were previously healthy and undergoing procedures under spinal anesthesia. These patients developed unanticipated cardiac arrest and subsequently died or experienced devastating neurologic injuries. The cases occurred between 1978 and 1986 (before routine pulse oximetry use), and common features among the patients included American Society of Anesthesiologists' physical status I or II; relative youth (36 ± 15 years); spinal anesthesia; and sufficient sedation to produce a comfortable-appearing, sleeplike state in which there was no spontaneous verbalization. Sedatives included fentanyl, diazepam, droperidol, and thiopental and were administered in reasonable doses. The cardiac arrests were commonly preceded by various combinations of bradycardia, hypotension, and cyanosis. Despite prompt recognition, the average duration of external cardiac massage was about 8 ± 4 minutes. Six patients died during that hospitalization, and 4 patients survived the initial hospitalization but never regained consciousness and subsequently died. Of the four patients who regained consciousness, all developed persistent cognitive defects and required assisted living. The authors proposed that a primary respiratory event producing hypoxia and hypercarbia and circulatory changes secondary to high sympathetic block were contributory factors in the patients' subsequent collapse. In an accompanying editorial, Keats[2] raised the issue of **deafferentiation** playing a role in modifying the respiratory response of sedatives in the setting of spinal anesthesia.

Describe the role of afferent spinal cord impulses on consciousness. Afferentiation theory states that consciousness is maintained in part through afferent stimulation. Peripheral sensory nerves and motor spindle fibers contribute sensory input into the reticular activating system, resulting in cerebral stimulation. Loss of this input, as through neuraxial anesthesia, may make a patient more prone to sedative-induced respiratory depression. Brainstem effects of neuraxially administered local anesthetics may play a part, although this has not been established definitively.

What is the effect of neuraxial anesthesia on volatile anesthetics? Numerous studies have shown the increased effects of sedatives and volatile anesthetics during spinal and epidural anesthesia. Ben-David et al[3] found that the doses of midazolam necessary to achieve loss of responsiveness to verbal stimuli during tetracaine spinal anesthesia were 50% of does required to achieve the same loss of response in patients without spinal anesthesia. Hodgson and Liu[6] found that lidocaine epidural anesthesia reduced by 34% the sevoflurane requirement to maintain a bispectral index reading of 50, a value showing adequate depth of anesthesia. A 50% reduction in the minimal alveolar concentration (MAC) of sevoflurane was noted during combined general and epidural anesthesia with lidocaine. The reduction of MAC was independent of systemic lidocaine levels. Sedative potentiation during regional anesthesia also has been noted with propofol, thiopental, and isoflurane.

Although neuraxial anesthesia clearly potentiates the effects of sedatives and volatile anesthetics, it is difficult to claim that this affect on either arousal or respiration results in cardiac arrest. Since the regular use of pulse oximetry, cardiac arrest during spinal anesthesia has been documented with oximetry saturations of 95% to 100%. Bradyarrhythmias and cardiac underfilling are likely more important. Spinal anesthesia results in blockade of cardiac accelerator fibers located from T1 to T4. Because sympathetic denervation is achieved two to six levels above sensory blockade, a T6 dermatomal sensory loss may be associated with total cardioaccelerator denervation. Loss of cardiac preload also may result in bradyarrhythmias. Reductions in right atrial pressure of 36% to 53% have been noted after spinal anesthesia. Although fluid augmentation is considered a necessity before instituting neuraxial blockade, lack of close attention in this regard has been documented. In association with decreased cardiac preload, cardiac slowing occurs as a result of neurally mediated cardiac reflexes (the Bezold-Jarisch reflex). Patients with high resting vagal tone may be particularly at risk for further heart rate reductions and cardiac arrest during neuraxial anesthesia.

Discuss the treatment of cardiac arrest during spinal (or epidural) anesthesia. Fluid administration before performing neuraxial anesthesia is important. Likewise, the need to replace intraoperative blood losses should not be underestimated. Cardiac underfilling may occur precipitously during periods of rapid blood loss, release of tourniquets, administration of vasodilators, and changes in positioning. If abrupt reductions in preload are suspected, rapid fluid administration and head-down positioning are appropriate to reestablish right atrial filling. Atropine or vasopressor administration (in escalating doses if necessary) should be considered.

A notable finding in Caplan's review was the average 8-minute delay before epinephrine was administered. When cardiac arrest is associated with loss of sympathetic tone, it is necessary to administer a potent α-adrenergic agonist quickly to reestablish acceptable organ perfusion. Rosenberg et al[4] showed significant reductions in coronary perfusion pressure during CPR in dogs having undergone spinal anesthesia and induced ventricular fibrillation compared with fibrillating dogs not having spinal anesthesia. The reductions in coronary perfusion pressure were believed to be below the threshold for successful resuscitation and required administation of epinephrine to improve. Rosenberg et al[4] suggested doses of 0.01 to 0.02 mg/kg of epinephrine during CPR, progressing rapidly to 0.1 mg/kg if lower doses are ineffective. The β-adrenergic effects of epinephrine also may be important by increasing heart rate.

The Present Patient

The present patient was returned immediately to the supine position and placed head-down. The patient was intubated, and chest compressions were initiated. Lactated Ringer's solution ran freely. Atropine, 0.5 mg, was administered without effect. Epinephrine, 0.5 mg, was administered with the second 0.5-mg atropine dose. A second dose of epinephrine (1 mg) was administered resulting in a sinus tachycardia and palpable radial pulse. Blood pressure was 140/90 mmHg. Fluid administration continued, and 1.5 L was administered after arrest. The patient regained consciousness, appeared in satisfactory condition, and was extubated. The surgical site was closed without completing the procedure. The patient was monitored in intensive care, found to be neurologically intact, and ruled out for a myocardial infarction. Three days later, the patient's procedure was completed without event under general anesthesia.

Clinical Pearls

1. Loss of afferent sensory and motor stimulation renders a patient sensitive to sedative medications secondary to deafferentiation.

2. For the same reason, neuraxial anesthesia decreases the MAC of volatile anesthetics.

3. Administration of supplemental oxygen when sedation accompanies neuraxial anesthesia is likely to maintain satisfactory oxygenation but may mask hypoventilation.

4. Vagal predominance suggests that a patient may be at risk for cardiovascular collapse during neuraxial anesthesia. Intraoperative bradycardia may be a sign of cardiac underfilling as a result of peripheral vascular dilation, surgical events, and inadequate intravenous fluid administration. Loss of cardioaccelerator innervation contributes to cardiac slowing as well.

5. Patients with sympathectomies require aggressive resuscitation, perhaps with unfamiliarly large doses of pressors, to reestablish myocardial perfusion after cardiac arrest. Atropine (at least 0.5 mg and repeat if needed) and epinephrine (0.2 to 0.3 mg and escalate if needed) should be administered. Ephedrine may be considered, but this is a relatively weak, indirect-acting pressor. IV fluids should be increased and the patient should be placed in a head-down position. Loss of consciousness or oxygen desaturation requires endotracheal intubation.

REFERENCES

1. Caplan RA, Ward RJ, Posner K, et al: Unexpected cardiac arrest during spinal anesthesia: A closed claims analysis of predisposing factors. Anesthesiology 68:5–11, 1988.
2. Keats AS: Anesthsia mortality: A new mechanism. Anesthesiology 68:2–4, 1988.
3. Ben-David B, Vaida S, Gaitini L: The influence of high spinal anesthesia on sensitivity to midazolam sedation. Anesth Analg 81:525–528, 1995.
4. Rosenberg JM, Wahr JA, Sung CH, et al: Coronary perfusion pressure during cardiopulmonary resuscitation after spinal anesthesia in dogs. Anesth Analg 82:84–87, 1996.
5. Hodgson PS, Liu SS, Gras TW: Does epidural anesthesia have general anesthetic effects? Anesthesiology 91:1687–1692, 1999.
6. Hodgson PS, Liu SS: Epidural lidocaine decreases sevoflurane requirement for adequate depth of anesthesia as measured by the bispectral index monitor. Anesthesiology 94:799–803, 2001.
7. Kinsella SM, Tuckey JP: Perioperative bradycardia and asystole: Relationship to vasovagal syncope and the Bezold-Jarisch reflex. Br J Anaesth 86:859–868, 2001.
8. Pollard JB: Cardiac arrest during spinal anesthesia: Common mechanisms and strategies for prevention. Anesth Analg 92:252–256, 2001.

James C. Duke, MD

PATIENT 13

A 22-year-old woman with a poorly functioning epidural catheter for cesarean section

A healthy 22-year-old gravida 1, para 0, Ab 0 woman (Height 153 cm, weight 84 kg) is admitted 2 weeks postdates for elective induction of labor. Her membranes are ruptured, and she is begun on an oxytocin (pitocin) infusion. When her cervix dilates to 5 cm, an epidural catheter is inserted to manage the pain of labor. With the patient in the lateral position, after povidone-iodine preparation, an epidural catheter is inserted atraumatically at the L3–4 level by the loss-of-resistance technique. The catheter advances easily, and a test dose of 3 mL of 1.5% lidocaine with 1:200,000 epinephrine is negative. After 1 L of normal saline is infused intravenously, bupivacaine 0.25%, 10 mL, is injected in divided doses and provides good pain relief. An infusion of bupivacaine 0.125% with fentanyl, 5 μg/mL, is started at 10 mL/h. Pain relief over the duration of labor is judged adequate, requiring occasional 5 to 10-mL top-up doses of bupivacaine 0.25%.

Approximately 24 hours after rupture of membranes, a cesarean section is elected because of arrest of descent, and the patient is taken to the operating room. The patient is placed supine with left uterine tilt, oxygen is administered by nasal cannula at 4 L/min, and monitors are placed. After 500 mL of normal saline is administered intravenously, the epidural catheter is dosed in a divided fashion with 20 mL of 0.5% bupivacaine. Testing at the planned incision site reveals incomplete anesthesia and an additional 10 mL of 0.5% bupivacaine is administered without satisfactory result. It is decided to proceed with spinal anesthesia, so the patient is placed in a lateral decubitus position, the epidural catheter is removed, and spinal anesthesia is administered in a technically unremarkable fashion with 1.5 mL of 0.75% hyperbaric bupivacaine. Before injection, cerebrospinal fluid is aspirated easily from the 24-G Sprotte needle. The patient is returned to a supine position with left uterine tilt in preparation for surgery; the operating table is maintained in a neutral position. Within 2 minutes, the patient complains of difficulty breathing and nasal stuffiness. She becomes agitated, aphonic, then unresponsive with dilated pupils. Blood pressure is 80/60 mmHg.

Questions: What has happened to this patient?

When is spinal anesthesia appropriate for a patient having insufficient epidural anesthesia?

Discuss the factors that may have contributed to this event.

What has happened to this patient? Central neurologic block (high spinal anesthetic).

Should time allow, owing to concerns for rapid oxygen desaturation, potential difficulty in securing the airway, and risk for pulmonary aspiration of gastric contents, regional anesthesia is the preferred technique in a pregnant patient requiring cesarean section. Acceptable regional techniques include spinal, epidural, and combined spinal-epidural anesthesia.

Pregnant patients regularly receive epidural catheters and weak local anesthetic solutions to ameliorate the pain associated with uterine contractions. Should necessity dictate operative delivery, more concentrated local anesthetic solutions can be administered to achieve the necessary dense anesthetic required for surgical delivery. Anesthesia may prove suboptimal, however, and require a change in technique to spinal or general anesthesia.

When is spinal anesthesia appropriate for a patient having insufficient epidural anesthesia? Especially with the introduction of atraumatic spinal needles (reducing the incidence of post–dural puncture headaches), spinal anesthesia has become a popular, effective, and safe anesthetic technique for cesarean section. Numerous descriptions (case reports and letters to the editor) of central neurologic blockade when spinal anesthesia was instituted after failed epidural anesthesia have put the safety of this technique in question, however. Typically, these patients had preexisting epidural catheters for labor pain and for obstetric reasons went on to require operative delivery. Catheters, although repeatedly dosed, failed to achieve adequate anesthetic levels and were discontinued. Spinal anesthesia was induced, either with bupivacaine or lidocaine, and in either a gradual or precipitous fashion, the patients developed upper extremity tingling and weakness associated with difficulty breathing. Some patients received general anesthesia and were intubated at this point, and some patients were intubated after they became unresponsive, often with pupillary dilation, suggesting central neurologic blockade. A summary of the reports describing this scenario is included in the Table. Because of ethical issues, a randomized controlled investigation of the phenomenon is likely never to occur.

Discuss the factors that may have contributed to this event. Numerous theories have been postulated as to why parturients in this setting are at risk. The volume of cerebrospinal fluid is reduced in late pregnancy, allowing for higher spread. There may be diffusion of epidural local anesthetic across the obligatory dural rent incurred during performance of the spinal anesthetic. The pressure within the intrathecal space becomes atmospheric when violated, and this may alter circulation of local anesthetics. Because epidural local anesthetics do diffuse across intact dura to some extent, a *subclinical* anesthetic state may exist before direct instillation of anesthetic solutions, resulting in a higher than anticipated

Summary of Reports Describing High Spinal Anesthetics After Epidural Anesthesia

Lead Author	Report Type	Age (yr)	Height (cm)	Weight (kg)	Epidural Volume (mL)	Spinal Dose (mg Bupiv)	Authors' Comments
Beck[2]	Case report	19	150	53	28 LA	10	"Advise
		33	150	70	15 Saline	12.5	caution"
Stone[1]	Case report	24	153	54	33 LA	8	"Demonstrates hazards"
Mets[5]	Case report	24	155	98	30 LA	11.25	"Cannot be recommended"
Gupta[7]	Case report	21	165	101	23 LA	12.5	"Relative
		24	162	88	Infusion	15	contraindication"
		27	172	80	Infusion	10	
Goldstein[6]	Letter	23	163	96	Not stated	40 mg Lido	"Strongly consider
		22	168	67	20 LA	30 mg Lido	the wisdom"
Dell[4]	Letter	26	158	78	45 LA	12.5	"Extreme caution"
Furst[9]	Case report	33	175	78	55 LA	12	"Reduce spinal
		20	165	71	>42 LA	9	dose by 20%"

LA, Local anesthetic; Bupiv, bupivacaine; Lido, lidocaine.

anesthetic level. The most convincing and well-supported argument is that the lumbar intrathecal sac collapses with epidural instillation of fluids (either local anesthetics or saline), resulting in cephalad displacement of cerebrospinal fluid and higher than anticipated spinal anesthetic levels. Blumgart et al[3] induced spinal anesthesia in a group of parturients, then administered either 10 mL of 0.5% bupivacaine or normal saline. In comparison to the control group that received no subsequent epidural injections, both study groups had similar progression of anesthetic levels. Similarly, Beck and Griffiths[2] injected 15 mL of saline into the epidural space of a patient in an attempt to open up the epidural space for passage of an epidural catheter (see Table). When this attempt failed, a spinal anesthetic was performed. The patient developed tingling in the hands; became hypotensive, dyspneic, and distressed; and received general anesthesia and endotracheal intubation. Takiguchi et al[11] showed extension of spinal anesthesia after instillation of 10 mL of normal saline into the epidural space (similar to Blumgart's experience) but also showed myelographically a 75% reduction in the diameter of the lumbar subarachnoid space as 20 mL of saline was incrementally infused epidurally.

Other factors that may put the parturient at risk include vena caval occlusion, which has been shown to transmit pressure to the epidural venous plexus. Distention of epidural veins increases the volume of this space and impinges on the volume of the intrathecal space. Additionally a high body mass index (i.e., short and fat) may predispose to high spinal anesthetics, although this is a matter of dispute. Orientation of nontraumatic spinal needles during local anesthetic injection may be a factor because higher anesthetic levels have been shown when the spinal needle lumen is oriented in a cephalad direction.

Numerous authorities reporting this phenomenon suggest that spinal anesthesia after failed epidural anesthesia is a questionable practice (see Table). Stoneham,[10] Waters,[8] and Furst[9] believe that spinal anesthesia can be administered safely if the spinal dose is reduced by 20%, the procedure is performed in the sitting position and allowed to "set up," the head and cervical spine are elevated, reverse Trendelenburg positioning is used, and uterine caval decompression is ensured. There is one important caveat. A patient with a potentially difficult airway is probably not a candidate for this practice. Should a total spinal ensue despite the most conscientious efforts to control the spinal anesthetic level, the urgent need to secure the airway may prove problematic and place the mother and child at risk. This is an interesting exception to some clinicians belief that patients with potential airway management difficulty are considered good candidates for regional anesthesia, other issues notwithstanding.

The Present Patient

A rapid sequence induction with cricoid pressure was instituted immediately using thiopental sodium, 175 mg and succinylcholine, 100 mg, intravenously. The airway was secured, and 0.5% isoflurane in 100% oxygen was administered. Ephedrine, 30 mg, was administered intravenously to correct the hypotension. A vigorous infant with Apgar score 9/10 was delivered expeditiously. At conclusion of the surgical procedure, the patient showed a 5-second head lift and strong grip and was extubated. She had no memory of any of the intraoperative events, and the residual spinal anesthetic regressed in an unremarkable fashion during routine postanesthetic care.

Clinical Pearls

1. In contrast to some anesthetic situations, spinal anesthesia after failed epidural anesthesia is contraindicated in the parturient with a difficult airway. A high spinal anesthetic may result in a "cannot ventilate, cannot intubate" scenario in a patient at high risk for gastric aspiration and oxygen desaturation.

2. Although many authorities believe spinal anesthesia is inappropriate after failed epidural anesthesia, some clinicians believe that spinal anesthesia with a 20% dose reduction is an acceptable anesthetic technique.

3. Should a spinal anesthetic be contemplated under these circumstances, the patient should be placed in a sitting position. The clinician should inject the dose with the lumen of the spinal needle directed caudad, inject slowly, elevate the head and neck when the patient is returned supine, and use reverse Trendelenburg positioning.

4. The clinician should not neglect uterine displacement because vena caval compression may increase the anesthetic level. Spinal anesthesia after failed epidural anesthesia might best be avoided in the remarkably obese patient for this reason.

5. The clinician should always be prepared to intubate and administer general anesthesia. Antacids should be administered preoperatively.

REFERENCES

1. Stone PA, Thorburn J, Lamb KSR: Complications of spinal anaesthesia following extradural block for Caesarean section. Br J Anaesth 62:335–337, 1989.
2. Beck GN, Griffiths AG: Failed extradural anaesthesia for Caesarean section: Complications of subsequent spinal block. Anaesthesia 47:690–692, 1992.
3. Blumgart CH, Ryall D, Dennison B, et al: Mechanism of extension of spinal anaesthesia by extradural injection of local anaesthetic. Br J Anaesth 69:457–460, 1992.
4. Dell RG, Orlikowski CEP: Unexpectedly high spinal anesthesia following failed extradural anaesthesia for Caesarean section (letter). Anaesthesia 48:641, 1993.
5. Mets B, Broccoli E, Brown AR: Is spinal anesthesia after failed epidural anesthesia contraindicated for Cesarean section? Anesth Analg 77:629–631, 1993.
6. Goldstein M, Dewan DM: Spinal anesthesia after failed epidural anesthesia (letter). Anesth Analg 79:1206, 1994.
7. Gupta A, Enlund G, Bengtsson M, et al: Spinal anaesthesia for caesarean section following epidural analgesia in labour: A relative contraindication. Int J Obstet Anaesth 3:153–156, 1994.
8. Waters JH, Leivers D, Hullander M: Response to spinal anesthesia after inadequate epidural anesthesia. Anesth Analg 78:1034, 1994.
9. Furst SR, Reisner LS: Risk of high spinal anesthesia following failed epidural block for Cesarean delivery. J Clin Anaesth 7:71–74, 1995.
10. Stoneham M, Souter A: Spinal anaesthesia for Caesarean section in women with incomplete extradural analgesia (letter). Br J Anaesth 76:476, 1996.
11. Takiguchi T, Okano T, Egawa H, et al: The effect of epidural saline injection on analgesic level during combined spinal and epidural anesthesia assessed clinically and myelographically. Anesth Analg 85:1097–1100, 1997.

Craig A. Andersen, CRNA, MS

PATIENT 14

A 49-year old man with postoperative hemorrhage

A 49-year-old man presents with postoperative hemorrhage. He had been evaluated for bilateral lower extremity radiculopathy; found to have degenerative disk disease; and scheduled for L4–5 laminectomy, decompression, and posterior instrumentation. He had a long history of smoking but was otherwise healthy. He had no prior surgeries. He denied chronic health problems and did not seek preventive health care on a regular basis. His medications included ibuprofen and an aspirin/oxycodone preparation. In addition to these medications, he took the following herbal preparations: *Allium sativum* (garlic), omega-3 fatty acids (fish oil), D-alpha tocopherol (Vitamin E), and *Panax ginseng* (ginseng). During preanesthetic evaluation (24 hours before surgery), he was advised to discontinue all herbal and prescription medications and to take only acetaminophen for pain.

The patient underwent general anesthetic induction and intubation with thiopental, fentanyl, and vecuronium. He was positioned prone on an Andrews frame. Anesthetic maintenance agents included desflurane, fentanyl, morphine, and vecuronium. Mean arterial pressure was maintained at about 60 to 65 mmHg. Throughout the procedure, the surgeons noted oozing from the wound. Hemostasis was obtained with electrocautery, absorbable gelatin sponge (Gelfoam), and topical thrombin. Before closure, the incision was inspected; no bleeding vessels were identified, and drains were placed. Estimated blood loss for the 6-hour procedure was 1,100 mL and was replaced with 3 L of Ringer's lactate. The patient was awakened and taken to recovery with a blood pressure of 116/70 mmHg and a heart rate of 80 beats/min.

In the postanesthesia care unit, the patient's lower back becomes discolored, and 350 mL of blood is noted in the surgical drains. He experiences throbbing lower back pain and decreased lower extremity strength. His hemoglobin and hematocrit decline to 10.3 g/dL and 24%.

Laboratory Findings: Hemoglobin 15.3 g/dL, Hct 45.3%, platelet count 223,000/μL. Prothrombin time 10.2 seconds, partial thromboplastin time 26.9 seconds, international normalized ratio 0.88.

Questions: What caused the patient's hemorrhage?
How does the Federal Food and Drug Administration (FDA) regulate herbal medications?
What is the incidence of the use of herbal/alternative medicine.
How can commonly used herbal medicines adversely affect the surgical patient?

What caused the patient's hemorrhage? Perioperative use of herbal medications.

Discussion: The societal use of herbal supplements is becoming widespread. Individuals use these medications to maintain a sense of control over their health care. Some distrust allopathic health care or Western medicine. The cost of conventional health care is beyond the means of some individuals, and self-medication with these readily available preparations is convenient. Although these supplements are considered *natural*, they are not free of harmful side effects, and they have the potential to inhibit coagulation or interact with prescription drugs.

How does the FDA regulate herbal medication? In 1994, the U.S. Food and Drug Administration (FDA) implemented the Dietary Supplement Health and Education Act (DSHEA), which outlines the regulation of dietary supplements. Under this act, manufacturers of alternative medications operate under less rigid guidelines than prescription pharmaceutical companies (or manufacturers of processed foods) for premarket determination of safety and efficacy of these supplements. The manufacturers must include the following information on product labeling:

1. Statement of identity (e.g., "ginseng").
2. Purpose or benefit derived from its use. The following statement also must be included: "This product has not been evaluated by the FDA. This product is not intended to diagnose, treat, cure, or prevent any disease."
3. Directions for use.
4. Supplement facts panel (serving size, amount, and active ingredients).
5. Other ingredients.

Notably absent from the DSHEA is a requirement for manufacturers to show efficacy, safety, quality or purity. Potency of herbal supplements may vary among manufacturers. Contamination with lead, mercury, arsenic, pollen, and mold has been reported.

What is the incidence of the use of herbal/alternative medicine. The use of herbal supplements in surgical patients has been reported to range from 17.4% to 61% and is higher in women than in men. Supplements most commonly used include vitamins (especially vitamins E and C), garlic, fish oil, *Gingko biloba* (gingko), ginseng, *Zingiber officinale* (ginger), *Hypericum perforatum* (St. John's wort), *Ephedra sinica, Echinacea angustifolia,* 2-amino 2-deoxyglucose sulfate (glucosamine), chondroitin 4-sulfate, chamomile, kava kava, and *Tanacetum parthenium* (feverfew). Vitamin E, garlic, fish oil, gingko, ginseng, ginger, and feverfew have anticoagulant potential. Herbal supplements have central nervous system and cardiovascular effects, but this discussion is limited to the anticoagulant effects of these agents.

How can commonly used herbal medicines adversely affect the surgical patient? Vitamin E is consumed for the prevention and treatment of cardiovascular disease, diabetes mellitus, and some forms of cancer. Vitamin E is an antioxidant that prevents the formation of free radicals, but high doses may increase bleeding secondary to antagonism of vitamin K–dependent coagulation factors and platelet aggregation. Concomitant use of vitamin E and anticoagulant or antiplatelet agents, including aspirin, clopidogrel (Plavix), dalteparin (Fragmin), enoxaparin (Lovenox), heparin, ticlopidine (Ticlid), and warfarin (Coumadin), may potentiate the risk of bleeding.

Fish oils are used primarily in the treatment of hyperlipidemia; hypertension; and chronic inflammatory states, such as rheumatoid arthritis and autoimmune disease. Fish oils contain two long-chain omega-3 fatty acids that compete with arachidonic acid in the cyclooxygenase and lipoxygenase pathways and have anti-inflammatory effects, likely secondary to the inhibition of leukotriene synthesis. Fish oils decrease blood viscosity and increase red blood cell deformability. The antithrombotic activity of fish oils results from prostacyclin inhibition, vasodilation, reduction in platelet count and adhesiveness, and prolongation of bleeding time. Concomitant use of fish oils and anticoagulant and antiplatelet drugs previously mentioned may increase the risk of bleeding.

Gingko is used for the treatment of dementia and Alzheimer's disease and conditions associated with cerebrovascular insufficiency, including memory loss, headache, tinnitus, vertigo, difficulty concentrating, mood disturbances, and hearing disorders. Active ingredients of gingko leaf and its extracts include flavenoids, terpenoids, and organic acids. Although the mechanism of action of gingko is only partially understood, there are several theories. Gingko may protect tissues from oxidative damage by preventing or reducing cell membrane lipid peroxidation, decreasing oxidative damage to erythrocytes, and may protect neurons and retinal tissue from oxidative stress. Extracts from the gingko leaf competitively inhibit platelet-activating factor, decreasing platelet aggregation, phagocyte chemotaxis, smooth muscle contraction, and free radical production, and prevent neutrophil degranulation. A case of bilateral spontaneous subdural hematomas has been linked to long-term ginko ingestion. Use of gingko may potentiate anticoagulant or antiplatelet agents.

Ginseng is a general tonic for improving well-being and stamina and may increase resistance to environmental stress. The active constituents of ginseng are ginsengosides, and these compounds may raise blood pressure and act as a central nervous system stimulant. Adrenal function and cortisol release may increase. Ginsengosides are reported to interfere with platelet aggregation and coagulation *in vitro,* but this effect has not been shown in humans.

Garlic decreases blood pressure and reduces plasma lipids. Garlic may produce smooth muscle relaxation and vasodilation by activation of endothelium-derived relaxation factor. Garlic also is believed to act as hydroxymethylglutaryl-coreductase inhibitor, reducing serum cholesterol. It has been shown to have antithrombotic properties by increasing thrombolytic activity secondary to plasminogen activation and decreasing platelet aggregation through inhibition of thromboxane B_2 formation. A spontaneous spinal epidural hematoma associated with excessive garlic ingestion has been reported.

Ginger is used for the treatment of arthritis, for a variety of gastrointestinal complaints, and as an antiemetic. Its active component is gingerol, and its mechanism of action is unclear, although gingerols are thought to inhibit prostaglandin and leukotriene synthesis. Ginger is believed to inhibit thromboxane synthetase, decreasing platelet aggregation.

Feverfew is used for fever, headache, and prevention of migraine headaches. At least 39 compounds within feverfew have been identified. It is not yet clear how feverfew works in the prevention of migraine. Laboratory evidence suggests that feverfew extracts might inhibit platelet aggregation and inhibit serotonin release from platelets and leukocytes. Feverfew may inhibit serum proteases and leukotrienes and block prostaglandin synthesis by inhibiting phospholipase, preventing the release of arachidonic acid.

The best means for detecting a coagulation defect caused by herbal medications is a properly taken clinical history. Especially important are questions related to the hemostatic response during previous surgeries. Questions regarding bleeding tendencies, such as easy bruising, gingival bleeding, or excessive bleeding after dental extractions, are important. Positive responses to these questions suggest the need for laboratory testing. The most commonly used measures of coagulation include the activated partial thromboplastin time, which evaluates the intrinsic system and the final common pathway; the prothrombin time, which evaluates the extrinsic pathway and the final common pathway; platelet count; and bleeding time. Bleeding time, the most commonly used measure of platelet function, is subject to many variables, however, and may not always be reliable. More reliable tests of platelet function are available but are expensive, are time-consuming, and are not appropriate for routine screening.

Perioperative use of herbal supplements in surgical patients may predispose them to an increased risk of bleeding. Although published adverse reactions are rare, anecdotal reports of unusual bleeding after surgery exist. Patients taking multiple herbal preparations probably should discontinue use of these agents 2 to 3 weeks before surgery.

The present patient was returned to the operating suite for surgical reexploration and evacuation of hematoma. Induction of anesthesia was with etomidate, fentanyl, and vecuronium. Mean arterial pressure was 50 to 55 mmHg, and heart rate was 110 beats/min. Blood pressure improved after administration of phenylephrine (500 μg in divided doses) and crystalloid infusion. The surgical incision was opened, and the hematoma was evacuated. With liberal use of electrocautery, Gelfoam, and topical thrombin, hemostasis was obtained. Blood loss from the second procedure was estimated at 100 mL with replacement with 2 L of crystalloid. On arrival in the postanesthesia care unit, his blood pressure was 108/60 mmHg, and his heart rate was 108 beats/min. The remainder of his postoperative recovery was unremarkable. His hemoglobin stabilized at 8.5 g/dL, and he had no residual neurologic deficit. He was discharged on the fourth postoperative day.

Clinical Pearls

1. Few controlled scientific data exist on the risks and benefits of herbal and alternative medications. Their effects in the immediate perioperative period are unknown.

2. The clinician always should ask patients about herbal and alternative medications that they may be taking. Patients should not be expected to volunteer such information.

3. *Herbal* does not mean safe. It is prudent for the anesthesia care provider to interview patients carefully preoperatively to establish the use of herbal and alternative medicines. In situations in which excessive bleeding may prove especially problematic or in a patient taking multiple supplements thought to have anticoagulant potential, it may be best to discontinue these medication for 2 to 3 weeks before surgery.

4. Coagulation defects secondary to herbal and alternative medicines may not be evident using standard laboratory studies.

REFERENCES

1. Rose KD, et al: Spontaneous spinal epidural hematoma with associated platelet dysfunction from excessive garlic ingestion: A case report. Neurosurgery 26:880–882, 1990.
2. Newall CA, Anderson LA, Philpson JD: Herbal Medicine: A Guide for Healthcare Professionals. London, The Pharmaceutical Press, 1996.
3. Rowin J, Lewis SL: Spontaneous bilateral subdural hematomas with chronic Gingko biloba ingestion. Neurology 46:1775–1776, 1996.
4. Ernest E: Harmless herbs? A review of recent literature. JAMA 104:170–177, 1998.
5. McLesky CH, Meyer TA, Baisden CE, et al: The incidence of herbal and selected nutraceutical use in surgical patients. Anesthesiology 91:A1168, 1999.
6. Weintraub PS, Jones DM: Anesthesiologists warn: If you are taking herbal products tell your doctor before surgery (press release). American Society of Anesthesiologists, Park Ridge, IL, May 1999.
7. Heck AM, DeWitt BA, Lukes AL: Potential interactions between alternative therapies and warfarin. Am J Health Syst Pharm 57:1221–1227, 2000.
8. Kaye AD, Clark RC, Subar R, et al: Herbal medicines: Current trends in anesthesiology practice—a hospital survey. J Clin Anesth 12:468–471, 2000.
9. Norred CL, Finlayson CA: Hemorrhage after the preoperative use of complementary and alternative medicines. AANA J 68: 217–220, 2000
10. Norred CL, Zamudio S, Palmer S: Use of complimentary and alternative medicines by surgical patients. AANA J 68:13–18, 2000.
11. Paskawicz J, Chatwan A: Herbal medicine use in surgical patients. Am J Anesth 27:538–543, 2000.

Howard J. Miller, MD

PATIENT 15

A 52-year-old woman with incomplete epidural analgesia

A 52-year-old woman presented with chronic thoracic pain secondary to previous herpes zoster infection. With the exception of a smoking history, she was otherwise healthy. She had undergone treatment with various analgesic drug regimens over the previous 6 months without success. Her current drug regimen included amitriptyline and a fentanyl patch. In consideration of future analgesic strategies, the patient was admitted for a trial of continuous thoracic epidural analgesia. Standard monitors were applied, and an intravenous catheter was inserted. While in the sitting position, an 18G Tuohy needle was placed paramedian, on a single pass at the T7–8 interspace, to loss of resistance to air at 5 cm. No cerebrospinal fluid, blood, or paresthesias were obtained. A 20G multiorifice epidural catheter was passed easily 4 cm into the epidural space, and the Tuohy needle was removed. The epidural catheter was secured (9 cm at the skin), and a 3-mL test dose of 2% lidocaine with epinephrine 1:200,000 was injected after negative aspiration of the catheter for cerebrospinal fluid or blood. After 5 minutes, the test dose failed to produce evidence of a subarachnoid block or intravascular injection.

The epidural catheter is dosed incrementally with a total of 10 mL of 2% lidocaine. After 15 minutes, the patient reports little relief of thoracic pain. Sensory blockade assessed by pinprick is patchy, and a distinct level is unattainable. An additional 5 mL of 2% lidocaine is injected, and the patient subsequently reports only mild relief. Again, sensory blockade level is indistinct and patchy. To establish why epidural analgesia is ineffective, a thoracic computed tomography (CT) scan is obtained after contrast dye injection of the epidural catheter (see Figure).

Questions: What does the CT scan demonstrate?
Why did the epidural catheter fail to produce sensory blockade, and what recommendations do you have for continuing to use this catheter?

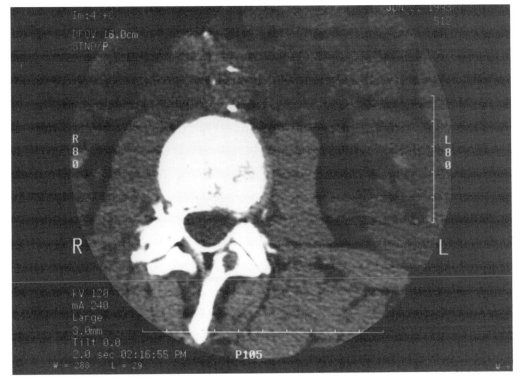

What does the CT scan demonstrate? Subdural catheter

Why did the epidural catheter fail to produce sensory blockade and what recommendations do you have for continuing to use this catheter? The subdural space has been shown clearly within the cerebral meninges, is seen less at the spinal meningeal level, but has been shown during myelography and at postmortem examination. In a postmortem study, Blomberg[1] easily separated dura from arachnoid with injection of fluid during spinaloscopy in 10 of 15 cadavers. The extraarachnoid subdural space contains serous fluid, continues for a short distance along cranial and spinal nerves, and is larger in the cervical region than the lumbar region (which may explain the sacral sparing and tendency toward high blocks, to be discussed later) (see Figure).

A subdural block as defined by Lubenow et al[2] is an extensive neural block out of proportion to the amount of local anesthetic injected in the absence of a subarachnoid puncture. A complication of planned epidural block, subdural catheterization was found retrospectively by these investigators to occur in roughly 1% of attempted epidural procedures. It may be more common than this because the incidence of inadvertent injection of contrast medium into the subdural space during myelography has been reported to be 13%. Although an extensive subarachnoid blockade might be observed within 1 to 2 minutes, there may be some delay after dosing before the excessive blockade of a subdural catheter manifests (≥20 minutes).

Characterization of subdural blockade has come about through anecdotal reports. Patterns that suggest subdural blockade include delayed but extensive sensory blockade, atypical spread with great variability in onset, asymmetric and patchy blockade, sparing of sacral dermatomes, and variable but often prolonged motor blockade. Subdural catheters may explain dramatic events after negative test doses or events heretofore attributed to catheter migration.

Many cases in parturients have been reported. Typically, epidural catheters were inserted uneventfully for labor analgesia, and dilute local anesthetic solutions provided adequate analgesia. When cesarean section became necessary, and the catheters were dosed with conventional volumes of more concentrated local anesthetics, the patients developed extremely high sensory levels, including central neurologic blockade, requiring emergent tracheal intubation. Such cases show the need for vigilance when epidural catheters used for the management of labor pain (with dilute local anesthetics) are subsequently dosed for surgical procedures (greater volumes of concentrated local anesthetics).

Contrast-enhanced CT is used regularly to determine the position of suspected subdural catheters. The contrast material circumferentially may outline the thecal sac, suggesting subdural catheter placement. There also may be extensive and irregular spread of contrast material. Dye injected through an epidurally positioned catheter would show contrast material along the anterior portion of the thecal sac only.

Tsui et al[7] described a technique whereby electrical stimulation was used to identify the position of epidural catheters. Stimulation of an epidurally positioned catheter resulted in a segmental motor

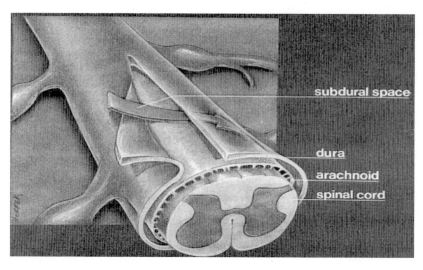

Anatomic relationship of dura and arachnoid. The subdural space is a potential space encircling the arachnoid membrane and contained within the dura. (From Lubenow et al,[2] with permission.)

response. Ordinary stimulating currents ranged from 1 to 10 mA. Tsui et al[1] subsequently used this technique to discriminate epidural from subdural catheter positioning. As opposed to the segmental epidural response, a diffuse and vigorous motor response with little electrical stimulation (0.3 mA) was observed in a patient suspected of having a subdural catheter. The diffuse response was due to considerable spread of conducting fluid within the subdural space, easily conducting current to multiple spinal nerve roots. Subdural placement later was confirmed radiographically.

The Present Patient

The catheter was removed and replaced at the T6–7 interspace using loss-of-resistance technique. After a negative test dose, the catheter was injected incrementally with 10 mL of 2% lidocaine. The patient reported excellent pain relief, and an appropriate sensory blockade level of T3–8 was obtained. An infusion of 0.1% bupivacaine with fentanyl, 5 μg/mL, was started at 10 mL/h. Having shown excellent relief of her herpetic pain, the patient was scheduled for placement of a long-term indwelling epidural catheter.

Clinical Pearls

1. Subdural injection of medications may result in markedly atypical and unexpected clinical findings. Examples include unusually extensive blocks, delay in onset of blockade, and patchy and asymmetric patterns.

2. Catheter aspiration and test doses do not detect subdural catheters.

3. If unusual clinical responses occur, the clinician should consider elucidating the exact position of the catheter by CT or electrical stimulation.

4. The current practice of using dilute local anesthetics for the management of labor-associated pain may obscure catheter malpositioning. Should surgical anesthesia be required subsequently, these catheters need to be dosed with vigilance. Unanticipated high blockade, including central neurologic blockade, may require emergent airway intervention.

5. Because of delays in presentation of subdural local anesthetic injection, patients who receive epidural local anesthetics as an outpatient (e.g., in association with epidural steroid administration) should be observed for at least 1 hour postinjection before release.

6. Suspected subdural catheters should be replaced because of the unpredictable nature of local anesthetic behavior within the subdural space.

REFERENCES

1. Blomberg RG: The lumbar subdural extraarachnoid space of humans: An anatomical study using spinaloscopy in autopsy cases. Anesth Analg 66:177–180, 1987.
2. Lubenow T, Keh-Wong E, Kristof K, et al: Inadvertent subdural injection: A complication of an epidural block. Anesth Analg 67:175–179, 1988.
3. Miller DC, Choi WW, Chestnut DH: Subdural injection of local anesthetics and morphine: A complication of attempted epidural anesthesia. South Med J 82:87–89, 1989.
4. Gershon RY: Surgical anaesthesia for caesarean section with a subdural catheter. Can J Anaesth 43:1068–1071, 1996.
5. Forrester DJ, Mukherji SK, Mayer DC, et al: Dilute infusion for labor, obscure subdural catheter, and life-threatening block at cesarean delivery. Anesth Analg 89:1267–1270, 1999.
6. Orbegozo M, Sheihk T, Slogoff A: Subdural cannulation and local anesthetic injection as a complication of an intended epidural anesthetic. J Clin Anesth 11:129–131, 1999.
7. Tsui BC, Gupta S, Emery D, Finucane B: Detection of subdural placement of epidural catheter using nerve stimulation. Can J Anaesth 47:471–473, 2000.

James C. Duke, MD

PATIENT 16

A 33-year-old man with chest pain and tachycardia after a motor vehicle accident

A 33-year-old man presents with chest pain and tachycardia after a motor vehicle accident. He struck a tree head-on with his automobile. Paramedics who freed him commented that the steering wheel had been deformed. In the emergency department, the patient complains of pain on inspiration, abdominal discomfort, and right leg pain. He is otherwise healthy and has a negative medical history. He is scheduled for open reduction and internal fixation of the right femur.

Physical Examination: Pulse 140, respirations 20, blood pressure 145/88. General appearance: Patient appears uncomfortable when breathing and is pale. HEENT: unremarkable. Neck: nontender. Chest: tender to palpation over sternum with bruising. Breath sounds clear and equal bilaterally. Cardiac: rapid regular heart rate without murmurs. Abdomen: tender left upper quadrant. Pelvis: stable. Extremities: swollen, tender right thigh, otherwise intact. Peripheral pulses and neurologic examination are unremarkable.

Laboratory Findings: Hematocrit 32%. Remainder of laboratory findings unremarkable. Oxygen saturation 98%. Abdominal ultrasound: small subcapsular splenic hematoma. Chest radiograph: unremarkable, displaced right femoral fracture. ECG: see Figure.

Questions: What is a likely cause of the abnormality on the ECG?
Discuss the value of ECG, cardiac enzymes and chest radiograph in this patient.
What is the value of echocardiography?
Should anesthesia be undertaken at this time? What potential intraoperative problems may occur?

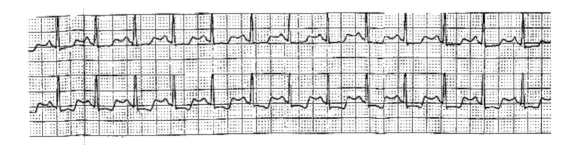

What is a likely cause of the abnormality on the ECG? Blunt cardiac injury.

Blunt cardiac injuries (BCI) are associated with motor vehicle accidents, falls, and blast injuries. A wide spectrum of injuries exists, including minimal concussion, focal cell death and necrosis (contusion), papillary muscle or valvular disruption, coronary artery thrombosis, and, in the extreme, septal or free wall rupture. The rate of coexisting injuries is high and includes great vessel injury, pulmonary contusion, head and intraabdominal injuries, and pelvic and long bone fractures. These associated injuries often are life-threatening.

Any patient experiencing blunt chest injury should be suspected of sustaining BCI. Patients may complain of chest pain or shortness of breath. Physical examination may reveal tenderness, bruising, or crepitance secondary to rib or sternal fractures. Auscultation may reveal a friction rub, gallop, murmur, or rales. Hemodynamic instability may be secondary to hypovolemia from associated injuries, tension pneumothorax, valvular disruption, cardiac rupture, or tamponade. BCI also may present with minimal or absent signs of chest trauma.

Discuss the value of ECG, cardiac enzymes and chest radiography. No gold standard exists to identify with high specificity and sensitivity patients who have sustained BCI. ECGs, chest radiographs, biochemical markers of cardiac injury, echocardiography, and radionuclide scanning have been used to identify patients so injured, yet all these modalities suffer from the lack of ability to identify accurately all patients sustaining BCI and exclude patients not sustaining BCI. Also, it is difficult to determine which patients will go on to have BCI-associated complications.

An ECG is indicated in any patient sustaining blunt chest injury. Dysrhythmias that have been associated with BCI include paroxysmal supraventricular tachycardia, multiple premature ventricular contractions, atrial fibrillation, ventricular tachycardia and fibrillation, second-degree and third-degree atrioventricular blocks, and complete heart block. Sinus tachycardia and nonspecific ST segment abnormalities are the most common dysrhythmias noted (35% to 80% of patients), but these are nonspecific rhythm disturbances. A significant portion of BCI involves the right ventricle, which is evaluated poorly by conventional ECG. Patients with normal ECGs 24 hours after injury have not been noted to develop pump failure or dysrhythmias resulting from BCI.

The value of chest radiography is detection of associated thoracic injuries. Of patients suspected of having BCI, 60% have coexisting injuries detected by chest radiograph. Although advocates of various radionuclide examinations (e.g., radionuclide ventriculography, multiple gated acquisition [MUGA], technetium pyrophosphate scanning) can be found, the cost, complexity, and time required to complete the examination limits their utility.

It was hoped that biochemical markers of cardiac injury might assist in establishing a diagnosis and offer prognostic value, but these hopes have not been realized. Creatine kinase (CK) has proved insensitive and nonspecific for evaluating BCI because it also is found in skeletal muscle. Patients with crush injuries or devascularization of extremities have CK elevation. Biffl et al[2] identified many patients with normal CK-MB who went on to have BCI-related problems. Cardiac troponins are specific to cardiac injury when elevated but are not always elevated when BCI-related complications are observed (i.e., insensitive and of low predictive value).

What is the value of echocardiography? Echocardiographic abnormalities do not seem to predict clinical complications reliably. Detectable abnormalities include regional wall motion abnormalities, intramyocardial hyperlucency (contused myocardium), chamber dilation, mural thrombi, valvular abnormalities, shunts, myocardial rupture, and tamponade. Echocardiography seems particularly valuable before an urgent surgical procedure when the patient's full clinical picture remains confusing or incomplete.

Should anesthesia be undertaken at this time? Most reports suggest general anesthesia is safe in patients with BCI, although some have noted an increased incidence of hypotension and dysrhythmias. Essential surgery need not be delayed, but invasive hemodynamic monitoring is appropriate, predicated on the planned procedure and the patient's condition. It cannot be said that any particular anesthetic technique is better or worse than any other. The anesthetic should be conducted in a familiar and comfortable manner (i.e., "do what you do best"). Dysrhythmias and pump failure should be treated conventionally.

Interpretation of pulmonary artery catheter data may be difficult. If pulmonary contusion is associated with BCI, it may be particularly difficult to separate the effects of increased pulmonary vascular resistance from right ventricular pump failure. The pulmonary artery catheter data may characterize left ventricular loading conditions poorly and obscure hypovolemia in need of treatment. Precipitous cardiovascular collapse may be caused by cardiac rupture, cardiac tamponade, acute valvular decompensation, air embolism, unappreciated hypovolemia, malignant ventricular arrhythmias, or tension pneumothorax.

The Present Patient

A 12-lead ECG of the present patient showed an acute inferior myocardial infarction. The orthopedic procedure was delayed for cardiac evaluation. The transthoracic echocardiogram showed right ventricular dyskinesia with an akinetic inferior segment. Cardiac catheterization revealed thrombosis of the right coronary artery. Overnight the patient showed no further deterioration in cardiac rhythm or hypotension. Open reduction and internal fixation was undertaken on the second hospital day. Intraarterial and central venous pressure monitors were instituted before anesthetic induction. The surgical procedure and the anesthetic proceeded unremarkably, and the patient experienced no episodes of hypotension or dysrhythmias. Postoperatively the patient had 24 hours of intensive care unit observation followed by 24 hours of telemetry. A repeat echocardiogram 5 days after admission showed resolution of the right ventricular wall motion abnormalities.

Clinical Pearls

1. The value of a diagnosis of cardiac contusion in the absence of any clinical abnormalities is of questionable clinical importance. Most patients with significant BCI have evidence of such injury at presentation (usually ECG abnormalities).

2. Patients having BCI frequently have other major injuries (head, chest, and abdominal injury; pelvic and long bone fractures). The outcome of these injuries usually is more significant than the BCI.

3. There is no gold standard for the evaluation of BCI. A diagnostic battery with high sensitivity, specificity, and predictive value has not been identified yet. Cardiac enzymes and radionuclide scans are insensitive and nonspecific. Echocardiography may prove valuable if the patient has unexplainable instability.

4. General anesthesia has been found to be safe in numerous, although not all, clinical studies. No anesthetic technique is intrinsically superior to any other. Invasive monitoring should be individualized. Dysrhythmias and pump failure are treated with standard pharmacologic therapy.

REFERENCES

1. Voyce SJ, Becker RB: Diagnosis, management, and complications for nonpenetrating cardiac trauma: A perspective for practicing clinicians. J Intensive Care Med 8:275–288, 1993.
2. Biffl WL, Moore FA, Moore EE, et al: Cardiac enzymes are irrelevant in the patient with suspected myocardial contusion. Am J Surg 169:523–528, 1994.
3. Maenza RL, Seaberg D, D'Amico F: A meta-analysis of blunt cardiac trauma: Ending myocardial confusion. Am J Emerg Med 14:237–241, 1996.
4. Hiatt JR, Yeatman LA, Child JS: The value of echocardiography in blunt chest trauma. J Trauma 28:914–922, 1998.
5. Barach P: Perioperative anesthetic management of patients with cardiac trauma. Anesthesiol Clin North Am 17:197–209, 1999.

James C. Duke, MD

PATIENT 17

A 56-year-old man with postoperative acute renal failure

A 56-year-old man with prostate cancer was scheduled for a suprapubic prostatectomy. With the exception of this malignancy, his medical history was significant only for hypertension, for which he took triamterene/hydrochlorothiazide (Dyazide), 50 mg daily.

Physical Examination: Temperature normal, heart rate 82, respirations 16, blood pressure 148/89. General appearance: Healthy-looking man except for his weight, 121 kg (height 6 feet, 3 inches). Pulmonary, cardiac, and abdominal examinations unremarkable. All other examinations unremarkable.

Laboratory Findings: Hct 48%. Sodium 139 mEq/L, potassium 4.3 mEq/L, chloride 110 mEq/L, CO_2 22 mEq/L. BUN 16 mg/dL, creatinine 1.0 mg/dL. Prostate-specific antigen 5.2. Urinalysis showed an occasional red blood cell.

Hospital Course: The patient refused placement of an epidural catheter for postoperative pain management but consented to an intrathecal dose of morphine; 1 mg of preservative-free morphine sulfate was administered intrathecally before general anesthesia. The patient underwent a balanced general anesthetic without significant hypotension. Central venous access was established by the right subclavian route, and central venous pressure ranged between 7 and 12 mmHg throughout the procedure. Blood loss was estimated at 1,600 mL. He received 4 L of lactated Ringer's solution, 0.5 L of hetastarch, and 2 U of autologous packed red blood cells. Because of the prostatectomy, there were periods when urine output could not be followed, but when the dissection was completed, urine output was measured at about 0.8 mL/kg/h. Near case conclusion, ketorolac, 60 mg, was administered intravenously. The patient was extubated, pain was managed easily during early postanesthetic care, and the patient was discharged to the floor with a Hct of 35% and stable vital signs. Because he received intrathecal morphine, oxygen was administered postoperatively, and oxygen saturations were monitored. In an attempt to limit the need for postoperative opioids, ketorolac, 30 mg intramuscularly every 6 hours, was ordered .

On the first postoperative day, the patient appeared puffy, and urine output had diminished remarkably. Repeated intravenous fluid boluses failed to improve urine output. Central venous pressure was 8 mmHg. Vital signs were as follows: temperature normal; heart rate 18, respirations 18, blood pressure 106/65.

Repeat Laboratory Findings: Hct 31%. Sodium 135 mEq/L, potassium 5.8 mEq/L, chloride 100 mEq/L, CO_2 19 mEq/L, magnesium 0.8 mEq/L. BUN 22 mg/dL, creatinine 2.0 mg/dL. Fractional excretion of sodium (FENa) 0.5%.

Questions: What is the cause of the patient's oliguria?
Describe the mechanisms that maintain renal blood flow and glomerular filtration rate.
Discuss the impact of nonsteroidal antiinflammatory drugs (NSAIDs) on renal function.
How is FENa calculated and how is it interpreted?
What are the treatment options?
What are the contraindications to administration of ketorolac?

What is the cause of the patient's oliguria?
Oliguric renal failure caused by ketorolac, a non-steroidal antiinflammatory drug.

A reasonable expectation of the surgical patient is adequate postoperative analgesia. Modalities suitable for the present patient include epidural or intrathecal administration of local anesthetics or opioids, intravenous opioids (patient-controlled analgesia would be excellent), and administration of NSAIDs as an adjuvant to opioids. Particularly in this patient, in whom intrathecal opioids were administered, the opioid-sparing effect of NSAIDs offers the advantage of reducing the likelihood of impaired central respiratory drive. The analgesic action of NSAIDs is due to inhibition of cyclooxygenase, a major enzyme in the biosynthesis of prostaglandins.

Discuss the mechanisms that maintain renal blood flow and glomerular filtration rate.
Prostaglandins are autocoids, or *local hormones,* substances that exert their physiologic effect at their site of synthesis. The kidney is extremely active in the synthesis of the vasodilatory prostaglandins PGE_2 and PGI_2, where they participate in autoregulation of renal blood flow and glomerular filtration. The role of prostaglandins in maintaining renal perfusion does not become important until the kidneys become underperfused. Renal hypoperfusion is a stimulus for the release of renin and angiotensin II, resulting in generalized vasoconstriction to maintain systemic perfusion. Because renal vasoconstriction is an undesirable side effect, local prostaglandin release results in renal vasodilation, improving renal blood flow and glomerular filtration. Other renal prostaglandin effects include inhibition of sodium chloride reabsorption in the ascending limb of Henle's loop and collecting duct, inhibition of urea reabsorption in the collecting duct, and inhibition of antidiuretic hormone.

Discuss the impact of NSAIDs on renal function. NSAIDs may be administered orally, rectally, or parenterally (intravenously or intramuscularly). Ketorolac is a parenterally administered NSAID with efficacy similar to moderate doses of parenteral morphine. Ketorolac may produce serious adverse effects, however, including allergic reactions, gastrointestinal bleeding (even when administered parenterally), impaired platelet aggregation, and decreased renal function. Renal effects of ketorolac include sodium and water retention; hyperkalemia; acute renal failure (ARF); and parenchymal disorders, such as interstitial nephritis, nephrotic syndrome, and papillary necrosis.

Numerous perioperative conditions may lead to renal hypoperfusion, including hypovolemia, shifting of intravascular fluid to extravascular compartments (i.e., third spacing), increased catecholamine and renin release, decreased cardiac output, and anesthesia-induced peripheral vasodilation. Similarly, certain medical conditions may place patients at greater risk, including congestive heart failure, cirrhosis, preexisting renal disease, diabetes mellitus, hypertension, and diuretic therapy. Age >65 years is another risk factor. When superimposed on the described perioperative events, administration of NSAIDs may lead to ARF. The table on the next page summarizes clinical characteristics of patients reported to experience ketorolac-induced ARF.

Overall, ARF associated with ketorolac is thought to be a rare event, with an incidence between 1 in 1,000 to 100,000. Feldman et al[11] retrospectively examined the medical records of 35 hospitals and found patients administered ketorolac to be no more likely than patients administered parenteral opioids to develop ARF (both groups had an incidence of ARF of approximately 1%). The patients who received ketorolac and developed ARF tended to do so after 5 days of therapy, and the authors suggested the risk of ARF was greater after prolonged administration. A meta-analysis by Lee et al[13] of postoperative patients receiving NSAIDs for 3 postoperative days found patients with normal preoperative renal function to have at most only brief and clinically unimportant reductions in renal function. There are case reports, however, describing episodes of renal failure after brief courses of ketorolac, even after a single dose.

How is FENa calculated and how is it interpreted? NSAID-induced ARF tends to be acute, oliguric, and prerenal in characteristics. Serum hyponatremia may be noted because water is retained out of proportion to sodium. As proximal sodium reabsorption is increased, less is delivered to the distal collecting ducts to exchange for potassium. Additionally, prostaglandin inhibition decreases renin release and leads to hyporeninemic hypoaldosteronism. The net effect of hyperkalemia is produced. Magnesium may be excreted leading to hypomagnesemia. Microscopic urinalysis in prerenal ARF is usually unremarkable, although hyaline casts occasionally may be observed, and does not aid in diagnosis. Analysis of urine electrolytes is valuable and is necessary to determine the FENa, a measure of the ability of the kidney to concentrate urine. The FENa measures how actively the kidney is reabsorbing sodium. This calculation requires mea-

Clinical Characteristics of Patients Developing Ketorolac-Induced Acute Renal Failure

Author	Age,Sex	Indication	Ketorolac Dose	Manifestation	Risk Factors
Schock[3]	71, F	Compression fracture	90 mg, 1 day	ARF	Cirrhosis, diuretics, gastrointestinal bleeding, renal insufficiency
Rotenberg[2]	59, M	Postthoracotomy	30 mg, 1 dose	Hyperkalemia only	Malignancy (bronchial adenocarcinoma)
Boras-Uber[1]	61, F	Replace mitral valve	90 mg, 1 day	ARF, anuria	HTN, DM, Mitral Insufficiency, CHF
Perazella[6]	32, M	Peritoneovenous shunt	150 mg, 1 day	Oliguric ARF	Alcoholic cirrhosis, portal hypertension, ascites, diuretics
Perazella[6]	76, F	Pacemaker placement	60 mg , 1 day	ARF	HTN, DM, ACE inhibitors, renal insufficiency, hypotension
Perazella[6]	65, M	Cholecystectomy	360 mg, 4 days	Nonoliguric ARF	HTN, IV contrast dye, obstructive cholecystitis, gentamicin
Fong[5]	76, M	Multiple surgeries	540 mg, 5 days	Oliguria, azotemia	HTN, uncertain volume status, hypoalbuminemia
Haragism[8]	57, W	Hepatic lobectomy	480 mg, 4 days	Oliguric ARF	Major intraabdominal procedure
Haragism[8]	66, W	ORIF hip	300 mg, 2 days	Nonoliguric ARF	Prior nephrectomy, chronic renal insufficiency, HTN
Haragism[8]	62, M	Partial colectomy	600 mg, 5 days	Nonoliguric ARF	Heart failure, dysrhythmias, mild renal insufficiency
Corelli[4]	59, M	S/P CABG, MI	120 mg, 2 days	ARF	Major surgical procedure
Corelli[4]	40, M	CHF	60 mg, 1 day	ARF	Dilated cardiomyopathy, CHF
Corelli[4]	50, F	Axillofemoral bypass	225 mg, 5 days	ARF	HTN, major surgical procedure
Corelli[4]	92, M	ORIF hip	90 mg, 3 days	ARF	Aortic stenosis, S/P cerebrovascular accident
Corelli[4]	60, F	Hepatic infusion pump	270 mg, 4 days	ARF	Liver cancer
Corelli[4]	20, M	Not mentioned	1,350 mg, 12 days	ARF	None mentioned
Smith[7]	29, F	D&C, tubal laparotomy	30 mg, 1 dose	ATN	Renal contrast

continued

Clinical Characteristics of Patients Developing Ketorolac-Induced Acute Renal Failure (*Continued*)

Author	Age,Sex	Indication	Ketorolac Dose	Manifestation	Risk Factors
Smith[7]	53, M	Total knee arthroplasty	240 mg, 2 days	ATN	Gentamicin, permanent renal impairment
Kelley[10]	50, M	Vertebrectomy	300 mg, 8 days	ARF	Major surgical procedure, no other factors mentioned
Quan[9]	44, M	AICD	60 mg, 1 dose	ARF, anuria	Cardiomyopathy, renal infarct, atrial flutter, hypovolemia

HTN, hypertension; DM, diabetes mellitus; CHF, congestive heart failure; ACE, angiotensin-converting enzyme; IV, intravenous; ORIF, open reduction and internal fixation; S/P, status post; CABG, coronary artery bypass graft; MI, myocardial infarction; D&C, dilation and curettage; ATN, acute tubular necrosis; AICD, automatic implantable cardioverter-defibrillator.

suring serum and urine creatinine and sodium (S_{Cr}, S_{Na}, U_{Cr}, U_{Na}) and is calculated as follows:

$$FENa\ (\%) = (U_{Na} \times S_{Cr})/(U_{Cr} \times S_{Na})$$

During renal hypoperfusion, sodium is actively reabsorbed to reestablish intravascular volume, and FENa is usually low (<1%). In intrinsic renal failure or postrenal failure, there is usually a defect in concentrating urine, and FENa is elevated >2% and often >3%. Diuretic therapy, especially loop diuretics, impairs sodium resorptive capacity and falsely elevates FENa in the setting of hypovolemia. There may be overlaps in the value of FENa between prerenal failure and acute tubular necrosis (ATN). An important point when interpreting FENa, as shown by the present patient, is that ARF caused by drug-mediated vasoconstriction may be mistaken for hypovolemia in the surgical patient and lead to incorrect therapy. ARF owing to radiocontrast dye, amphotericin B, angiotensin-converting enzyme inhibitors, and cyclosporine also may be associated with FENa <1%. In this patient, re-

peated courses of volume resuscitation were instituted, and the role of ketorolac was not appreciated initially. FENa always should be interpreted during clinical investigation. The Table below offers useful laboratory guidelines to distinguish prerenal ARF from ATN.

What are the treatment options? Treatment of NSAID-induced ARF includes discontinuing the offending agent, avoiding nephrotoxic agents, and ensuring adequate perfusion pressures and intravascular volume. Severe hyperkalemia may require treatment (options include loop diuretics, dietary potassium restriction, sodium bicarbonate, insulin and glucose, calcium chloride, β-2-adrenergic agonists, and potassium-binding resins; the extent of treatment depends on the degree of potassium elevation and ECG changes). If recognized promptly and treated adequately, renal function usually improves in days, although it could last several weeks. Smith et al[7] noted a case in which renal function was impaired perma-

Laboratory and Urinary Indices to Distinguish Prerenal Acute Renal Failure From Acute Tubular Necrosis*

Measurement	Prerenal ARF	ATN
Urine sodium	<10 mEq/mL	>20 mEq/mL
Specific gravity	>1.020	Approx. 1.010
FENa (%)	<1%	>2%
Urine/serum osmolality	>1.8	<1.1
Urine osmolality	>500 mOsm	<350 mOsm
Serum BUN/creatinine ratio	>20	<15
Microscopic sediment	Benign or hyaline casts	Granular casts or epithelial cells

*Considerable variation in the values of these indices was noted between sources.

nently, and at the time of that publication, hemodialysis was being considered.

What are the contraindications to administration of ketorolac? Ketorolac was introduced in 1990, and most reported cases of renal dysfunction occurred during early use and led subsequently to revised guidelines for dosages and duration of therapy (see Table). It also became clear that appropriate patient selection is essential, and hypovolemic patients or patients with congestive heart failure or hepatic or renal disease should be considered carefully before ketorolac is administered (if at all). Ketorolac is an *adjuvant* to opioid therapy, not a replacement. Ketorolac should be used for the shortest time possible in the smallest doses necessary, and renal function should be monitored regularly for the duration of therapy.

The Present Patient

The present patient received a total of 90 mg of ketorolac; the drug was discontinued when renal dysfunction was recognized by laboratory analysis. The Foley catheter was irrigated for clots to rule out postrenal (obstructive) causes of renal failure. Because of the patient's generalized edematous state, he was only modestly fluid challenged. When urine output improved and serum potassium decreased, serum magnesium was repleted. Serum creatinine normalized after 48 hours of supportive therapy.

Dosage Guidelines for Ketorolac

Patient Characteristics	Intramuscular Use	Intravenous Use
Age <65 y	60 mg (SD) or 30 mg q6h NTE 120 mg/d for ≤5 days	30 mg q6h NTE 120 mg/d for ≤5 days
Age >65 y Renal impairment Body weight <50 kg	30 mg (SD) or 15 mg q6h NTE 60 mg/d for ≤5 days	15 mg q6h NTE 60 mg/d for ≤5 days

SD, single dose; NTE, not to exceed.

Clinical Pearls

1. Although NSAIDs are excellent analgesic adjuvants, they should be avoided in patients with preexisting hepatic or renal dysfunction, congestive heart failure, sepsis, hypovolemia, and other hypoperfusion states.

2. NSAIDs should be used with great caution (if at all) in patients undergoing surgery with large intravascular volume loss or third-space accumulation.

3. Low perfusion states, hypovolemia, and medications that produce renal vasoconstriction have a FENa <1%. The treatment for these conditions differs. FENa should be interpreted within the clinical context. Medications always should be reviewed when evaluating oliguria.

4. Laboratory analysis suggesting NSAID-induced oliguric ARF includes increasing BUN and creatinine, hyponatremia, hyperkalemia, hypomagnesemia, and FENa <1%. NSAID-induced ARF should be treated by stopping the offending agent, avoiding other nephrotoxins, establishing adequate intravascular volume if depleted, ensuring adequate perfusion pressure, and treating associated electrolyte abnormalities when renal function begins to improve.

5. Preliminary data suggest cyclooxygenase-2-selective inhibitors share the renal effects of NSAIDs, and similar recommendations to NSAIDs are made for these agents.[12]

REFERENCES

1. Boras-Uber LA, Bracket NC: Ketorolac-induced acute renal failure. Am J Med 92:450–452, 1992.
2. Rotenberg FA, Giannini VS: Hyperkalemia associated with ketorolac. Ann Pharmacother 26:778–779, 1992.
3. Schock PH, Ranno A, North DS: Acute renal failure in an elderly woman following intramuscular ketorolac administration. Ann Pharmacother 26:1233–1235, 1992.
4. Corelli RL, Gericke KR: Renal insufficiency associated with intramuscular administration of ketorolac tromethamine. Ann Pharmacother 27:1055–1057, 1993.
5. Fong J, Gora ML: Reversible renal insufficiency following ketorolac therapy. Ann Pharmacother 27:510–512, 1993.
6. Perazella MA, Buller GK: NSAID nephrotoxicity revisited: Acute renal failure due to parenteral ketorolac. South Med J 86:1421–1424, 1993.
7. Smith K, Halliwell RMT, Lawrence S: Acute renal failure associated with intramuscular ketorolac. Anaesth Intensive Care 21:700–703, 1993.
8. Haragism L, Dalal R, Bagga H, et al: Ketorolac-induced acute renal failure and hyperkalemia: Report of three cases. Am J Kidney Dis 24:578–580, 1994.
9. Quan DJ, Kayser SR: Ketorolac induced acute renal failure following a single dose. Clin Toxicol 32:305–309, 1994.
10. Kelley M: Ketorolac-induced acute renal failure and hyperkalemia. Clin Nephrol 44:276–277, 1995.
11. Feldman HI, Kinman JL, Berlin JA, et al: Parenteral ketorolac: The risk for acute renal failure. Ann Intern Med 126:193–199, 1997.
12. Brater DC: Effects of nonsteroidal anti-inflammatory drugs on renal function: Focus on cyclooxygenase-2-selective inhibition. Am J Med 107:65S–71S, 1999.
13. Lee A, Cooper MG, Craig JC, et al: The effects of nonsteroidal anti-inflammatory drugs on postoperative renal function: A meta-analysis. Anaesth Intensive Care 27:574–580, 1999.
14. Reinhart DJ: Minimizing the adverse effects of ketorolac. Drug Safe 22:487–497, 2000.

Kathryn King MD

PATIENT 18

A 54-year-old man with extreme cardiovascular instability postoperatively

A 54-year-old man with a prior history of myocardial infarction, insulin-dependent diabetes mellitus, and prostate cancer underwent radical retropubic prostatectomy and periaortic lymph node dissection. Preoperative evaluation revealed good exercise tolerance (walks 2 miles daily) and mild hypertension (160/90 mmHg). The intraoperative course was complicated by hypertension on intubation (200/120 mmHg) and intraoperative hypotensive episodes (70–90/40–60 mmHg) during periods of vigorous blood loss. Intraoperative fluids included 3.4 L of Ringer's lactate, 1 L of normal saline, and 2 U of packed RBCs. Estimated blood loss was 3.2 L, and urine output was 540 mL.

At case conclusion, he is extubated and transferred to the postanesthesia care unit in satisfactory condition. He has periods of hypotension (80 to 90 mmHg systolic) that respond to fluid challenge. His heart rate gradually increases to 120 beats/min, and he appears anxious, although he denies chest pain.

Physical Examination: Pulse 122, respirations 20, blood pressure 89/56, oxygen saturation 94 on 3 L/min nasal cannula, central venous pressure 5 mmHg. Skin pale and cool. Chest auscultation: rales along dependent bases. Cardiac examination: Rapid rate with occasional irregular beat; no gallops, rubs, or murmurs. Surgical site unremarkable.

Preoperative Laboratory Findings: Hematology, chemistry, coagulation parameters all normal, Hct 42%. ECG: evidence of old inferior myocardial infarction with left ventricular hypertrophy and left axis deviation.

Further fluid boluses are ordered and a hematocrit is drawn. Soon thereafter, the nursing staff notes a prolonged audible alarm at the patient's bedspace; the cardiac monitor shows the following rhythm (Figure). The patient is obtunded, and a pulse cannot be detected.

Questions: Diagnose this arrhythmia.
What treatment is immediately necessary?
What is the recommended drug therapy?

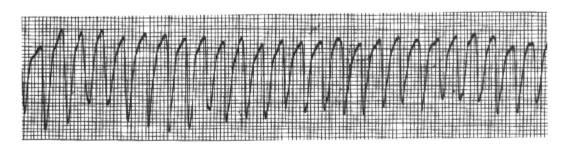

Diagnose this arrhythmia. Pulseless ventricular tachycardia.

Discussion: The recommendations for **advanced cardiac life support (ACLS)** as published by the American Heart Association were developed by international experts on the basis of evidence-based methodology. Based on the strength of the scientific evidence, every intervention receives a recommendation for clinical applicability. The levels of recommendation are as follows: Class I (excellent, definitive evidence), Class IIa (good evidence of effectiveness and safety), Class IIb (fair-to-good evidence), Class Indeterminate (insufficient evidence to support a final recommendation), and Class III (suggests or confirms probability of harm). ACLS guidelines have been modified in view of the strength of evidence supporting or refuting the efficacy of any intervention, and the treatment recommendations that follow reflect these most current recommendations.

Differential diagnosis of the rhythm in the Figure should include stable, unstable, and pulseless VT. These distinctions determine whether the patient will be treated with drugs, urgent cardioversion, or defibrillation.

Stable VT implies there are no symptoms or clinical evidence of tissue hypoperfusion or shock, and there may be sufficient time to allow for drug therapy. QRS morphology is often monomorphic but may be polymorphic and responds to such agents as procainamide, sotalol, amiodarone, and β-blockers. Synchronized cardioversion also may be an option. Choice of agent is contingent on underlying cardiac function and length of the Q-T interval.

In unstable VT, the heart rate is usually >150 beats/min, there is evidence of tissue hypoperfusion, and the rhythm often quickly degenerates to ventricular fibrillation (VF). Immediate synchronized cardioversion is indicated to reestablish a perfusing rhythm. Hemodynamically unstable polymorphic VT should be treated as VF/pulseless VT.

What treatment is immediately necessary?
If a defibrillator is immediately available, in the setting of VF/pulseless VT, defibrillation takes priority over all other interventions, including cardiopulmonary resuscitation (CPR) and drugs (see Figure). Every minute of delay decreases by 10% the chance of successful conversion to a hemodynamically favorable rhythm. Three sequential shocks are recommended if needed as the rhythm persists without pausing for pulse checks. Prompt defibrillation is essential because as myocardial adenosine triphosphate rapidly depletes, the rhythm becomes refractory to therapy as it deteriorates from coarse to fine VF then to asystole.

What is the recommended drug therapy?
After defibrillation with three consecutive shocks, supportive measures are begun, including CPR, securing IV access when none previously exists, establishing a patent airway with an endotracheal tube or airway adjunct such as laryngeal mask airway, and pharmacologic therapy. The first class of drug to be used with any pulseless rhythm is a *vasoconstrictor*. Although in the past epinephrine traditionally was used in cardiac arrest scenarios, there is a paucity of evidence to show it improves outcome in humans. Additionally, although high-dose epinephrine results in a higher rate of return of spontaneous circulation, it leads to myocardial dysfunction and a toxic hyperadrenergic state, and no improvement in the rate of survival to hospital discharge has been realized. Research has shown vasopressin (Class IIB evidence) to be equivalent or superior to epinephrine in resuscitation from VF cardiac arrest. Vasopressin produces intense peripheral vasoconstriction through stimulation of V1 receptors and has no β-adrenergic activity; it increases coronary perfusion without increasing myocardial oxygen consumption. Vasopressin is administered as a single supraphysiologic dose of 40 IU and has a half-life of 10 to 20 minutes. Should the patient not respond to vasopressin, epinephrine, 1 mg, is administered intravenously and repeated every 3 to 5 minutes, although no specific human data exist to support this recommendation. Epinephrine has received a Class Indeterminate assignment.

Successive interventions include alternating drugs with electrical shocks, with pulse checks between all interventions after the initial defibrillation attempts. Should defibrillation and vasoconstrictor therapy fail, the next pharmacologic treatment indicated would be an *antiarrhythmic agent*.

Old standbys, such as lidocaine (Indeterminate evidence), bretylium, and procainamide (Class IIb evidence), have less solid endorsement than previously. Bretylium is no longer recommended, in part because of adverse side effects but also because the natural resources to manufacture bretylium are diminishing.

Amiodarone (Class IIB evidence) is the only antiarrhythmic agent that has been proved in a randomized, placebo-controlled trial to improve survival to hospital admission in out-of-hospital arrest. Amiodarone prolongs repolarization, blocks sodium channels at rapid pacing frequencies, has noncompetitive antisympathetic action, blocks calcium channels, and is used in the treatment of supraventricular tachycardias. Amiodarone has vasodilatory and negative inotropic effects that are often a function of dose and rate of infusion, although its negative inotropic effects are less than those of

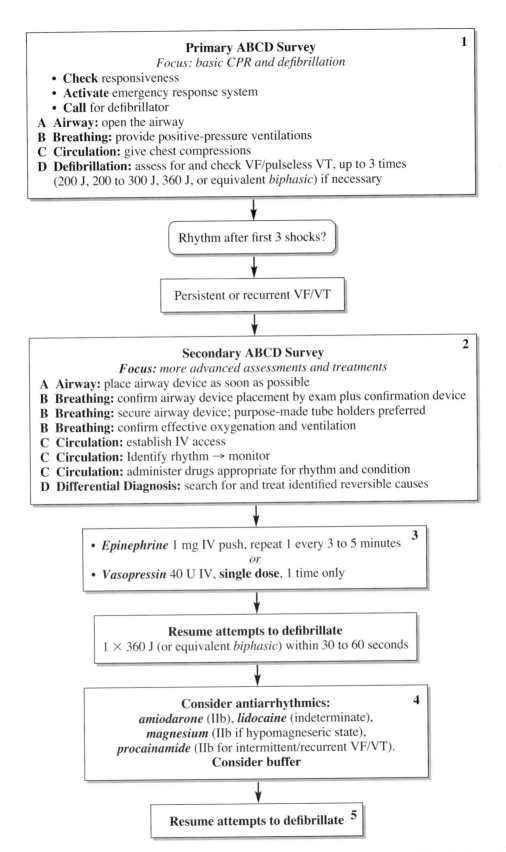

Primary ABCD Survey
Focus: basic CPR and defibrillation
- **Check** responsiveness
- **Activate** emergency response system
- **Call** for defibrillator

A **Airway:** open the airway
B **Breathing:** provide positive-pressure ventilations
C **Circulation:** give chest compressions
D **Defibrillation:** assess for and check VF/pulseless VT, up to 3 times (200 J, 200 to 300 J, 360 J, or equivalent *biphasic*) if necessary

1

Rhythm after first 3 shocks?

Persistent or recurrent VF/VT

Secondary ABCD Survey
Focus: more advanced assessments and treatments
A **Airway:** place airway device as soon as possible
B **Breathing:** confirm airway device placement by exam plus confirmation device
B **Breathing:** secure airway device; purpose-made tube holders preferred
B **Breathing:** confirm effective oxygenation and ventilation
C **Circulation:** establish IV access
C **Circulation:** Identify rhythm → monitor
C **Circulation:** administer drugs appropriate for rhythm and condition
D **Differential Diagnosis:** search for and treat identified reversible causes

2

- *Epinephrine* 1 mg IV push, repeat 1 every 3 to 5 minutes
or
- *Vasopressin* 40 U IV, **single dose**, 1 time only

3

Resume attempts to defibrillate
1 × 360 J (or equivalent *biphasic*) within 30 to 60 seconds

Consider antiarrhythmics:
amiodarone (IIb), *lidocaine* (indeterminate),
magnesium (IIb if hypomagneseric state),
procainamide (IIb for intermittent/recurrent VF/VT).
Consider buffer

4

Resume attempts to defibrillate **5**

Ventricular fibrillation/pulseless ventricular tachycardia algorithm. (From International Consensus on Science,[4] with permission of American Heart Association)

most antiarrhythmics. The initial dose is 300 mg intravenously. A repeat dose, 150 mg, may be administered if the pulseless rhythm persists. Infusions are not begun until after the patient regains a pulse. After initial bolus dosing, 150 mg of amiodarone is infused over 10 minutes, followed by 360 mg over the next 6 hours, and finally 540 mg over the next 18 hours. The maximum dose of amiodarone is 2.2 gm over 24 hours. Hypotension and bradycardia are common adverse effects and may be related to rate of infusion.

Amiodarone has several features that complicate administration. Because it is absorbed by plastic, it is distributed in 6-mL glass vials and must be filtered and diluted to 20 mL before being administered. Amiodarone is stable in plastic bags only for 2 hours; prolonged infusions require glass bottles. Defibrillation should not be delayed while the drug is prepared.

Failure to respond to electrical or pharmacologic therapy should precipitate a search for other potentially treatable events. Although found in algorithms addressing asystole or pulseless electrical activity, VF may be a result of the five Hs (hypoxia, hypovolemia, hydrogen ion acidosis, hyperkalemia/hypokalemia, and hypothermia/hyperthermia) and the five Ts (toxins/tablets, tamponade, tension pneumothorax, thrombosis–coronary, and thrombosis–pulmonary).

Other new developments include evolution in defibrillation technology. Electrical therapy delivered in biphasic waveform impulses may produce less myocardial damage compared with standard monophasic waveforms. Biphasic countershocks at nonescalating doses of 150 to 200 J offer comparable outcomes compared with escalating shocks at 200 J, 300 J, and 360 J, using a conventional monophasic defibrillator. (*Note:* American Heart Association authorities are still undecided about the *optimal* level of delivered biphasic energy.[4]) Most automatic external defibrillators use biphasic technology; conventional manual defibrillators using biphasic waveforms should become readily available as older devices are replaced.

The Present Patient

Recognizing the patient had unstable ventricular tachycardia, immediate defibrillation was instituted. The patient responded on the second defibrillation attempt, returning to a sinus tachycardia. The patient received further support along ACLS guidelines. Further evaluation revealed he had sustained a second inferior myocardial infarction.

Clinical Pearls

1. Clinicians should appreciate that the scientific evidence for efficacy of ACLS drug recommendations is at best usually only fair to good.

2. After determination of apnea and pulselessness, rhythm analysis and determination of whether the rhythm is susceptible to countershock are of utmost importance. Susceptibility to countershock decreases 10% with every passing minute; defibrillation should be the first treatment for VF/pulseless VT and should not be delayed for any reason other than availability of equipment and operator or bystander safety.

3. The first line of pharmacologic treatment for VF/pulseless VT is a vasoconstrictor; consider either vasopressin (40 IU intravenously) or epinephrine (1 mg intravenously). Vasopressin is a potent vasoconstrictor, produces no β-adrenergic effects, and maintains coronary perfusion pressure while not increasing myocardial oxygen consumption.

4. The evidence supporting the efficacy of lidocaine and procainamide in shock-refractory VF and pulseless VT is weak. The evidence supporting use of amiodarone in these settings is much stronger and justifies its use as a first-line antiarrhythmic for shock-resistant and vasoconstrictor-resistant VT/VF.

5. Although usually associated with non-VF/VT arrest (pulseless electrical activity and asystole), potentially correctable causes of acute cardiopulmonary deterioration include hypoxia, hypovolemia, tension pneumothorax, cardiac tamponade, hypoxia, hyperkalemia or hypokalemia, acidosis, hypothermia, or drug overdose. These cause should be considered in nonresponding patients.

6. New defibrillation technology delivering biphasic waveform energy may produce less myocardial damage compared with standard monophasic waveform defibrillators. Alhough the optimal energy level has yet to be determined, biphasic countershocks at nonescalating doses of 150 to 200 J offer comparable outcomes in ventricular fibrillation compared with escalating shocks at 200 J, 300 J, and 360 J using a conventional monophasic defibrillator. Technology should be updated as existing equipment approaches end of useful life.

REFERENCES:

1. Lindner KH, Dirks B, Strohmenger H-U, et al: Randomized comparison of epinephrine and vasopressin in patients with out-of hospital ventricular fibrillation. Lancet 349:535–537, 1997.
2. Cummins RO, Hazinski MF, Kerber RE, et al: Low-energy biphasic waveform defibrillation: Evidence-based review applied to emergency cardiovascular care guidelines. Circulation 97:1654–1667, 1998.
3. Kudenchuk PJ, Cobb LA, Copass MK, et al: Amiodarone for resuscitation after out-of-hospital cardiac arrest due to ventricular fibrillation. N Engl J Med 341:871–878, 1999.
4. International Consensus on Science: Guidelines 2000 for cardiopulmonary resuscitation and emergency cardiovascular care. Circulation 102(suppl):I-86–I-171, 2000.

Scott Schartel, D.O.

PATIENT 19

A 28-year-old man with a difficult airway requiring single-lung ventilation

A 28-year-old man was an unrestrained passenger in a multivehicle accident. He sustained multiple left-sided rib fractures; left pulmonary contusion; and fractures of the zygomatic arch, maxilla, left tibia, and left fibula. He was intubated in the emergency department and subsequently underwent fixation of tibial and facial fractures. The patient remained intubated postoperatively. On the second postoperative day, he developed a left-sided pneumothorax that was treated with tube thoracostomy and suction drainage. Over the next 24 hours, blood drained at 200 mL/h from the thoracostomy tube, and a persistent air leak was noted. The patient received 2 U of packed RBCs in response to a Hct of 20%. Completion cervical spine studies have not been performed, and the patient remains in a Philadelphia collar. He is scheduled for a left thoracoscopy to address persistent bleeding and close a bronchopleural fistula. Single-lung ventilation will be required.

Physical Examination: Temperature 37.0° C, pulse 122, respirations 18, blood pressure 105/65. Marked facial edema and ecchymosis and 2.5-cm edematous tongue laceration. An 8.5 mm oral endotracheal tube is in place. Patient is sedated and unable to cooperate with examination; passive mouth opening is limited. Cardiac: chest auscultation, heart tones regular, and no murmur heard. Coarse rhonchi noted over left hemithorax.

Laboratory Findings: Hct 28%. ABG: pH 7.45, $PaCO_2$ 34 mmHg, PaO_2 155mmHg, oxygen saturation 98% (Volume-cycle, assist control mode, tidal volume 750 mL, respiratory rate 16, FIO_2 0.55, PEEP 7.5 cm H_2O). Chest radiograph: moderate left-side pulmonary contusion and rib fractures. Right lung appears normal.

Questions: How does the pulmonary contusion affect decision making for the planned procedure?
What factors make single-lung ventilation problematic?
What options exist for instituting one-lung ventilation, and what procedure may be the best, given the patient's pattern of injury?

How does the pulmonary contusion affect decision-making for the planned procedure? Pulmonary contusion may limit tolerance to one-lung ventilation. Evidence of impaired alveolar-capillary diffusion in the present patient includes a decreased PaO_2/FIO_2 ratio and increased alveolar-arterial (A-a) gradient. The PaO_2/FIO_2 ratio is a predictor of outcome in patients with pulmonary contusion.[2] Besides the lung affected by contusion, there also can be impairment of the noncontused lung caused by the systemic inflammatory response initiated by the trauma.[3,6] Pathologic changes include increased pulmonary capillary permeability, diapedesis of WBCs, and decreased surfactant activity. Fluid resuscitation and the effects of shock also may worsen the acute lung injury.

What factors make single-lung ventilation problematic? The extent of injury to the nonoperative lung is an important determinant of the patient's tolerance of single-lung ventilation. The contused left lung, the likely source of the large A-a gradient, will be collapsed during surgery, and this may improve ventilation-perfusion matching. Although one-lung ventilation initially induces an increase in pulmonary shunt, gravitational forces while in the lateral decubitus position increase perfusion to the dependent (uninjured) right lung. Positional changes have been shown to be beneficial in some patients with unilateral lung injury, probably resulting from improvement in ventilation-perfusion matching. Because impairment in oxygenation is only moderate, and there is no radiographic evidence of right pulmonary involvement, single-lung ventilation is likely to be successful.

What options exist for instituting one lung ventilation, and what procedure may be the best, given the patient's pattern of injury? Options for pulmonary isolation include replacing the existing endotracheal tube with a double-lumen endobronchial tube, deliberate right mainstem bronchial intubation with the existing endotracheal tube, or use of an endobronchial blocker with a single-lumen endotracheal tube or a Univent tube. Achieving pulmonary isolation in a patient with a traumatized airway and an uncleared cervical spine is problematic, however, and the decision to perform airway exchange must be made with caution. The margin of safety for endotracheal tube exchange is decreased as the increased A-a gradient virtually guarantees rapid oxygen desaturation. An airway exchange catheter may provide an additional safeguard for successful airway exchange, but this technique is not foolproof. Exchange catheters may become dis-

lodged from the trachea during use, especially during insertion of the long double-lumen tubes. Edematous tissues may make tube insertion difficult despite a well-placed exchange catheter. Exchange catheters may traumatize the distal tracheobronchial tree or lung parenchyma and may extend the bronchopleural fistula. If jet ventilation is used temporarily, barotrauma is a risk. At case conclusion, tubes must be reexchanged. For these reasons, use of a double-lumen endotracheal tube is not ideal.

Advancing the existing endotracheal tube into the right main stem bronchus with fiberoptic bronchoscopic guidance could be considered; however, obstruction of the right upper lobe bronchus increases the likelihood of intraoperative hypoxemia. A typical cuff length for an 8-mm endotracheal tube is 40 mm. The distance from the carina to the right upper lobe bronchial lumen averages 19 ± 6 mm in men and 15 ± 5 mm in women, the risk of obstruction by the endotracheal tube cuff is great.[1]

Another approach to pulmonary isolation is to place an endobronchial blocking catheter into the left main stem bronchus. The Univent tube has a bronchial blocking catheter in the wall of the tube but requires airway exchange. Fogarty embolectomy catheters have been used for bronchial blocking but may be difficult to place, especially into the left main stem bronchus. The Arndt endobronchial blocker (Cook Critical Care, Bloomington, IN) allows pulmonary isolation without the risks of airway exchange (see Figure on next page).[7] A multiport airway adapter allows the introduction of the bronchial blocker and a fiberoptic bronchoscope into the endotracheal tube (an ≥ 8.0 endotracheal tube is recommended), while maintaining the ability to ventilate the patient during the placement of the blocker. The balloon-tipped bronchial catheter has a central lumen through which a nylon guide passes. The bronchoscope and the bronchial blocker are introduced through the multiport adapter, and the bronchoscope is passed through the nylon guide loop. The bronchoscope and blocker are introduced into the endotracheal tube, and the multiport adapter is connected to a 15-mm endotracheal tube connector. The bronchoscope is advanced into the main stem bronchus to be blocked. The endobronchial blocker is advanced over the bronchoscope and positioned in the main stem bronchus, and the bronchoscope is retracted above the carina. The position of the endobronchial blocker is adjusted until the inflated blocker cuff fills the entire lumen of the main stem bronchus but does not herniate into the trachea. The nylon guide loop is removed from the blocker, making the area of the central lu-

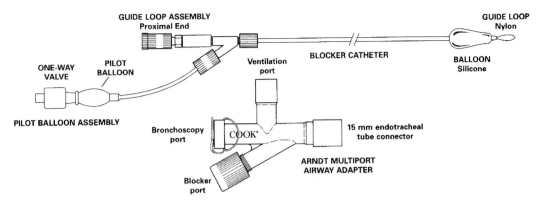

Arndt endobronchial blocker and multiport airway adapter. (Courtesy of Cook Critical Care, Bloomington, IN.)

men larger. Deflation of the lung is facilitated by ceasing ventilation, deflating the blocker cuff, and having the surgeon compress the lung. The blocker is reinflated, and ventilation is resumed. At the conclusion of the surgical procedure, the cuff of the blocker is deflated, the blocker is withdrawn, and the difficulties of airway exchange have been avoided.

Any endobronchial blocker, including the Arndt catheter, has some limitations compared with a conventional double-lumen endobronchial tube. A bronchial blocker does not allow secretions to be suctioned from the nonventilated lung, and it cannot provide postoperative differential lung ventilation. If both lungs require surgery, the requirement to reposition the blocker limits its practicality. Application of continous positive airway pressure to the nondependent lung during single-lung ventilation may be more difficult, although oxygen insufflation through the central lumen of an Arndt endobronchial blocker has been described.[8]

Despite these limitations, use of an endobronchial blocker provides advantages in the patient with an existing endotracheal (or tracheostomy) tube when one-lung ventilation is required and airway exchange may be dangerous. It is also a satisfactory choice when awake fiberoptic intubation is necessary.

The Present Patient

An Arndt endobronchial blocker was placed in the patient. During single-lung ventilation, the bronchopleural fistula was oversewn, and a bleeding intercostal vein was ligated. Using combinations of PEEP to the dependent lung, occasional continuous positive airway pressure to the nondependent lung, and high FIO_2, satisfactory oxygenation was maintained throughout the operation. The intubated patient was returned to intensive care. Pulmonary status improved, maxillofacial swelling subsided, and the patient was extubated 6 days postoperatively.

Clinical Pearls

1. The potential for loss of a patent airway should be considered carefully in any patient in whom airway exchange is being considered.

2. Even when standard cervical radiographs are normal, cervical spine precautions should be maintained until the patient can cooperate with a physical examination or flexion/extension radiographs rule out ligamentous injury.

3. The Arndt endobronchial blocker is good choice for achieving one-lung ventilation when safe airway exchange is thought to be difficult or impossible.

4. During one-lung ventilation using an endobronchial blocking catheter, lung deflation can be facilitated by deflating the cuff of the bronchial blocker and having the surgeon compress the lung while the patient is apneic. The bronchial cuff is reinflated before resuming ventilation.

REFERENCES

1. Benumof JL, Partridge BL, Salvatierra C, Keating J: Margin of safety in positioning modern double-lumen endotracheal tubes. Anesthesiology 67:729–738, 1987.
2. Kollmorgen DR, Murray KA, Sullivan JJ, et al: Predictors of mortality in pulmonary contusion. Am J Surg 168:659–664, 1994.
3. Hellinger A, Konerding MA, Malkusch W, et al: Does lung contusion affect both the traumatized and the noninjured lung parenchyma? A morphological and morphometric study in the pig. J Trauma 39:712–719, 1995.
4. Benumof JL: Difficult tubes and difficult airways. J Cardiothorac Vasc Anesth 12:131–132, 1998.
5. Hagihira S, Takashina M, Tahkahik M, Yoshiya I: One-lung ventilation in patients with difficult airways. J Cardiothorac Vasc Anesth 12:186–188, 1998.
6. Obertacke U, Neudeck F, Majetschak M, et al: Local and systemic reactions after lung contusion: An experimental study in the pig. Shock 10:7–12, 1998.
7. Arndt GA, DeLessio ST, Kramner PW, et al: One-lung ventilation when intubation is difficult—presentation of a new endobronchial blocker. Acta Anaesthesiol Scand 43:356–358, 1999.
8. Arndt GA, Kranner PW, Valdes-Mura H: Reversal of hypoxemia using insufflation of oxygen during one-lung ventilation with a wire-guided endobronchial blocker. J Cardiothorac Vasc Anesth 15:144, 2001.

John D. Lockrem, MD

PATIENT 20

A 75-year-old man with intraoperative deterioration in oxygenation and ventilation

A 75-year-old man was scheduled for urgent laparoscopic cholecystectomy. He had been admitted to the intensive care unit with the diagnosis of cholelithiasis. Medical history was significant for chronic obstructive pulmonary disease and hypertension. Medications included albuterol and atropine metered-dose inhalers and metoprolol, 50 mg twice a day.

Physical Examination: Temperature 37.8° C, pulse 84, blood pressure 150/94, SpO_2 96 on 2 L/min nasal cannula. Patient cachectic and dyspneic at rest. He was not using accessory muscles of ventilation but had difficulty finishing sentences without taking an extra breath. Multiple attempts at left subclavian venous catheterization had failed. Chest: breath sounds equal but distant bilaterally. Cardiac: heart sounds normal.

Laboratory Findings: Hct 53%, WBC 14,000/µL, electrolytes normal. ABG on 2 L/min oxygen by nasal cannula: pH 7.38, PCO_2 45 mmHg, PO_2 85 mmHg, HCO_3 26 mEq/L. Vital capacity 2.4 L, forced expiratory volume in 1 second 1.35 L. Chest radiograph: hyperlucent lung fields, no infiltrates, and no pneumothorax. Initial chest radiograph after attempts at catheter insertion showed only hyperlucent lung fields. ECG: sinus rhythm with no ischemic changes.

Hospital Course: Anesthesia was induced with etomidate and maintained with desflurane and fentanyl. Intubation of the trachea was facilitated with vecuronium. After 70 minutes of stable vital signs, the following changes were noted: SpO_2 decreased from 98 to 89, blood pressure decreased gradually to 85/70 mmHg, central venous pressure increased from 8 to 14 mmHg, heart rate decreased to 60 beats/min, and inspiratory peak pressures increased from 18 to 42 cm H_2O. Breath sounds were distant but present bilaterally with faint expiratory wheezing. The diaphragm was not noted to be bulging as seen through the laparoscope. To assist in diagnosis, a chest radiograph was taken (see Figure).

Questions: What is the diagnosis?
Discuss the differential diagnosis?
What is the significance of the chest radiograph?
What clinical maneuvers may have contributed to the condition?

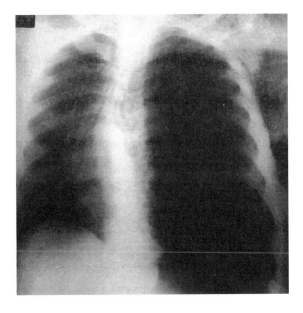

What is the diagnosis? Tension pneumothorax from attempts to place a central catheter, exacerbated by laparoscopy.

Discuss the differential diagnosis. The combination of respiratory and circulatory collapse could be caused by many processes. Bronchospasm, left ventricular failure, endobronchial intubation, anaphylaxis, pulmonary embolism, and tension pneumothorax all could present in this manner. Left ventricular failure may result in hypotension, elevated central venous pressure, hypoxia from poor lung perfusion, and increased ventilatory pressure from the reduced compliance of pulmonary edema. Frothy edema fluid may become apparent. Anaphylaxis produces bronchospasm and decreased peripheral resistance and may result in right heart failure from pulmonary vasoconstriction. Pulmonary embolism could present as circulatory and ventilatory collapse and may be associated with bronchospasm. Endobronchial intubation can cause overdistention of the lung with ventilation-perfusion mismatch and decreasing oxygen saturation and, in its most severe form, could impede venous return.

Pneumothorax may be due to alveolar rupture, visceral pleural violation, or parietal pleural disruption. Alveolar rupture could occur spontaneously because of weakened tissue in chronic destructive pulmonary disease, a ruptured bleb, or mechanical ventilation. The escaping gas passes into the lung tissue and dissects along blood vessels to the mediastinum, where it enters the pleural space. The visceral pleura may have been punctured during subclavian catheterization attempts. The incidence of pneumothorax after subclavian or internal jugular venous catheterization varies from about 0.5% to 4%.

What is the significance of the chest radiograph? The negative chest radiograph after the procedure does not rule out a pleural violation. Pneumothorax has been known to develop 48 hours after the procedure. Pneumothorax also may be missed if the radiograph was taken with the patient recumbent.

What clinical maneuvers may have contributed to the condition? Tension pneumothorax results when gas enters the pleural space and accumulates under pressure. Spontaneous breathing may not develop a large enough pressure gradient to cause a significant pneumothorax, but positive-pressure ventilation may increase the extent of pneumothorax dramatically. The pressurized gas employed during laparoscopy has been known to violate the parietal pleura and cause pneumothorax; this can occur from inadvertent trauma to the diaphragm or from gas tracking through the diaphragm along the esophagus. During open abdominal procedures, as the volume of the tension pneumothorax increases, the diaphragm may be observed protruding under pressure into the abdominal cavity. In the present case, the diaphragm may not have changed configuration because of the pressurized gas in the abdomen, however, counterbalancing the increased pressure in the chest.

The classic description of tension pneumothorax is hypotension in the setting of unilaterally decreased breath sounds and tracheal deviation. Some important points should be made, however. First, detecting differences in breath sounds may be difficult, especially in a patient with distant breath sounds in a noisy operating room, and tracheal deviation may be a late, preterminal finding. Second, animal studies examining the physiologic effects of tension pneumothorax challenge the traditional assumptions concerning the mechanical effects of tension pneumothorax on hemodynamics. A pig model of progressive tension pneumothorax found decreasing oxygen saturation to precede decreases in cardiac output and blood pressure. A related study performed in sheep showed early tachycardia and significant compensation in spontaneously breathing animals by generating large intrapleural pressure gradients. When ventilation was converted from spontaneous to positive pressure, compensatory mechanisms quickly diminished. The practitioner should be cognizant of these early changes because earlier diagnosis and treatment may be facilitated.

The Present Patient

Tension pneumothorax was suspected and a device as depicted in the Figure on the next page was inserted in the second intercostal space at the midclavicular line on the left side. A rush of air was detected by bubbling through the saline in the syringe barrel. The vital signs normalized quickly. The procedure was finished within minutes, and a left tube thoracostomy was performed in the operating room. Postoperative recovery was uneventful, and the chest tube was removed the following day.

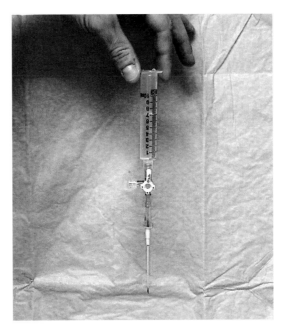

Emergency pneumothorax detection device made from readily available equipment. The syringe plunger has been removed and the barrel filled with saline to detect gas escaping from the chest. The catheter is inserted in the midclavicular line of the second intercostal space, and the stopcock is turned to allow the gas to flow through the device.

Clinical Pearls

1. Precipitous hemodynamic collapse may be due to tension pneumothorax, pulmonary embolus, left ventricular failure, anaphylaxis, and cardiac tamponade.

2. Delayed pneumothorax can develop after a negative postprocedure radiograph. Recumbent radiographs are notorious for missing small pneumothoraces.

3. Findings associated with a pneumothorax can be nonspecific. It can be difficult to localize a pneumothorax, especially in the operating room. Pneumothorax should be considered if cardiac performance or oxygenation deteriorate acutely after central catheter placement, especially if catheter placement was difficult.

4. The traditional triad of hypotension, unilateral absence of breath sounds, and tracheal deviation may be late, preterminal findings and may be preceded by tachycardia, decreasing oxygen saturation, and dyspnea.

5. Many central catheters are started in the operating room without the benefit of immediate postprocedural radiographs. Immediate postprocedural radiographs are strongly recommended if catheter placement is difficult.

6. A spontaneously breathing patient without significant chronic pulmonary disease may be able to compensate for a pneumothorax but may decompensate rapidly when positive-pressure ventilation is instituted.

7. With a high index of suspicion, tension pneumthorax should be relieved without radiographic confirmation. Evacuation of air under pressure can be lifesaving.

REFERENCES

1. Gustman P, Yerger L, Wanner A: Immediate cardiovascular effects of tension pneumothorax. Am Rev Respir Dis 127:171–174, 1983.
2. Denlinger JK: Pneumothorax. In Gravenstein N, Kirby R (eds): Complications in Anesthesiology. Philadelphia, Lippincott-Raven, 1996, pp 241–249.
3. Barton ED, Rhee P, Hutton KC, et al: The pathophysiology of tension pneumothorax in ventilated swine. J Emerg Med 15:147–153, 1997.
4. Coulter T, Wiedemann H: Complications of hemodynamic monitoring. Clin Chest Med 20:249–266, 1999.

James C. Duke, MD

PATIENT 21

A 64-year-old woman with new onset of arrhythmia postoperatively

A 64-year-old woman was scheduled for a laparoscopic-assisted hemicolectomy for polyps. She has a history of hypertension, diabetes mellitus, and hypercholesterolemia. She occasionally consumes alcohol and is a light cigarette smoker. Exercise tolerance is two flights of stairs. Medications include lisinopril, aspirin, metformin, atorvastatin (Lipitor), and insulin.

Physical examination: Pulse 68, respirations 16, blood pressure 144/63. General appearance: A slightly obese woman in no acute distress. Lungs: clear. Cardiac: regular rhythm without murmurs or gallops. Abdomen: benign. No peripheral edema.

Laboratory Findings: Sodium 141 mEq/L, potassium 4.4 mEq/L, chloride 107 mEq/L, Glucose 213 mg/dL, BUN 13 mg/dL, creatinine 0.8 mg/dL. Hct 37.4%, hemoglobin 12.6 g/dL, platelets 132,000/μL. Oxygen saturation 90%. ECG: sinus rhythm.

The patient received a balanced endotracheal anesthetic for the procedure. Oxygenation and ventilation were unremarkable intraoperatively, even during laparoscopy. Because she received a bowel preparation preoperatively, lactated Ringer's solution was administered generously, totaling 4 L over the 90-minute procedure. Blood loss was 250 mL, and urine output averaged about 1 mL/kg/h. The patient was extubated at case conclusion and taken to recovery. Early in the recovery phase, a rapid, irregular cardiac rhythm was noted (see Figure). At the time, the patient was being medicated for abdominal pain but denied chest pain or shortness of breath. She appeared uncomfortable. Her blood pressure was 132/91 mmHg; on 3 L oxygen by nasal cannula, oxygen saturation was 92%.

Questions: What is the diagnosis?
What are predisposing factors for this dysrhythmia?
Suggest a course of therapy.
What factors determine the aggressiveness of therapy?

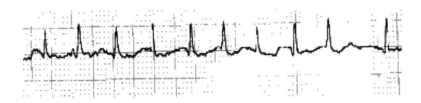

What is the diagnosis? Atrial fibrillation (AF) with rapid ventricular response (approximately 150/min).

AF is a most common arrhythmia in elderly patients. The topic is extensive, so of necessity this discussion focuses on treatment in the perioperative period only. Not included in the discussion is long-term treatment of AF, including numerous medications administered primarily in this context, and anticoagulation.

What are predisposing factors for this dysrhythmia? AF may be considered a primary arrhythmia in the absence of structural heart disease, an arrhythmia secondary to structural heart disease, or an arrhythmia secondary to noncardiac systemic abnormalities. Causes of AF include acute myocardial ischemia or infarction, congestive heart failure, hypoxemia, chronic pulmonary disease, electrolyte abnormalities, pulmonary embolism, thyrotoxicosis, alcohol abuse, and digoxin or quinidine toxicity. Cholinergic medications may produce AF. AF often is noted postoperatively, especially after coronary artery bypass graft surgery (10% to 40%), valvular surgery (50%), pneumonectomy, and other intrathoracic procedures.

The mechanism of AF is microreentry, frequently from multiple propagating impulses (multiple wavelet hypothesis). Increased age, hypertension, diabetes mellitus, coronary artery disease, left ventricular dysfunction, concomitant valvular disease (often rheumatic in origin), and prior history of AF are risk factors. Increased parasympathetic tone predisposes otherwise normal hearts to AF. Muscarinic atrial tissue receptors, when stimulated by acetylcholine, shorten the refractory period. Increased sympathetic activity, as often occurs in the perioperative period, also is a factor in AF.

The ventricular rate, duration of tachydysrhythmia, and cardiac function are important determinants of the patient's ability to tolerate AF. Because atrial systole contributes ≥20% to left ventricular preinjection volume (*atrial kick*), loss of organized atrial activity may impair cardiac output significantly. Patients at risk for reductions in cardiac output include those with impaired diastolic filling, resulting from stenotic valvular lesions, cardiomyopathy, ventricular hypertrophy, diastolic dysfunction, or pericardial disease. Elevated heart rates also reduce the time for diastolic chamber filling. Persistence of AF for >24 hours may result in development of atrial thrombi; systemic embolization may occur when sinus rhythm is reestablished unless anticoagulation has been instituted.

Suggest a course of therapy. The goals of therapy include controlling ventricular rate, reestab-lishing sinus rhythm, and preventing thromboembolism. The degree of hemodynamic embarrassment determines therapy for acute AF. If the patient is hypotensive or showing myocardial ischemia or pulmonary edema, immediate synchronized cardioversion at 100 to 200 J is indicated. Although sedation during cardioversion is desirable, hemodynamic status determines its risk and benefit.

Medications that rapidly slow ventricular response include calcium channel blockers, β-adrenergic blocking agents, and amiodarone (see Table on next page). These medications prolong the refractory period and decrease the conduction velocity of atrial tissue and the atrioventricular node. Diltiazem is the drug of choice for many and usually results in less myocardial depression and hypotension than verapamil. β-Blockers, including esmolol, propranolol, atenolol, and metoprolol, are effective and are the drugs of choice when thyrotoxicosis is thought to cause AF. Digoxin may be useful when impaired systolic function is contributing to congestive heart failure; its effect on the atrioventricular node is indirect, vagally mediated, and slow in onset. Digoxin is less effective for rate control in young or active patients and others with high adrenergic tone. Agents that depress atrioventricular conduction, when administered in combination, may result in severe bradycardia. Under these circumstances, usual dose recommendations may be excessive, and these medications always should be titrated to effect.

Patients with Wolff-Parkinson-White syndrome require special attention because extremely rapid ventricular excitation by accessory pathways may lead to precipitous clinical detrioration, including ventricular fibrillation and sudden cardiac death. Digitalis, calcium channel blockers, and β-adrenergic blockers may accelerate conduction over the accessory pathway and are contraindicated. Procainamide is the drug of choice for hemodynamically stable patients with Wolff-Parkinson-White syndrome. Unstable patients require cardioversion.

Ventricular slowing often is followed by spontaneous conversion to sinus rhythm. If not, specific therapy may be administered to produce pharmacologic conversion. Digitalis, verapamil, propranolol, and esmolol rarely terminate AF. Amiodarone, procainamide, sotalol, and ibutilide are effective for restoring sinus rhythm, although cardioversion may be necessary after the patient is drug-loaded. Other drug options include propafenone, flecainide, quinidine and disopyramide.

Some patients with AF may have a normal ventricular rate (50 to 100 beats/min); this is presumptive evidence of atrioventricular nodal disease, high vagal tone, or both. Nodal slowing agents generally are not needed and might produce

Suitable Antiarrhythmia Medications for Acute Treatment of Atrial Fibrillation

Medication	Class	Typical IV Dose*	Precautions
Diltiazem	Calcium channel blocker	0.25 mg/kg over 2 min Infusion 5–15 mg/h	Caution in setting of accessory pathways
Verapamil	Calcium channel blocker	0.075–0.15 mg/kg over 2 min	Caution in setting of accessory pathways and in combination with other nodal blockers
Esmolol	β-blocker	0.5–1.0 mg/kg over 1 min 50–200 μg/kg/min by infusion	Worsen heart failure, may aggravate atrioventricular nodal conduction disorders[†]
Propranolol	β-blocker	0.15 mg/kg	Bronchospasm, heart failure, impair atrioventricular conduction
Metoprolol	β-blocker	2.5–5 mg over 2 mins. May repeat up to 3 doses	Same as propranolol
Amiodarone	Vaughan Williams class III[‡]	150 mg over 10 min Infuse 360 mg over 6 h, then 540 mg over 18 h	May potentiate hypotensive or bradycardic effects of other drugs; atrioventricular block; worsens heart failure
Digoxin	Glycoside/inotrope	0.5 mg, the 0.25 mg every 4 h for 2 doses 0.125–0.25 mg daily	Not effective quickly, may worsen AF with WPW syndrome
Procainamide	Vaughan Williams class IA	10–15 mg/kg initial dose 2–4 mg/min infusion	Useful for AF associated with WPW syndrome May produce hypotension or worsen atrioventricular block; normalize electrolytes before administration; avoid with prolonged Q-T interval

*Medications should be titrated to effect. Elderly patients may show the expected effect with small doses. Patients with left ventricular dysfunction may become hypotensive.

[†]Administration of multiple medications with atrioventricular nodal blocking effects should be undertaken carefully because severe and refractory bradycardia may ensue.

[‡]Amiodarone has properties of all Vaughan Williams class antiarrhythmics.

AF, atrial fibrillation; WPN, Wolff-Parkinson-White.

---

severe bradycardia. Some patients also may have sinus node dysfunction (bradycardia-tachycardia syndrome) and have significant bradycardia with chemical or electrical therapy.

What factors determine the aggressiveness of therapy? It is highly desirable to reestablish sinus rhythm in postoperative patients within 48 hours. Failure to reestablish sinus activity after 24 hours of drug therapy might be an indication for cardioversion. It is important to review (by prior records, ECGs and discussion of symptoms) whether AF has occurred previously, however. If the timing of onset is unclear, it might be best to assume that AF has occurred before and to institute 3 to 4 weeks of anticoagulation before cardioversion. Echocardiography often is indicated to search for evidence of structural heart disease.

Many of these patients should be treated acutely with heparin, but this decision must be made in light of the patient's surgery and other medical problems. Patients at high risk for stroke (the elderly and patients with left ventricular dysfunction of hypertrophy, hypertension, diabetes mellitus, coronary artery disease, mitral valve disease, hyperthyroidism, and prior stroke) should be considered for heparin therapy. If mural thrombi are ruled out by transesophageal echocardiography, this period of anticoagulation before cardioversion may be reduced. Cardiologists debate the benefit of antiarrhythmic loading before cardioversion. Some experts believe the small but real risk of antiarrhythmic toxicity is reason enough to avoid these agents in otherwise healthy patients. Because atrial electrical activity precedes atrial mechanical activity, anticoagulation should be continued after cardioversion for at least 3 weeks.

The Present Patient

The present patient was administered diltiazem, 15 mg intravenously over 10 minutes, and placed on a diltiazem infusion at 5 mg/h. The ventricular response promptly decreased to 70 to 80 beats/min (see Figure). Blood pressure was 151/70 mmHg. Within 24 hours, the patient's rhythm reverted to sinus rhythm. Sinus rhythm was noted at postoperative visits 2 and 4 weeks later.

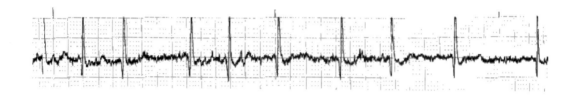

Clinical Pearls

1. Postoperative arrhythmias are frequent, especially after coronary artery bypass graft surgery, valvular replacement, and other intrathoracic procedures.

2. The aggressiveness of therapy is predicated on the patient's stability. Often patients with AF are relatively stable, and medical therapy is reasonable. Patients with hemodynamic instability or evidence of end-organ hypoperfusion are candidates for cardioversion.

3. Pharmacologic therapy focuses on slowing ventricular response, reestablishing sinus rhythm, and preventing atrial clot formation. Suitable agents include diltiazem, β-adrenergic blockers, amiodarone, and digoxin. Electrolytes, acid-base status, and adequacy of oxygenation and ventilation also should be assessed because acute abnormalities may contribute to the new rhythm disturbance. A 12-lead ECG should be reviewed for new onset of ischemia, and a myocardial infarction should be ruled out. Echocardiography may detect structural heart disease.

4. Atrial clots may develop quickly, and the benefits of heparin therapy must be considered in light of the patient's recent surgical procedure and other comorbidities, especially risk of stroke.

5. Administration of multiple agents that depress atrioventricular function should be undertaken with care because severe and refractory bradyarrhythmias may result.

REFERENCES

1. Atlee JL: Perioperative cardiac dysrhythmias, diagnosis and management. Anesthesiology 86:1397–1424, 1997.
2. Prystowsky EN, Benson W, Fuster V, et al: Management of patients with atrial fibrillation. American Heart Association Executive Summary, 1996. Available at www.americanheart.org/scientific/statements/1997.html.
3. Balser JR: Perioperative management of arrhythmias. Probl Anesth 10:197–214, 1998.
4. Delle Karth G, Geppert A, Neunteufl T, et al: Amiodarone versus diltiazem for rate control in critically ill patients with atrial tachyarrhythmias. Crit Care Med 29:1149–1153, 2001.
5. Fuster V, Ryden LE, Asinger RW, et al: ACC management of patients with atrial fibrillation. J Am Coll Cardiol 38:1–70, 2001.

Eric Zeeb, MD

PATIENT 22

A 27-year-old woman with multiple injuries and metabolic acidosis

A 27-year-old, 60-kg, otherwise healthy woman was hit by a car. On arrival at the emergency department, she was hypotensive and complaining of low back and pelvic pain. She received an initial 2 L of normal saline (NS) bolus.

Initial Laboratory Findings: WBC 9,200/μL, hemoglobin 9.8 g/dL, Hct 30%, platelets 348,000/μL. Na 138 mEq/L, K 3.3 mEq/L, Cl 100 mEq/L, HCO_3 20.8 mEq/L. BUN 16 mg/dL, creatinine 1.1 mg/dL. Radiographs: an open book pelvic fracture.

Continued occult blood loss was shown by declines in serial Hct measurements. She was taken to the operating room for vaginal repair and external pelvic fixation. She had received 10 L of NS and 5 U of packed RBCs before arrival in the operating room. After a standard rapid-sequence induction and intubation, a radial arterial catheter was inserted.

Physical Examination: Pulse 110, respirations 20, blood pressure 92/50, oxygen saturation 98% on 3 L O_2/min via nasal cannula. Lower abdomen: tender; Pelvic: severe pain with manipulation; blood in the vaginal vault.

Repeat Laboratory Findings: Hct 28%. Na 134 mEq/L, K 4.0 mEq/L, Cl 116 mEq/L, HCO_3 14 mEq/L. BUN 19 mg/dL, creatinine 1.1 mg/dL, lactate 1.5 mg/dL, glucose 225 mg/dL. ABG on F_IO_2 of 1.0: pH 7.18, $PaCO_2$ 35 mmHg, PaO_2 348 mmHg, HCO_3 15 mEq/L, SpO_2 99%, base excess −13.

Question: What is the cause of the patient's metabolic acidosis?
What is the etiology of dilutional acidosis?
What are the differences among commonly available intravenous solutions?
What are the clinical implications of dilutional acidosis?

What is the cause of the patient's metabolic acidosis? Hyperchloremic metabolic acidosis associated with aggressive NS administration.

What is the etiology of dilutional acidosis? The concept of dilutional acidosis (an acidosis traditionally thought to be caused by dilution of HCO_3 from aggressive intravenous fluid therapy) was proposed many decades ago. Shires and Holman first studied the concept in 1948. They infused dogs with NS at 300 mL/min over 5 minutes, observed a progressive acidosis, and hypothesized the mechanism to be a dilution of HCO_3. This was the generally accepted view until 1969, when further research challenged the validity of these findings. Rosenbaum et al[2] studied the effects of saline infusion on nephrectomized dogs and found large saline infusions produced only transient acid-base changes. They criticized Shires and Holman for not measuring acid-base changes beyond the initial infusion time and hypothesized that compensatory renal and cellular buffers were adequate to offset the effects of dilution. Garella et al[3] corroborated these findings, concluding "an acute volume expansion of a degree capable of causing marked hemodynamic alterations would still be insufficient to result in a clinically appreciable degree of metabolic acidosis."

Several more recent case reports and controlled studies have renewed interest in dilutional acidosis but with a new appreciation of the etiologic importance of hyperchloremia. Goodkin et al[5] described the first case report involving an 84-year-old woman treated for sepsis complicated by myocardial infarction. Her initial resuscitation included 6 L of NS. She remained acidotic after resuscitation with a pH of 7.18, an increase in chloride from 106 to 120 mEq/L, and a decrease in HCO_3 from 22 to 10 mEq/L. Saline-induced hyperchloremic metabolic acidosis subsequently has been observed or studied in many clinical situations: ileal bladder augmentation, nephrectomy, gynecologic surgery, acute normovolemic hemodilution, trauma resuscitation, prolonged vascular and intraabdominal surgery, management of right ventricular infarction, and surgery with cardiopulmonary bypass. Prough[10] commented that **dilutional acidosis** is currently the best descriptive term for this phenomenon but stated that further clarification is needed regarding the actual mechanism.

Many authors have challenged the belief that dilution of HCO_3 is the cause of this acidosis, instead citing hyperchloremia as the major culprit. Rapid volume expansion with NS, which contains a supraphysiologic concentration of chloride (154 mEq/L), is thought to induce a hyperchloremic

metabolic acidosis; this was shown by Waters et al and Bernstein[11] in a prospective crossover study design. They alternatively infused two groups of healthy volunteers with 15 mL/kg of either 6% Hespan (hetastarch constituted in NS) or 5% albumin over 30 minutes. Each group showed an approximately 25% increase in plasma volume (calculated based on changes in hematocrit), but only the Hespan group showed significant acid-base changes (significantly decreased HCO_3, base excess, and albumin). The Hespan group became hyperchloremic. It was determined that chloride elevation was the major determinant of the acid-base changes, not the degree of volume expansion.

To understand how hyperchloremia results in metabolic acidosis, a review of acid-base physiologic modeling as proposed by Stewart[4] is necessary. Stewart challenged traditional concepts of acid-base physiology by mathematically modeling biologic fluids as complete physicochemical systems. According to Stewart,[4] the Henderson-Hasselbalch approach to acid-base physiology, in which acidosis is seen as an aberration of CO_2 and HCO_3 concentration, is an oversimplification and misrepresentation of the true nature of acid-base physiology. Stewart's approach to acid-base modeling relies on three independent variables as the sole determinants of acid-base status: PCO_2, strong ion difference (SID), and the nonvolatile weak plasma acids. HCO_3 concentration is a dependent variable, a function of the relative values of the independent variables, and not a principal determinant of overall acid-base balance. The metabolic acid-base disturbances are induced by changes in the nonvolatile weak acids or the strong ions. Principal nonvolatile weak acids include the inorganic phosphates and serum proteins (mainly albumin), which dissociate only partially in solution. Strong ions dissociate completely in solution and include primarily sodium, potassium, and chloride. The mathematical difference between the strong cations and strong anions is the SID. A normal SID is approximately 40, reflecting unmeasured anions. A more negative SID induces a metabolic acidosis, whereas a more positive SID causes a metabolic alkalosis. Administration of large volumes of NS induce a hyperchloremic metabolic acidosis by decreasing the SID. This approach to acid-base balance negates the possibility of HCO_3 dilution as the cause of acidosis.

What are the differences among commonly available intravenous solutions? The ionic contents of commonly used IV solutions are shown in the Table. NS use should be limited to the dilution of packed RBC for transfusion and use in patients at

Composition of Commonly Available Solutions

Solution	pH	Osmolarity (mOsm)	Sodium	Potassium	Chloride	Calcium	Magnesium	HCO$_3$, Source
Plasma	7.4	280–295	134–145	3.4–5	98–108	2.25–2.65	0.7–1.1	22–32
0.9% Saline	5.0	308	154	0	154	0	0	0
Lactated Ringer's	6.5	273	130	4	109	3	0	28, lactate
Plasma-Lyte 148	7.4	294	140	5	98	0	3	27, acetate; 23, gluconate
Plasma-Lyte R	5.5	312	140	10	103	5	3	47, acetate; 8, lactate
Normosol-R		295	140	5	98	0	3	0
5% albumin			140	0.2	105	0.22		
Hespan (6% hetastarch in NS)			154	0	154	0	0	0
Hextend (6% hetastarch in LR)	5.9	307	143	3	124	5	0.9	28, lactate

NS, normal saline; LR, lactacted Ringer's.

risk for cerebral edema (owing to its higher osmolarity). The American College of Surgeons recommends the use of lactated Ringer's solution for initial fluid resuscitation in the resuscitation of shock.

What are the clinical implications of dilutional of acidosis? The significance of saline-induced hyperchloremic metabolic acidosis is a subject of ongoing debate. Severe acidosis causes myocardial depression, arrhythmogenicity, altered catecholamine responsivity, and other end-organ dysfunction. Hyperchloremia itself also may be harmful. Hyperchloremia is known to produce renal vasoconstriction, decreasing renal blood flow, glomerular filtration rate, and urine output. Decreased urine output has been noted in numerous studies when NS has been compared with other, more physiologic, crystalloid solutions. Wilkes et al[13] showed decreased gastric mucosal perfusion to be associated with NS administration, suggesting hyperchloremia may reduce splanchnic perfusion. Waters et al[6] found increased blood product requirements in patients undergoing elective aortic aneurysm repair who received NS in comparison with lactated Ringer's solution. Although these observations suggest clinical implications of hyperchloremia, further research is needed to establish its significance definitively.

Perhaps the greatest risk of hyperchloremic acidosis associated with NS administration is a failure to recognize it. A frequent cause of metabolic acidosis in the perioperative setting is lactic acidosis associated with cellular hypoperfusion. If it is not recognized that NS administration, not hyperlactacidemia, is the cause of acidosis, continued NS will only worsen the acidosis and confuse the clinical picture. Recognition also prevents potential clinical mismanagement.

Saline-induced hyperchloremic metabolic acidosis is an easily preventable clinical entity. Whenever massive volume resuscitation is ongoing, the clinician must choose a resuscitation fluid rationally. When faced with a metabolic acidosis, measuring serum lactate can be beneficial in ruling out hypoperfusion-related lactic acidosis. Additionally, measuring electrolytes and calculating an anion gap (AG = Na − Cl − HCO$_3$ [normal AG = 12–16]), can distinguish between an elevated and a normal AG acidosis. Hyperchloremic metabolic acidosis has a normal anion gap. Additionally, furosemide (Lasix) administration may be considered when hyperchloremia is encountered because it is chlorouretic. Only in situations of life-threatening acidosis should sodium bicarbonate therapy be considered.

The Present Patient

The patient had a significant metabolic acidosis without respiratory component (pH 7.18, HCO$_3$ 15 mEq/L, base excess −13, PCO$_2$ 35 mmHg).

Laboratory evaluation revealed hyperchloremia (Cl 116 mEq/L), a normal anion gap (8), and normal serum lactate (lactate 1.5 mg/dL). Saline-induced hyperchloremic metabolic acidosis was the diagnosis, caused by massive volume resuscitation with a poorly chosen solution (NS). IV fluids were changed to lactated Ringer's solution, and the acidosis resolved without sequelae.

Clinical Pearls

1. A rational approach to fluid choice is paramount, especially when large volumes are to be infused.
2. NS has limited indications.
3. Aggressive NS administration may result in a hyperchloremic metabolic acidosis.
4. While the debate over the etiology of dilutional acidosis continues, recent research supports an aberration of the SID as the etiology, rather that a dilution of HCO_3^-.
5. The clinical significance of saline-induced hyperchloridemic metabolic acidois has yet to be definitively established, but recognition is vital.

REFERENCES

1. Shires GT, Holman J: Dilutional acidosis. Ann Intern Med 28:557–559, 1948.
2. Rosenbaum BJ, Makoff DL, Maxwell MH: Acid-base and electrolyte changes induced by acute isotonic saline infusion in the nephrectomized dog. J Lab Clin Med 74:427–435, 1969.
3. Garella S, Tzamaloukas AH, Chazan JA: Effect of isotonic volume expansion on extracellular bicarbonate stores in normal dogs. Am J Physiol 225:628–636, 1973.
4. Stewart PA: Modern quantitative acid-base chemistry. Can J Physiol Pharmacol 61:1444–1461, 1983.
5. Goodkin DA, Raja RM, Saven A: Dilutional acidosis. South Med J 83:354–355, 1990.
6. Waters JH, Gottlieb A, Schoenwald P, et al: Normal saline versus lactated Ringer's solution for intraoperative fluid management in patients undergoing abdominal aortic aneurysm repair: An outcome study. Anesth Analg 93:817–822, 1991.
7. Fencl V, Leith DE: Stewart's quantitative acid-base chemistry: Applications in biology and medicine. Respir Physiol 91:1–16, 1993.
8. Mathes DD, Morell RC, Rohr MS: Dilutional acidosis: Is it a real clinical entity? Anesthesiology 86:501–503, 1997.
9. Scheingraber S, Rehm M, Sehmisch C, et al: Rapid saline infusion produces hyperchloremic acidosis in patients undergoing gynecologic surgery. Anesthesiology 90:1265–1270, 1999.
10. Prough, DS: Acidosis associated with perioperative saline administration: Dilution or delusion? (editorial). Anesthesiology 93:1167–1169, 2000.
11. Waters JH, Bernstein CA: Dilutional acidosis following hetastarch or albumin in healthy volunteers. Anesthesiology 93:1174–1183, 2000.
12. Ho AMH, Karmakar MK, Contardi LH, et al: Excessive use of normal saline in managing traumatized patients in shock: A preventable contributor to acidosis. J Trauma 51:173–177, 2001.
13. Wilkes NJ, Woolf R, Mutch M, et al: The effects of balanced versus saline-based hetastarch and crystalloid solutions on acid-base and electrolyte status and gastric mucosal perfusion in elderly surgical patients. Anesth Analg 93:811–816, 2001.

Philip Vercio MD

PATIENT 23

An 80-year-old woman with rapid heart rate after pneumonectomy

An 80-year-old woman with a history of smoking, emphysema, and primary lung cancer is scheduled for left-sided pneumonectomy. Preoperative evaluation reveals a thin, 50-kg woman in no acute distress. She reports her emphysema limits her exercise tolerance because of shortness of breath with exertion. She sleeps on three pillows at night. She denies any history of myocardial infarction. She states she has had high blood pressure for 15 years treated with enalapril, 5 mg twice a day, and her primary care physician started furosemide (Lasix), 20 mg per day about 6 months ago for swelling in her ankles. Other medications include prednisone, 5 mg daily, and albuterol and beclomethasone metered-dose inhalers. She has a 100-pack-year smoking history; she denies alcohol or other substance abuse.

For anesthetic management, a left 37F double-lumen endotracheal tube is placed. A left radial artery catheter is placed after induction with propofol, fentanyl, and rocuronium. Muscle relaxation is maintained during the case and reversed with neostigmine and glycopyrrolate. She is extubated at case conclusion without difficulty. Perioperative blood loss was estimated at 850 mL with intraoperative crystalloids totaling 1,000 mL. She refused epidural placement preoperatively, and pain control is achieved with patient-controlled analgesia with fentanyl during an uneventful 90-minute postanesthesia care unit stay. She is transferred to the intensive care unit in good condition. Three hours later, she complains of her chest fluttering. She denies dizziness but states her breathing is a little difficult.

Physical Examination: Temperature 37° C; pulse 136, respirations 28, blood pressure 100/55, SpO2 90%. Skin: pale. HEENT: normal. Chest: rapid shallow breathing pattern, clear but minimal air movement with breath sounds more prominent on the right than left side. Cough effort poor and nonproductive. Cardiac: rapid, regular rhythm. Abdomen: normal. Extremities: clubbing of fingers, 1 to 2+ lower extremity edema without cyanosis. Neurologic: arouses easily and is appropriately oriented.

Preoperative Laboratory Findings: CBC: hemoglobin 12 g/dL, Hct 36%, other values normal. NA 145 mEq/L, K 3.4 mEq/L, Cl 95 mEq/L, CO_2 27 mEq/L. BUN 25 mg/dL, creatinine 1.3 mg/dL, glucose 130 mg/dL. Prothrombin time, partial thromboplastin time, international normalized ratio all normal. ECG: normal sinus rhythm with nonspecific T wave abnormalities. Spirometry values: forced expiratory volume in 1 second (FEV_1) 2.4 L (76% of predicted), FEV_1 forced vital capacity (FVC) 60%. FEV_1 and FEV_1/FVC improved to 80% and 65% after bronchodilator treatment. ABG: pH 7.4, $PaCO_2$ 49 mmHg, PaO_2 68 mmHg, SaO2 93%.

Postoperative Laboratory Findings: CBC: Hct 25%, remaining values normal. NA 142 mEq/L, K 3.0 mEq/L, Cl 96 mEq/L, CO_2 27 mEq/L. BUN 24 mg/dL, creatinine 1.3 mg/dL. ECG: see Figure. ABG (room air): pH 7.38, $PaCO_2$ 52 mmHg, PaO_2 56 mmHg, base deficit -12, SaO_2 89%. Chest radiograph: mild left-sided mediastinal shift, hyperlucent right lung field with flattened right hemidiaphragm, otherwise unremarkable.

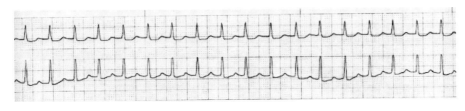

Questions What is the cardiac rhythm?
What are the likely predisposing causes of the rhythm in this patient?
What are the diagnostic considerations?
What is the appropriate treatment?
What are the side effects and risks of pharmacologic treatment?

What is the cardiac rhythm? Paroxysmal supraventricular tachycardia (SVT).

What are the likely predisposing causes of the rhythm in this patient? Paroxysmal supraventricular tachycardia (SVT). Narrow-complex tachycardia is a frequent perioperative complication with a 20% to 40% incidence after cardiac surgery. Likewise, patients undergoing large abdominal and noncardiac intrathoracic surgical procedures (pulmonary or esophageal resections) are at an increased risk. There is a 10% to 20% incidence of SVT after pneumonectomy. Patients having large vascular procedures also are at increased risk. The most common narrow-complex tachycardia observed in these settings is atrial fibrillation.

Patients may have preexisting conditions or intraoperative events that serve as arrhythmia substrates. Preexisting conditions include advanced age, coronary artery disease, cardiomyopathies and valvular disease, congestive heart failure, hypertension, chronic pulmonary disease, sick sinus syndrome, and Wolff-Parkinson-White (WPW) syndrome. Patients >60 years old seem particularly prone to SVT. Intraoperative events include hypomagnesemia, hypokalemia and hyperkalemia, hypoxemia, hypercarbia and acidosis, hypothermia, hypotension and myocardial ischemia, pulmonary embolus, elevated catecholamine states, and insufficient depth of anesthesia.

What are the diagnostic considerations? The accurate diagnosis of a rapid rhythm is important and challenging. Especially with extremely fast heart rates, the diagnosis may be uncertain based on rhythm strips, and obtaining a 12-lead ECG frequently is essential to differentiate the cause. A crucial first step is determining cardiovascular stability. Patients with coronary artery disease or left ventricular dysfunction may develop myocardial ischemia or pump failure quickly. When associated with hemodynamic instability, chest pain, or alterations in mental status, aggressive therapy is indicated and takes precedence over obtaining a 12-lead ECG. Synchronized cardioversion should be considered under such circumstances. Although the appropriate initial energy level is a function of the underlying rhythm, an initial energy setting of 100 J is reasonable (atrial flutter may respond to lower energy levels). Stepwise increases in energy of 100 J are reasonable if the patient fails to respond. Sedation before cardioversion is desirable, although the patient's circulatory status would determine the advisability of sedative therapy.

Assuming cardiovascular stability, the next step in characterizing the rhythm is determining whether the QRS is narrow or wide complex. Although a wide QRS complex may be aberrantly conducted SVT, a wide QRS tachycardia is likely to be ventricular tachycardia in 90% of patients with structural heart disease. The treatment is dramatically different (see later). If the rhythm appears to be a narrow-complex tachycardia, the next assessment is whether the rhythm is regular or irregular. An irregular tachycardia is most likely rapid atrial fibrillation, although atrial flutter with variable block and multifocal atrial tachycardia are possibilities. At least three different atrial morphologies are necessary to make the diagnosis of multifocal atrial tachycardia. This rhythm often is associated with chronic lung disease.

A regular narrow-complex tachycardia may be sinus tachycardia, atrial tachycardia (an ectopic rhythm that comes from atrial tissue, not primarily involving the atrioventricular [AV] node), atrial flutter with regular block, or one of the classic reentrant forms of SVT that involve the AV node. Sinus tachycardia is important to recognize. Before drug therapy is considered, sinus tachycardia should prompt a search for reversible, potentially life-threatening causes, such as hemorrhage, pulmonary embolus, hypoxemia, and myocardial ischemia. Light anesthesia also should be considered. In contrast to other narrow-complex tachycardias, sinus tachycardia tends to be gradual, rather than abrupt, in onset and termination.

SVTs are a family of rhythms that have several elements in common. Because these rhythms involve a reentrant loop that includes the AV node, they tend to respond to vagal maneuvers and to drugs that block the AV node (adenosine, digoxin, β-blockers, and certain calcium blockers). There are two main types of SVT: (1) AV nodal reentrant tachycardia (AVNRT), in which the microreentrant circuit is confined to the vicinity of the AV node, and (2) atrioventricular reentrant tachycardia, (AVRT), in which macroscopic reentrant circuit travels from the atria to the ventricles via the AV node, then conducts back to the atria through an accessory pathway. Even though an accessory pathway is involved in the circuit, because the AV node and His-Purkinje system is activated initially, the QRS complex is narrow rather than wide. In contrast, in WPW syndrome, the ventricles may be activated initially through the accessory pathway (resulting in a wide QRS complex) with retrograde conduction back through the AV node to the atria.

As mentioned, a 12-lead ECG obtained during tachycardia (in a stable patient) can be helpful. If the P wave is close to the next QRS complex (a *long R-P tachycardia*), atrial tachycardia should be strongly considered. With reentrant forms of SVT, the P wave is retrograde and close to the previous QRS, and a *short R-P tachycardia* is generally present. With AVNRT, the end of the QRS may be deformed by the P wave or not seen at all, whereas with AVRT, the P wave often deforms the ST segment. In each case, comparison of the 12-lead ECG during tachycardia with the patient's baseline tracing suggests the correct diagnosis.

What is the appropriate treatment? When stable SVT is encountered, an initial attempt to increase vagal tone by encouraging a Valsalva maneuver may terminate the rhythm. In patients without bruits or a history of carotid artery disease, unilateral carotid sinus massage may terminate the rhythm. Should these maneuvers fail, pharmacologic options include adenosine, calcium channel blockers, esmolol, and other β-blockers. Adenosine is usually the first drug of choice for a regular SVT because of its short duration of action (6 to 10 seconds), relative cardiovascular stability, and ability to slow AV nodal conduction. Adenosine takes advantage of the difference in resting action potentials between atrial and ventricular cardiac tissue (-90 mV) and nodal conducting tissue (-70 mV). Adenosine preferentially hyperpolarizes nodal tissue as potassium channels open, rendering this tissue refractory to electrical conduction. The rhythm either is terminated or is slowed sufficiently that P-wave morphology becomes evident and aids in diagnosis. Adenosine is ineffective for terminating irregular tachycardias such as atrial fibrillation, the electrical origin of which is in atrial, not conducting, tissue. When adenosine is administered by way of a peripheral vein, 6 mg is given, followed by a saline push. A second dose of 12 mg may be administered in 1 to 2 minutes if the initial dose was insufficient to achieve sustained rhythm slowing. If given through central venous access, a 50% dose reduction is suggested.

What are the side effects and risks of pharmacologic treatment? Possible negative effects of adenosine include inducing hypotension, atrial fibrillation, and concerning bradyarrhythmias. Adenosine can initiate polymorphic and monomorphic ventricular tachycardia (i.e., it is proarrhythmic) and produce transient asystole, especially in patients receiving calcium channel blockers or β-blockers. Ventricular arrhythmias may result if adenosine is given to patients with WPW syndrome and atrial fibrillation because AV conduction may be accelerated, putting the patient at risk for ventricular fibrillation. Adenosine also may produce bronchospasm, particularly in patients with a history of reactive airway disease. Despite the short half-life of adenosine, patients with reactive airway disease have required endotracheal intubation after severe bronchospasm. Facial flushing, dyspnea, and chest discomfort are common and transient events.

When the QRS complex is narrow and adenosine fails to terminate the rapid rhythm, verapamil may be considered for patients with satisfactory left ventricular function. The dose is 2.5 to 5.0 mg administered intravenously over 1 to 2 minutes. A second dose of 5 to 10 mg may be given intravenously in 15 minutes if needed. Hypotension and excessive bradycardias are a risk, especially when the patient has taken or been administered other cardiodepressant medications. Calcium channel antagonists also prolong the AV nodal refractory period. Verapamil should not be administered in the setting of a wide QRS tachycardia because if the rhythm is of ventricular origin, cardiovascular collapse or ventricular fibrillation may result. In most wide QRS tachycardias, calcium channel antagonists or β-blockers are best avoided.

The Present Patient

As the patient was not in hemodynamic distress, aggressive coughing and Valsalva maneuvers were tried initially but without success. The next approach was pharmacologic treatment with rapid IV administration of adenosine, 6 mg, then 12 mg. Her heart rate slowed, revealing underlying P waves and 1 to 2-mm ST depression in the inferior and lateral leads. She was administered oxygen by mask and transfused with packed RBCs to a hematocrit of 30%. Additionally she was given potassium to correct to normal serum levels. With this treatment, the ST depression on the ECG normalized, and follow-up troponin levels were negative for myocardial injury. Her further postoperative course was uneventful, and she was discharged home 4 days later.

Clinical Pearls

1. SVT is a common perioperative complication that requires prompt evaluation and appropriate treatment. Causes of SVT include electrolyte abnormalities, acidosis, hypoxemia, myocardial ischemia, hypotension, light anesthesia, congestive heart failure, pulmonary embolus, and elevated catecholamine levels.

2. The underlying rhythm may be difficult to ascertain in the setting of extremely fast rates. A 12-lead ECG or multichannel rhythm strips often are necessary to make the diagnosis. If the patient is unstable, synchronized cardioversion should not be delayed awaiting the 12-lead ECG.

3. Adenosine is first-line therapy for treatment of narrow-complex stable SVT. An important feature rendering this medication safe for administration is its short duration of action. It should not be administered to patients with WPW syndrome and atrial fibrillation because it may accelerate AV conduction and put the patient at risk for ventricular fibrillation. By slowing the rate in narrow-complex tachycardias, adenosine may be valuable in diagnosing the underlying rhythm.

4. Although the short half-life of adenosine makes it an attractive medication to use, the potential to induce life-threatening bronchospasm in patients with reactive airway disease should be recognized. In addition, profound, transient bradycardia is common.

5. Calcium channel blockers are second-line therapy for patients with stable narrow-complex SVT.

6. The diagnosis of the underlying rhythm of a wide QRS tachycardia is difficult, and treatment is potentially perilous. It is prudent to consider a wide-complex rhythm ventricular in origin, rather than attribute it to SVT with aberrancy. Approximately 90% of wide QRS tachycardias are ventricular tachycardias when the patient has structural heart disease. Treating a wide QRS tachycardia with verapamil may result in cardiovascular collapse.

REFERENCES

1. White RD: Supraventricular tachyarrhythmias. In Faust R (ed): Anesthesiology Review, 3rd ed. New York, Churchill Livingstone, 2002.
2. Atlee JL: Perioperative cardiac dysrhythmias. Anesthesiology 86:1397–1424, 1997.
3. Balser JR, Martinez EA, Winters BD, et al: Beta-adrenergic blockade accelerates conversion of postoperative supraventricular tachyarrhythmias. Anesthesiology 89:1052–1059, 1998.
4. Mathew J, Hunsberger S, Fleg J, et al: Incidence, predictive factors, and prognostic significance of supraventricular tachyarrhythmias in congestive heart failure. Chest 118:914–922, 2000.
5. Tan HL, Spechorst HH, Peters RJ, et al: Induced ventricular arrhythmias with adenosine. Pacing Clin Electrophysiol 24:450–455, 2001.

Rita Agarwal, MD

PATIENT 24

A 4-week-old infant with bloody stools and hemodynamic instability

A 4-week-old boy, born at 26 weeks' gestation, presents with abdominal distention and bloody stools and is scheduled for exploratory laparotomy. The infant's hospital course had been complicated by respiratory distress syndrome requiring intubation for 2 weeks. He had been started on strength feeds approximately 1 week before this event. He had had one episode of sepsis 2 days before this event. His symptoms seemed to be improving before the development of the abdominal distention. The infant was placed on dopamine, 5 μg/kg/min to maintain perfusion pressure; 15 mL of 5% albumin, 25 mL of packed RBCs, and 25 mL of normal saline had been administered in the past 4 hours.

Physical Examination: Temperature 35.6° C, heart rate 170, blood pressure 65/30, weight 1,100 g. General appearance: acutely ill appearing infant. The infant was mechanically ventilated with the following settings: respirations 35, PIP 28, PEEP 8, FIO$_2$ 100%. Abdomen: tense, distended. Skin: mottled. Cardiac: heart sounds regular with a 1–2/6 systolic murmur.

Laboratory Findings: ABG: pH 7.29, CO$_2$ 50 mmHg, PO$_2$ 65 mmHg, oxygen saturation 86%, base deficit 6.8. Potassium 5.9 mEq/L. Hct 26%. Prothrombin time 17 seconds, partial thromboplastin time 42 seconds. These represented remarkable deterioration from laboratory values of earlier that day. Abdominal radiograph: pneumatosis intestinalis and free air.

Questions: What is the likely cause of the infant's clinical presentation?
Describe the risk factors for this illness.
Describe differences in neonatal and adult physiology?
What other problems can premature infants experience?
What are the principal intraoperative concerns?

What is the likely cause of the infant's clinical presentation?   Necrotizing enterocolitis (NEC).

Describe the risk factors for this illness. NEC is a life-threatening condition usually seen in premature infants, although occasionally full-term infants may be affected. Its cause is not fully understood, but it seems to be caused by bowel ischemia resulting from decreased mesenteric blood flow. Sepsis, congenital heart disease, arrhythmias, hypotension, hypoxemia, fetal asphyxia, heart failure, bacterial infection, intestinal infection, and feeding with hyperosmolar formula are among the predisposing factors leading to NEC. Patients present with abdominal distention, bloody stools, and bilious vomiting. Worsening pulmonary function, hypoxia, hypercarbia, acidosis, hypothermia, electrolyte imbalance (particularly hyperkalemia), hypotension, and shock ensue. Coagulopathy, thrombocytopenia, and anemia are common. These infants usually are moribund, are toxic in appearance, and are among the most challenging patients to treat. Exploratory laparotomy is required in patients in whom there is evidence of bowel perforation or necrosis.

Describe differences in neonatal and adult physiology. Adult and neonatal physiology differ remarkably. Neonates have a higher incidence of airway obstruction and greater tendency to desaturate on induction of anesthesia. A faster respiratory rate, higher alveolar ventilation-to-functional residual capacity ratio, and increased oxygen consumption quickly lead to hypoxia. Oxygen consumption may be >6 mL/kg/min (twice that of adults). Cardiac output depends on heart rate and ventricular diastolic filling. Myocardial performance is near maximum, and augmentation of myocardial contractility is limited, and decreases in intravascular volume are poorly tolerated. Parasympathetic innervation to the heart is fully developed at birth, whereas the sympathetic supply continues developing for 6 weeks. Neonates are susceptible to bradycardia without a subsequent increase in contractility. Neonates may have a patent ductus arteriosus or foramen ovale; left-to-right shunt may persist, and right-to-left shunt may develop in the presence of elevated pulmonary vascular resistance. The presence of a possible shunt can increase the patient's risk for paradoxical air embolus and increase myocardial work, predisposing the infant to pulmonary vascular hypertension and making him or her more susceptible to desaturation. Fetal hemoglobin is not as efficient at unloading oxygen at the tissues as hemoglobin A (i.e., a left-shifted oxyhemoglobin dissociation curve). Newborns have small nephrons, decreased glomerular filtration rate, and limited concentrating ability. Because they are obligate sodium excretors, they cannot compensate for acute or chronic volume changes as well as older infants and children can. Neonates have limited ability for gluconeogenesis, so exogenous glucose should be provided, especially under stressful conditions. Premature and full-term infants have limited abilities for thermogenesis. They have a large surface area relative to their weight, thin skin, and few fat stores. They are unable to maintain temperature by shivering and resort to metabolism of brown fat (nonshivering thermogenesis).

What other problems can premature infants experience?   Premature infants have many other associated problems that must be taken into consideration when preparing to administer anesthesia (see Table).

What are the principal intraoperative concerns?   To determine abnormalities requiring intraoperative management, the clinician should review ABGs, electrolytes, and hematology and coagulation profiles. These values can change rapidly, and frequent review is necessary. Volume status should be optimized as much as possible by administering fluid and blood based on body weight. Fluid boluses (either 5% albumin or normal saline) are administered in 10-mL/kg increments. Packed RBCs, 10 mL/kg, should increase the hematocrit by approximately 3% to 6% if there is no ongoing blood loss. Fresh frozen plasma and platelets also are administered in 10-mL/kg increments. A decreasing heart rate and increasing blood pressure are helpful guides to adequate volume replacement. An attempt should be made to start correcting any laboratory abnormalities. Normothermia must be ensured aggressively, and a warm room, warming lights, forced air warming blanket, warm fluids, warm preparation solutions, and humidifiers can help minimize hypothermia. Adequate IV access is mandatory; central catheters lines or surgical cutdown may be required. Arterial pressure monitoring is useful; cutdowns may be required.

If the patient is not intubated, a rapid-sequence induction and endotracheal intubation should be performed expeditiously and carefully. Awake intubation should be considered in unstable patients. Anesthetic maintenance usually consists of opioids, muscle relaxants, and low doses of inhalation agent as tolerated. Ventilation can be problematic because these infants often require high respiratory rates, high peak inspiratory pressures, and careful management of tidal volume.

Problem	Cause and Significance
Respiratory distress syndrome	Surfactant deficiency causes alveolar collapse, hypercarbia, hypoxia, pneumothorax, pneumomediastinum, pulmonary interstitial emphysema
Bronchopulmonary distress	Chronic obstructive lung disease accompanied by interstitial fibrosis, cysts, impaired ventilation and oxygenation, and reactive airways
Apnea and bradycardia	Absence of breathing for 15–30 seconds; bradycardia may occur quickly after apnea and worsen hypoxia
Patent ductus arteriosus	Increasing incidence with greater degrees of prematurity. Left to right shunt can lead to fluid overload, congestive heart failure, and respiratory distress
Intraventricular hemorrhage	Posthemorrhagic hydrocephalus or periventricular leukomalacia is a significant source of neurologic dysfunction and disability
Retinopathy of prematurity	Proliferation of retinal blood vessels occurs in the presence of high concentrations of oxygen. Decreased visual acuity and blindness may result
Necrotizing enterocolitis	Ischemic injury to bowel, bowel necrosis, perforation, and postinflammatory strictures can occur

The infant's intensive care unit ventilator may be superior to anesthesia ventilators. Intermittent Ambu-bag ventilation may improve oxygen saturation. Aggressive fluid therapy with crystalloid, colloids, and blood should continue; insensible fluid loss resulting from gut exposure should figure into estimation of fluid needs. These infants have massive third-space losses and bleeding. Fluid requirements of 100 to 200 mL/kg are common. The use of inotropes for hemodynamic support is common. Hyperkalemia is common because of blood transfusion and bowel necrosis. Hypocalcemia may occur secondary to transfusion. Metabolic acidosis and hypercarbia are common and refractory to treatment. Postoperatively patients should be returned to the neonatal intensive care unit, intubated, ventilated, and provided with ongoing cardiovascular support.

These infants may need to return at a later date for further surgical interventions (stricture, closure of enterostomies).

The Present Patient

A central catheter was placed in the present patient in the operating room for additional IV access. An exploratory laparotomy revealed several large areas of bowel necrosis. These were resected, and enterostomies were performed. The patient was hemodynamically unstable throughout the procedure and required packed RBCs, plasma, and platelet transfusions. Dopamine was increased to $10 \mu g/kg/min$ to maintain a systolic blood pressure >60 mmHg. Bicarbonate, 2 mEq/kg, was administered intravenously. Calcium gluconate, 20 mg/kg, was given intravenously in response to hyperkalemia.

Clinical Pearls

1. Patients with NEC are severely ill. Maintaining oxygenation and ventilation can be challenging. The practitioner should be prepared to use a ventilator other than the standard anesthesia machine ventilators.

2. Adequate IV access is mandatory and often difficult to achieve. The surgeons may have to be recruited to help by establishing central venous access or cutting down on appropriate vessels.

3. Metabolic derangements and coagulopathies are common and require aggressive therapy. Frequent laboratory analysis is required because metabolic deterioration may be precipitous.

4. Volume resuscitation is ongoing and massive. Volume requirements of 100 to 200 mL/kg/h may be necessary.

5. Hypothermia should be avoided aggressively with use of high ambient temperatures, warming lights, fluid, circuit, and forced-air warming,

6. Inotropic support is uncommon but is not a substitute for volume resuscitation.

REFERENCES

1. Gregory GA: Anesthesia for premature infants. In: Gregory G (ed): The Practice of Anesthesia for Infants and Children, 3rd ed. New York, Churchill Livingstone, 1994, pp 351–374.
2. Newborn physiology and development. In: Bell C, Kain ZN (eds): The Pediatric Anesthesia Handbook. Mosby, St. Louis, 1997, pp 401–414.
3. Holland RM, Bensard DB: Neonatal surgery. In: Merentstein GB, Gardner SL (eds): Handbook of Neonatal Intensive Care, 4th ed. St. Louis, Mosby, 1998, pp 625–646.
4. Agarwal R: Neonatal anesthesia. In: Duke J (ed): Anesthesia Secrets, 2nd ed. Philadelphia, Hanley & Belfus, 2000, pp 299–304 .

Howard J. Miller, MD

PATIENT 25

A 28-year-old paraplegic man with hypertension and bradycardia during cystoscopy

A 28-year-old paraplegic man underwent cystoscopy for hematuria. He had complete sensory and motor loss below the level of T6, secondary to a motor vehicle accident 2 years prior. The accident resulted in complete spinal cord transection at the level of T6. He was otherwise healthy and had no known drug allergies. Immediately after his accident, he underwent thoracic spine fusion, under general anesthesia, without complication. Other surgeries included two cystoscopies, under local anesthesia with monitored anesthesia care (MAC), without incident. The current cystoscopy is performed under local anesthesia and MAC. He receives 2 mg of midazolam for sedation and oxygen per nasal cannula. Thirty minutes into the procedure, the patient's blood pressure is 220/110 mmHg with a heart rate of 49 beats/min.

Physical Examination (preoperative):   Heart rate 67, blood pressure 118/62.

Questions   What is the diagnosis?
Who is at risk?
Describe the pathophysiology.
What could have been done to prevent the extremes in his vital signs?

What is the diagnosis? Autonomic hyperreflexia (AH).

Who is at risk? AH is observed in patients with a history of spinal cord injury. The response can occur 1 to 3 weeks postinjury or after resolution of spinal shock and return of spinal cord reflexes, but is noted more frequently as the patient develops sequelae of the spinal cord injury. Distention of a hollow viscus (rectum or bladder), management of urologic disease associated with chronic spinal cord injury (e.g., lithotripsy, cystoscopy, or percutaneous stone removal), and treatment of decubitus ulcers all have been described as triggering episodes of AH. Approximately 65% to 85% of patients with transections at or above T7 have an AH episode in response to cutaneous or visceral stimulation below the level of the lesion. The stimulus can result from daily activities but more commonly occurs during surgical stimulation. Patients with transections below T10 rarely have AH.

Describe the pathophysiology. Pathologically, a stimulus below the level of the spinal cord injury sends afferent impulses to the spinal cord that are not inhibited by higher central nervous system influences. This stimulus results in massive unopposed reflex sympathetic discharge, manifested as severe vasoconstriction and hypertension. The aortic arch and carotid sinus receptors respond reflexively to the elevation in blood pressure with increased parasympathetic and decreased sympathetic outflow. The area of the body below the transection remains neurologically isolated, however, and does not have the influence of higher centers. Vasodilation above and vasoconstriction below the level of transection occur, along with a reflex bradycardia.

Associated symptoms include nasal stuffiness, headache, visual changes, nausea, confusion, and difficulty breathing. Sudden and sustained hypertension may lead to seizures, intracerebral bleeding, and subarachnoid hemorrhage. Cardiopulmonary complications include left and right ventricular failure, pulmonary edema, myocardial ischemia, and dysrhythmias.

What could have been done to prevent extremes in the patient's vital signs? Despite an apparent absence of sensation below the level of spinal cord injury, AH is an autonomic response independent of the patient's ability to perceive pain, and such patients require anesthesia while undergoing surgical and diagnostic procedures. Topical anesthesia unreliably prevents AH, but general and regional anesthetics have been proved to prevent AH. For perineal or bladder surgery, spinal anesthesia is more reliable than epidural anesthesia because sacral roots are more completely blocked.

Immediate treatment of AH, once suspected, is critical. The surgeon should be asked to stop operating immediately and desist from any potential stimulating event. Deepening the plane of general anesthesia or raising the level of an epidural may be beneficial. An added-advantage of epidural catheters is they can be used to prevent postoperative AH episodes. Pharmacologic intervention includes vasodilators, calcium channel blockers, and ganglionic blocking agents. The vasodilator sodium nitroprusside is most useful because it is easily titrated, but an arterial catheter should be placed to monitor blood pressure continuously. α-Adrenergic blocking drugs are not useful because they block the effect of circulating norepinephrine rather than blocking norepinephrine that is released at neuronal junctions.

The Present Patient

In the present patient, the stimulus of the cystoscopy and a distended bladder resulted in an episode of AH. The surgeon immediately halted the procedure and emptied the bladder. An infusion of sodium nitroprusside was begun, and an arterial catheter was placed. The sodium nitroprusside was titrated until the patient's blood pressure normalized. The patient was transported to the postanesthesia care unit, where he remained for several hours until the sodium nitroprusside infusion could be discontinued safely. The patient returned to the operating room 2 days later and underwent an uneventful cystoscopy under general anesthesia.

Clinical Pearls

1. Patients with spinal cord transections at or above the level of T7 are at high risk for AH. An anesthetic plan that reasonably would be expected to prevent such an event should be instituted. Sedation with topical anesthesia most likely will prove insufficient and, owing to the significant morbidity associated with an AH episode, should be discouraged. Patients with spinal cord transections below the level of T10 have a small risk of AH.

2. If general anesthesia is selected or a change in anesthetic plan is indicated requiring endotracheal intubation, succinylcholine should be avoided because of concerns for massive hyperkalemic response in paraplegics.

3. An arterial catheter and medications to treat severe hypertension should be made readily available before any procedure performed on a patient at risk for AH.

4. AH may occur postoperatively; close monitoring should continue for a reasonable postprocedural period.

REFERENCES

1. Lambert DH, Deane RS, Mazuzan Jr JE: Anesthesia and the control of blood pressure in patients with spinal cord injury. Anesth Analg 61:344–348, 1982.
2. Diseases of the central nervous system. In Stoelting RK, Dierdorf SF, McCammon L (eds): Anesthesia and Coexisting Disease, 2nd ed. New York, Churchill Livingstone, 1988, pp 325–329.
3. Amzallag M: Autonomic hyperreflexia. Int Anesthesiol Clin 31:87–102, 1993.
4. Bishop ML: Autonomic hyperreflexia. In Faust RJ, Cucchiara RF, Rose SH, et al (eds): Anesthesiology Review, 2nd ed. New York, Churchill Livingstone, 1994, pp 407–408.
5. Hambly PR: Anaesthesia for chronic spinal cord lesions. Anaesthesia 53:273–289, 1998.
6. Murphy DB, McGuire G, Peng P: Treatment of autonomic hyperreflexia in a quadriplegic patient by epidural anesthesia in the postoperative period. Anesth Analg 89:148–150, 1999.

Sunil Kumar, M.D.

PATIENT 26

A 45-year-old morbidly obese man with precipitous
hemodynamic collapse during endotracheal tube change

A 45-year-old morbidly obese man is being treated in the intensive care unit for respiratory failure. The anesthesiologist is requested to change the endotracheal tube (ETT) because of a cuff leak. Anticipating a potentially difficult airway, the anesthesiologist decides to use a Cook airway exchange catheter (AEC). A medium-size AEC is inserted into the 7-mm I.D. ETT until resistance is felt, which is interpreted as carina. In preparation for removal of the indwelling ETT, jet ventilation with 50 lb/in.^{2} (psi) oxygen source is initiated through the exchange catheter. After 4 to 5 jet ventilation breaths, just as the ETT is about to be withdrawn, there is a precipitous decrease in blood pressure associated with oxygen desaturation. Crepitance is detected over the patient's neck and face.

Questions: What is the diagnosis?

Explain the precipitous decline in the patient's hemodynamic status.

What steps can be taken to minimize the risk of barotrauma while using an ETT exchanger?

What is the diagnosis? Pneumothorax with subcutaneous emphysema secondary to barotrauma.

What steps can be taken to minimize the risk of barotrauma while using an ETT exchanger? Changing an ETT in a patient with a known or potentially difficult airway can be a hazardous procedure. AECs can be used to increase the safety of changing ETTs. An AEC is a long, small, hollow, semirigid catheter that is inserted through an *in situ* ETT before extubation. After the indwelling ETT is withdrawn over the AEC, it serves as a stylet for the new ETT and can provide a conduit to administer oxygen until the new tracheal tube is placed successfully. Although the concept of the AEC is simple, jet ventilation through these catheters has the potential to cause life-threatening complications unless some simple principles and clinical details are followed.

Placing an inappropriately sized stylet through the ETT can significantly reduce the annular air space available for passive exhalation. When air entry exceeds air egress, inevitable consequences are lung hyperinflation, tension pneumothorax, pneumomediastinum, and subcutaneous emphysema. Air entry should be limited by reducing the jet ventilator driving pressure to 25 psi, by using an inline pressure regulator, and by limiting the inspiratory time to <1 second. For even the smallest AECs, a 1-second inspiratory time at 25 psi provides sufficient ventilatory support for most clinical situations. Having an in-line regulator in the jet ventilator allows for adjustment of tidal volume when deemed necessary.

Exhalation is a passive process and depends on an airway of sufficient lumen and expiratory time of sufficient duration. If the equivalent annular air exit space that surrounds the AEC is less than a 4-mm I.D. ETT, ventilation is not possible because exhalation time is prolonged markedly. The Figure shows that there are only a limited number of ETT-AEC combinations in which the annular air space exceeds this minimal acceptable limit.

FUNCTIONAL SIZE EQUIVALENT > 4mm ID TUBE AND CLINICAL RECOMMENDATION FOR ETT/AEC STYLET COMBINATIONS

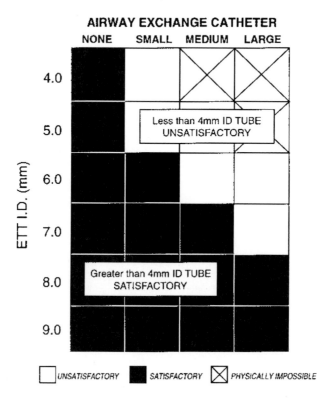

Recommendations for ETT-AEC combinations for functional size equivalent of annular space around the AEC when its inner diameter is > 4 mm. (Modified from Benumof,[5] with permission. Copyright © 1999 American Society of Anesthesiologists. All rigts reserved.)

106

When the ETT-AEC combination results in unacceptably small annular air space, as was the situation in the present case, the jet ventilation should not be used through the AEC. When ventilating a patient through an AEC that is placed inside the trachea alone (rather than inside an ETT), the natural airway must be kept maximally patent with jaw thrust and oropharyngeal or nasopharyngeal airways. An AEC that is inserted too deep can be especially dangerous; not only does increasing the depth of insertion increase the risk of perforation of the tracheobronchial tree, but also it progressively decreases annular air space surrounding the catheter. The depth of AEC insertion should never exceed 26 cm in an adult, and it should never be inserted when resistance is encountered.

Another risk with the use of an AEC is failure to pass the new ETT over the AEC. This risk can be minimized if a laryngoscope is used with the AEC whenever possible. Optimal laryngoscopy helps to clear the supraglottic pathway and may allow the anesthesiologist to see where resistance is being encountered. The risk that an ETT will fail to pass the laryngeal inlet is minimized when a relatively small ETT and a relatively large AEC are used.

The Present Patient

Auscultation of the chest revealed decreased breath sounds on the predominant side of subcutaneous emphysema. On inserting a 16G angiocatheter, a rush of air was detected. Improvements in oxygenation and hemodynamics soon followed. A tube thoracostomy was performed, a large ETT was placed with use of an AEC, and, after a course of respiratory failure the patient improved.

Clinical Pearls

1. An AEC must be selected that is proportional to the size of the ETT such that the annular air space is sufficient to allow passive expiration.

2. AEC insertion should never exceed 26 cm in an adult, and the AEC should never be advanced when resistance is encountered.

3. Consideration should be given to providing a low flow of oxygen (1 to 2 L/min) via the lumen of the AEC. This may provide adequate apneic oxygenation.

4. Whenever jet ventilation is used, the risk of barotrauma is minimized by limiting the jet ventilator driving pressure to ≤25 psi, limiting the inspiratory time <1 second, and allowing sufficient time for expiration.

5. Chest movements should be monitored closely, and jet ventilation should be discontinued the moment incomplete chest deflation is recognized. In most cases, rapid rates of jetting are unnecessary. One or two jet pulses per 30 to 60 seconds may be all that is necessary.

6. Precipitous declines in blood pressure or oxygen saturation may be due to tension pneumothorax and require emergent decompression by needle, then tube thoracostomy.

REFERENCES

1. Dworkin R, Benumof JL, Benumof R, Karagianes TG: The effective tracheal diameter that causes air trapping during jet ventilation. J Cardiothorac Vasc Anesth 4:731–736, 1990.
2. Gaughan SD, Benumof JL, Ozaki GT: Quantification of the jet function of a jet stylet. Anesth Analg 74:580–585, 1992.
3. Takata M, Benumof JL, Ozaki GT: Confirmation of endotracheal intubation over a jet stylet: In vitro studies. Anesth Analg 80:800–805, 1995.
4. Baraka AS: Tension pneumothorax complicating jet ventilation via a Cook airway exchange catheter. Anesthesiology 91:557–558, 1999.
5. Benumof JL: Airway exchange catheters, simple concept, potentially great danger. Anesthesiology 91:342–344, 1999.

Kenneth Swank, M.D.

PATIENT 27

A 44-year-old woman with dyspnea on recumbency

A previously healthy 44-year-old woman with mild asthma presents with progressively increasing dyspnea, pleuritic chest pain, dry cough, and chest pressure of 1 month's duration. She received empirical treatment for pneumonia 3 weeks prior, which was of no benefit. Her symptoms are not relieved by inhaled β_2-agonists. She reports increasing fatigue and a diminished exercise capacity over the last week but still is able to climb one flight of stairs without resting. Her dyspnea is worse when lying supine or on her left side, and she now sleeps semirecumbent on stacked pillows.

Physical Examination: Heart rate 97, respirations 18, blood pressure 136/85, SaO_2 on 2 L nasal cannula 93%. General appearance: A 75-kg woman in no distress and breathing comfortably while in a sitting position. She refused to position herself supine because of respiratory distress in that position. Chest auscultation: unremarkable except for mildly decreased breath sounds over the lung bases bilaterally. Head, neck, and airway examinations all normal. No upper body venous distention present.

Laboratory Findings: CBC, electrolytes, BUN, creatinine, liver functions all normal. ECG: normal. Chest CT: see Figure. Subsequent CT-guided needle biopsy nondiagnostic. Open biopsy required.

Questions: What is the diagnosis?
Describe the anatomy of the mediastinum.
What are common pathologies involving the mediastinum?
What are the pathophysiologic consequences of mediastinal masses?
Describe the preoperative evaluation of patients presenting with mediastinal masses.
Should symptomatic patients receive therapy to shrink the tumor mass before any surgical procedure?
Describe the anesthetic management of patients with a mediastinal mass.

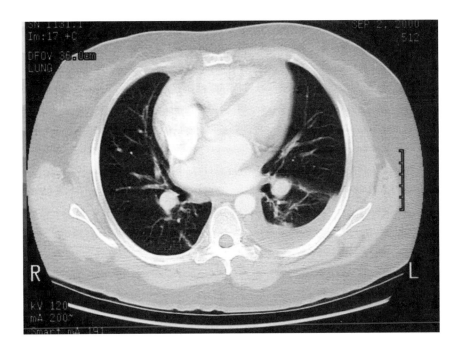

What is the diagnoses? Anterior mediastinal mass.

Describe the anatomy of the mediastinum. The mediastinum lies in the thorax between the left and right pleura, extending superiorly from the thoracic inlet to the diaphragm inferiorly and from the sternum anteriorly to the vertebral bodies posteriorly. It is divided into superior and inferior regions by an arbitrary plane through the sternal angle and fourth vertebral body. The inferior mediastinum is divided into anterior, middle, and posterior regions by the pericardium. Because the anterior/inferior mediastinum is contiguous with the superior mediastinum, these can be considered as one compartment, the anterosuperior mediastinum. Crucial anatomic structures, including the tracheal bifurcation, aorta, superior vena cava, pulmonary artery and superior surface of the heart lie at the junction of the superior and inferior mediastinum.

What are common pathologies involving the mediastinum? The position of a mass within the mediastinum depends on the tumor type. In adults, anterosuperior masses constitute two thirds of mediastinal masses, with thymomas being the most common. Of these tumors, 50% are malignant, and 50% are associated with myasthenia gravis (although not all tumors associated with myasthenia gravis are malignant). Other causes of anterior mediastinal masses are thyroid tumors, teratomas, and lymphomas. Middle mediastinal masses usually arise from metastatic involvement of the hilar lymph nodes by bronchogenic carcinoma or lymphomas. Nonneoplastic masses include vascular aneurysms and bronchogenic or pericardial cysts. Masses involving the posterior region are usually neurogenic.

What are the pathophysiologic consequences of mediastinal masses? Because of their close proximity to crucial thoracic structures, mediastinal masses of any type, especially anterosuperior masses, can cause dramatic pulmonary or cardiovascular compromise. Greater degrees of compression, especially with rapid expansion of the mass, usually result in severe pathophysiologic syndromes.

Tracheobronchial compression may cause respiratory distress. Common complaints include cough, dyspnea (often when recumbent), chest pain, and recurrent pulmonary infections. The degree of respiratory compromise may increase greatly during anesthetic induction and emergence, even in patients experiencing relatively mild preoperative symptoms. Airway obstruction perioperatively, leading to inability to ventilate, is a po-

tentially catastrophic event. Factors thought to play a role in this phenomenon include a decrease in thoracic volume, muscle relaxation, change from negative-pressure to positive-pressure ventilation, and redistribution of venous blood within the thorax, some or all of which occur during anesthetic induction.

Compression of the superior vena cava, right atrium, right ventricle, and pulmonary artery also may result in symptoms. Compression of the superior vena cava obstructs venous flow from the upper body, leading to venous engorgement and tissue and airway edema, known as **superior vena cava syndrome.** Intubation may be difficult because of significant airway edema. Compression of the right heart or pulmonary outflow tract may produce positional dyspnea, hypoxemia, syncope, and arrhythmias. Vascular compromise can lead to severe hypotension and cardiac arrest during anesthetic induction or sedation. Besides the intrathoracic mass effects associated with mediastinal tumors, particular tumors may have primary pathophysiologic consequences. Thymic hyperplasia or thymomas associated with myasthenia gravis may be associated with profound musculoskeletal weakness resulting from loss of competent neuromuscular junctions. Other mediastinal tumors, such as pheochromocytoma and parathyroid and thyroid adenomas, usually have systemic effects resulting from hormonal secretions.

Discuss the preoperative evaluation of patients presenting with mediastinal masses. Thorough preoperative evaluation is crucial, even in patients with seemingly mild symptoms. Detailed questioning should include a search for respiratory and cardiac symptoms, noting any changes in the degree of symptoms with position. Syncope, especially during Valsalva maneuvers, suggests vascular impairment. Symptoms of associated systemic disorders, such as myasthenia gravis, pheochromocytoma, and parathyroid and thyroid disease, should be determined.

Chest auscultation may reveal asymmetric breath sounds, stridor, and wheezing. Other important physical signs include an engorged, plethoric upper body and cervical lymphadenopathy. These are signs suggesting difficulty with tracheal intubation.

Valuable diagnostic studies include ECG, chest radiograph, sitting and supine pulmonary function tests including flow volume loops, CT or MRI, and echocardiography. Chest CT or MRI is necessary to delineate tumor size, position, and impingement on adjacent structures. Airway compression shown by CT is predictive of perianesthetic airway obstruction. Children with airway compression of 50% are virtually guaranteed to develop significant or total airway obstruction at anesthetic induction.

Airway compression of $\geq 35\%$ produces severe respiratory symptoms in nearly half of patients. Echocardiography provides information on the dynamic character of the mass and may be done with the patient in several positions to characterize cardiovascular competency. Sitting and supine pulmonary function tests quantify the degree of dynamic respiratory compromise and its positional nature and differentiates intrathoracic from extrathoracic obstruction. Spirometry does not characterize the nature or position of the airway obstruction and fails to predict perioperative airway obstruction, however, leading some authorities to question its value in preoperative evaluation of such patients.

Should symptomatic patients receive therapy to shrink the tumor mass before any surgical procedure? The preoperative use of radiation or high-dose steroid therapy in symptomatic patients without a tissue diagnosis is controversial. Although many mediastinal masses shrink dramatically with these therapies, and the incidence of perioperative airway difficulties is much less in patients so treated, these therapies result in cellular changes, making pathologic diagnosis more difficult. For this reason, radiation or steroid therapy rarely is instituted before a firm tissue diagnosis is established. This rationale should be kept in mind for the high-risk, symptomatic patient who absolutely requires general anesthesia for biopsy. Collimated radiotherapy, in which a small area of the mass is excluded from radiotherapy, preserving it for accurate biopsy, is an option in these situations. Discussion between the anesthesiologist, surgeon, oncologist, and pathologist is essential under these circumstances.

Describe the anesthetic management of patients with mediastinal masses. Every patient with a mediastinal mass should be considered a high-risk patient. If the procedure can be accomplished under local anesthesia, it should be done so in all circumstances. If local anesthesics are used, sedation should be minimal if used at all and titrated to effect.

If general anesthesia is necessary, thorough preoperative preparation is essential. Small-diameter and armored endotracheal tubes may be needed for bypassing tracheal obstructions. Microlaryngectomy tubes are useful because they are longer than standard small endotracheal tubes. All materials required for awake fiberoptic intubation should be at hand, including topical anesthetic delivery devices and a flexible fiberoptic bronchoscope. The presence of an individual skilled in rigid bronchoscopy is essential for patients with severe symptoms and and is advised

strongly for patients with lesser degrees of airway obstruction. Attention to proper patient positioning is a must. One or two large-bore intravenous catheters are essential; patients with superior vena cava syndrome should have lower extremity intravenous access. Preinduction intraarterial pressure monitoring should be considered.

In asymptomatic patients with small masses and no positive findings on sitting or supine spirometry, an intravenous anesthetic induction usually can be performed without difficulty. Before muscle relaxation, the ability to ventilate should be verified, and a short-acting muscle relaxant should be used. Even if induction and intubation seem routine, extubation should be undertaken with care because significant airway obstruction may occur even in patients with mild preoperative symptoms. Even patients with minimal preoperative symptoms require thorough preparation and vigilance.

Mildly to moderately symptomatic patients, patients with radiographic or spirometric evidence of airway compression, and patients having significant echocardiographic abnormalities require the airway to be secured before anesthetic induction. Because sedative agents are not advised, topical airway anesthesia should be meticulous, ensuring a comfortable and cooperative patient. During bronchoscopy, the airway should be examined for extent of compression and collapse and intraluminal tumor extension. If bronchoscopy reveals only minimal compression, intubation is followed by a careful inhalation induction while maintaining spontaneous respiration. Sevoflurane is preferred because it is nonirritating to the airways, and its concentration can be lowered quickly. Neuromuscular blockade should be avoided if possible because muscle relaxants may worsen airway obstruction secondary to a decrease in thoracic volume.

Inhalation induction by mask has been used in this group of patients, but this technique cannot be recommended. These patients are already at high risk for developing potentially life-threatening airway compromise without adding the additional risks that generally are associated with mask induction, such as laryngospasm. Awake intubation followed by inhalation induction should be used instead. Mask induction does not allow for a preinduction fiberoptic examination of the airway.

Severely symptomatic patients and patients with markedly abnormal preoperative diagnostic studies who require general anesthesia are at extreme risk for perioperative catastrophic airway obstruction and cardiovascular collapse. Empirical preoperative radiation or steroid therapy should be considered. Intubation should precede anesthetic induction, and muscle relaxants should be avoided. These patients should be prepared for femorofemoral cardiopulmonary bypass before any anesthetic activity. In this way, if severe cardiopulmonary difficulties do occur, the patient may be placed on immediate cardiopulmonary support.

Finally, as previously suggested, patients with mediastinal masses also may experience respiratory obstruction on anesthetic emergence, particularly patients having only diagnostic procedures. About 50% of patients with mediastinal masses experience some difficulty at emergence. Airway edema may be worsened after airway manipulation and intravenous fluid therapy.

The Present Patient

In the present patient, preoperative pulmonary function testing revealed a mildly reduced forced expired volume in 1 second with essentially normal flow volume loops. After a discussion with the surgeons, local anesthesia for open biopsy was deemed impractical, necessitating a general anesthetic. Although spirometry showed no findings, and only slight airway compression was noted on chest CT, the patient had significant symptoms, and an inhalation induction following awake fiberoptic intubation was planned. The patient was brought to the operating room and positioned in semisitting (semi-Fowler's) position. One large-bore intravenous catheter and radial arterial catheter were placed. The patient's airway was topically anesthetized, and fiberoptic bronchoscopy revealed no extrinsic compression. She was intubated over the fiberoptic bronchscope without difficulty, inhalation induction was achieved with sevoflurane, and spontaneous ventilation was continued throughout the procedure with good results. Emergence and extubation were uneventful.

Clinical Pearls

1. Patients with mediastinal masses undergoing general anesthesia are at high risk for potentially catastrophic cardiovascular and respiratory failure because of impingement of the mass on vital intrathoracic structures. In these patients, local anesthesia should be used if possible.

2. Careful preoperative planning is necessary to avoid such complications. Chest CT, pulmonary function tests with flow volume loops, and echocardiography are useful for developing a safe anesthetic plan for these patients. Evidence of any airway compression places the patient at an increased risk for severe respiratory complications on anesthetic induction and emergence.

3. Anesthesia for diagnostic biopsy of mediastinal masses may be troublesome because these patients usually have not received radiation or steroid therapy to shrink their masses. General anesthesia should be administered only when no other options exist.

4. Inhalation induction following awake bronchoscopy and intubation is recommended for moderately or severely affected patients. Paralysis should be avoided.

REFERENCES
1. Mackie AM, Watson CB: Anaesthesia and mediastinal masses. Anaesthesia 39:899–895, 1984.
2. Neuman GC: The anesthetic management of the patient with an anterior mediastinal mass. Anesthesiology 60:144–147, 1984.
3. Pullertis J, Holzmann R: Anaesthesia for patients with mediastinal masses. Can J Anaesth 36:681–688, 1989.
4. Ferrari L, Bedford R: General anesthesia prior to treatment of anterior mediastinal masses in pediatric cancer patients. Anesthesiology 72:991–995, 1990.
5. Goh MH, Liu XY, Goh YS: Anterior mediastinal masses: An anesthetic challenge. Anaesthesia 54:670–682, 1999.
6. Narang S, Harte BH, Body SC: Anesthesia for patients with a mediastinal mass. Anesthesiol Clin North Am 19:559–579, 2001.

Sunil Kumar, MD

PATIENT 28

A 68-year-old man requesting epidural analgesia for surgery

A 68-year-old man is scheduled for left total knee replacement surgery. He had received epidural anesthesia and postoperative epidural analgesia for right knee replacement years ago and had been quite satisfied and is requesting epidural analgesia for this surgery. The patient had been taking ibuprofen preoperatively until the day before surgery. The surgeon wishes to use enoxaparin postoperatively.

Questions: What are the concerns about concurrent use of neuraxial anesthesia and low-molecular-weight heparin?

Can a patient who has been given standard heparin receive neuraxial techniques?

What are the recommendations for neuraxial techniques when warfarin has been given?

How does the perioperative use of antiplatelet drugs influence the decision to use neuraxial anesthesia?

Review the recommendations for using neuraxial techniques when fibrinolytic or thrombolytic drugs have been given.

Should patients receiving multiple classes of anticoagulants simultaneously receive neuraxial techniques?

What are the concerns about concurrent use of neuraxial anesthesia and low-molecular-weight heparin? The use of epidural anesthesia and postoperative epidural analgesia has increased as a result of benefits including decreased postoperative pain, earlier mobilization, and, in some situations, decreased blood loss and incidence of deep venous thrombosis. Use of various anticoagulants to prevent deep venous thrombosis formation in the perioperative period also has increased. Concurrent use of anticoagulant medications and neuraxial techniques presents a challenge for anesthesiologists because of the risk of serious hemorrhagic complications.

Low-molecular-weight heparin (LMWH) has been used increasingly for thromboprophylaxis in perioperative patients. Before its introduction in the United States, LMWH had undergone extensive clinical testing and use in Europe. The European experience over 10 years did not show an increased risk of spinal hematoma in patients undergoing neuraxial anesthesia while receiving LMWH perioperative thromboprophylaxis. In the 5 years after the release of LMWH in the United States, however, >40 cases of spinal hematoma associated with neuraxial anesthesia administered in the presence of perioperative LMWH prophylaxis were reported. Many of these complications occurred when LMWH was given intraoperatively or postoperatively to patients receiving continuous epidural anesthesia. Concomitant antiplatelet therapy was present in several cases. The apparent difference in incidence in Europe compared with the United States may be a result of a difference in dose and dosage schedule. In Europe, the recommended dose of enoxaparin is 40 mg once daily, rather then 30 mg every 12 hours.

Anesthesiologists in the United States can draw on the European experience when developing their own practice guidelines for management of patients undergoing neuraxial blocks while receiving perioperative LMWH. Patients receiving preoperative LMWH can be assumed to have altered coagulation. Concomitant use of other drugs with potential to affect hemostasis, such as antiplatelet drugs, standard heparin, or dextran, should be avoided. A single-dose spinal anesthetic may be the safest neuraxial technique in patients receiving preoperative LMWH. The spinal anesthetic should be delayed until at least 10 to 12 hours after the last LMWH dose. Patients receiving larger thromboprophylactic doses of LMWH (e.g., enoxaparin, 1 mg/kg twice daily) require delays of at least 24 hours, however, before neuraxial anesthesia is contemplated. Neuraxial techniques should be avoided in patients given a dose of LMWH 2 hours preoperatively because needle placement would occur during peak anticoagulant activity. The presence of blood during needle and catheter placement does not necessitate postponing surgery. Initiation of LMWH therapy should be delayed, however, until 24 hours postoperatively. Traumatic needle or catheter placement may signify an increased risk of spinal hematoma when LMWH is administered, and a discussion with the surgeon is recommended regarding appropriate anticoagulant choices, timing of administration, and patient monitoring plans.

Patients with LMWH thromboprophylaxis initiated postoperatively may undergo safely single-dose and continuous catheter neuraxial anesthetic techniques. Epidural catheters usually should be removed before the first dose of LMWH, which should be administered no earlier than 24 hours postoperatively and only in the presence of adequate hemostasis. The decision to use LMWH thromboprophylaxis in the presence of an indwelling catheter must be made with caution. Vigilance regarding the patient's neurologic status is warranted. The timing of catheter removal is important. Catheter removal should be delayed for at least 10 to 12 hours after a dose of LMWH. Subsequent dosing should not occur for at least 2 hours after catheter removal.

Can a patient who has been given standard heparin receive neuraxial techniques? Low-dose standard (unfractionated) heparin is used frequently for deep venous thrombosis prophylaxis in general, orthopedic, and urologic surgical patients. Therapeutic and full anticoagulant doses of standard heparin are used intraoperatively and perioperatively in vascular and cardiac surgical patients. Planning neuraxial anesthetic techniques demands that the practitioner have a knowledge of the surgeon's operative plans.

The administration of subcutaneous heparin (minidose, 5000 units) is not a contraindication to neuraxial techniques. The risk of neuraxial bleeding may be reduced by delaying heparin injection until after the block. This risk may be increased in debilitated patients or after prolonged therapy. Combining neuraxial techniques with intraoperative heparin anticoagulation during vascular surgery has been practiced with good results, but with the following cautions:

- Neuraxial anesthesia should be avoided in patients with other coagulopathies.
- Concurrent use of drugs that affect other components of the coagulation mechanism may increase the risk of hemorrhagic complications.
- Heparin administration should be delayed for 1 hour after needle placement.
- The catheter removal should be timed to occur

1 hour before or 2 to 4 hours after heparin administration.

- The neurologic status of patients should be monitored closely and frequently (every 2 to 4 hours). To facilitate neurologic monitoring, epidural analgesic infusion solution should contain minimal or no local anesthetic.
- Although the occurrence of a bloody or difficult neuraxial needle placement may increase risk, there are no data to support mandatory cancellation of a case. Clinical judgment is needed. If a decision is made to proceed, full discussion with the surgeon and careful postoperative monitoring are warranted.

Currently, there are insufficient data and experience to determine whether the risk of neuraxial hematoma is increased when combining neuraxial techniques with the full anticoagulation of cardiac surgery. Prolonged therapeutic anticoagulation seems to increase risk of spinal hematoma formation, especially if combined with other anticoagulants or thrombolytics. Neuraxial blocks should be avoided in this clinical setting. If systemic anticoagulation therapy is begun with an epidural catheter in place, it is recommended to delay catheter removal for 2 to 4 hours after discontinuation of heparin therapy and evaluation of coagulation status.

What are the recommendations for neuraxial techniques when warfarin has been given? Anesthetic management of patients on warfarin therapy depends on dosage and timing of initiation of therapy. Patients on long-term oral anticoagulation require 3 to 5 days for normalization of their prothrombin time and international normalized ratio (INR) after discontinuation of the anticoagulant therapy. INR <1.5 should be documented before initiation of neuraxial anesthesia. Some surgeons use warfarin therapy for perioperative thromboprophylaxis, typically administering the initial dose of warfarin preoperatively. Initial studies evaluating the safety of epidural analgesia in association with oral anticoagulation used low-dose warfarin, with daily doses approximating 5 mg. If the initial dose was given >24 hours earlier, the prothrombin time and INR should be checked before starting a neuraxial procedure. Patients receiving low-dose warfarin therapy during postoperative epidural analgesia should have their prothrombin time and INR monitored on a daily basis and checked before catheter removal. Higher doses of warfarin may require more intensive monitoring of the coagulation status. An INR >3 should prompt the physician to withhold or reduce the warfarin dose. Clinical judgment must be exercised when considering removing catheters in patients experiencing excessive warfarin effects.

How does the perioperative use of antiplatelet drugs influence the decision to use neuraxial anesthesia? Antiplatelet drugs, such as aspirin and other nonsteroidal antiinflammatory drugs, by themselves seem to represent no added significant risk for the development of spinal hematoma in patients having neuraxial anesthesia. The concurrent use of other medications affecting clotting mechanisms, such as oral anticoagulants, standard heparin, and LMWH, may increase the risk of bleeding complications in these patients. There is no wholly accepted test, including the bleeding test, that guide antiplatelets therapy. Careful preoperative assessment of the patient to identify alterations of health that might contribute to bleeding is crucial.

Ticlopidine and clopidogrel are newer antiplatelet drugs. These agents interfere with platelet membrane function by inhibiting adenosine diphosphate (ADP)–induced platelet-fibrinogen binding and subsequent platelet-platelet interaction. There are not enough data to assess the safety of combining this therapy with neuraxial techniques or to recommend the systematic cessation of these agents before performing the block. Until further information becomes available, a cautious benefit/risk evaluation is warranted, and careful and prolonged follow-up of patients should be considered.

Review the recommendations for using neuraxial techniques when fibrinolytic or thrombolytic drugs have been given. Although based on limited case reports and extrapolation of data from patients receiving thrombolytic drugs and heparin for coronary thrombosis, such patients can be presumed to be at high risk of adverse neuraxial bleeding during spinal or epidural anesthesia. It should be clear from patient history whether these medications have been been administered recently, but it also must be considered whether these patients might receive lytic medications postoperatively and for many days to come. Inferring from the guidelines and contraindications for use of thrombolytic drugs (recommending avoidance of these drugs within 10 days of puncture of noncompressible vessels), neuraxial techniques may be contraindicated. There are no data to offer a recommendation as to the length of time neuraxial puncture should be avoided after discontinuing lytic therapy. Likewise, if epidural catheters were placed previously, there are no data to guide time of removal, although measurement of fibrinogen may be useful.

Should patients receiving multiple classes of anticoagulants simultaneously receive neuraxial techniques? Simultaneous use of more than one class of anticoagulants puts the patient at increased risk of hemorrhagic complications and may do so without influencing commonly used coagulation tests. Medications that may interact in this way include aspirin and other nonsteroidal antiinflammatory drugs, other antiplatelet drugs, dextrans, warfarin compounds, LMWH, and standard heparin. Education of the entire patient care team is necessary to avoid potentiation of the anticoagulant effects.

Close and regular assessment of sensory and motor function should be done when patients on multiple medications with some anticoagulant effect receive postoperative epidural analgesia. The most dilute local anesthetic solution that is effective in providing analgesia should be used. Neurologic assessment should be continued for at least 24 hours after catheter removal and longer if the coagulation tests are borderline at the time of catheter removal.

The Present Patient

A discussion was held with the surgeon of the present patient. The patient's strong preference for regional anesthesia was taken into consideration. The patient received epidural anesthesia and epidural analgesia for the first postoperative day. On the second postoperative day, the patient's pain was managed successfully with intravenous patient-controlled analgesia, and the epidural catheter was removed. After the appropriate interval, enoxaparin therapy was initiated.

Clinical Pearls

1. Neuraxial intervention in patients receiving perioperative anticoagulants requires careful consideration of potential benefits versus risks of spinal hematoma.

2. The patient's coagulation status should be optimized at the time of needle placement and catheter removal, and the coagulation status should be monitored while the epidural catheter is indwelling.

3. Simultaneous use of more than one class of anticoagulants increases the risk of hemorrhagic complications and may do so without influencing commonly used coagulation tests.

4. Communication between various clinicians involved in patient care is essential to reduce the risk of serious hemorrhagic complications.

5. Patients should be monitored closely for signs and symptoms of neurologic impairment. If neurologic compromise is noted, urgent treatment is necessary to preserve spinal cord function.

REFERENCES

1. Lumpkin MM: Reports of epidural or spinal hematomas with the concurrent use of low molecular weight heparin and spinal/epidural anesthesia or spinal puncture. FDA Public Health Advisory. U.S. Department of Health and Human Services B Public Health Service, December 1997.
2. Enneking KF, Benzon HT: Oral anticoagulants and regional anesthesia: A perspective. Reg Anesth Pain Med 23:140–145, 1998.
3. Umrey WF, Rowlingson JC: Do antiplatelet agents contribute to the development of perioperative spinal hematoma? Reg Anesth Pain Med 23:146–151, 1998.
4. Rosenquist RW, Brown DL: Neuraxial bleeding: Fibrinolytics/thrombolytics. Reg Anesth Pain Med 23:152–156, 1998.
5. Liu SS, Mulroy MF: Neuraxial anesthesia and analgesia in the presence of standard heparin. Reg Anesth Pain Med 23:157–163, 1998.
6. Horlocker TT, Wedel DJ: Neuraxial block and low molecular weight heparin: Balancing perioperative analgesia and thromboprophylaxis. Reg Anesth Pain Med 23:164–177, 1998.

Shawn Dufford, M.D.

PATIENT 29

A 36-year-old woman undergoing abdominal surgery with heavy blood loss

A 36-year-old woman is scheduled for a total abdominal hysterectomy for uterine fibroids. She is otherwise healthy, takes only supplemental iron, and has no allergies.

Physical Examination: Pulse 72, respirations 14, blood pressure 124/76, SpO_2 96% on room air. General appearance: Healthy woman in no apparent distress. Laboratory Findings: Hct 32%. All other tests normals. She is assigned an American Society of Anesthesiologists physical class II.

The patient is taken to the operating room with normal saline (0.9% sodium chloride) running freely through an 18G peripheral intravenous catheter. Midazolam, 2 mg IV, is given while automated blood pressure, ECG, and pulse oximeter are applied. The patient is preoxygenated with 100% oxygen, and a standard induction is performed with propofol, fentanyl, rocuronium, and desflurane. A 7.0 endotracheal tube is inserted easily with positive carbon dioxide return. An esophageal stethoscope with temperature probe, nasogastric tube, and an additional 16G peripheral intravenous catheter are inserted. A forced air heater is placed over the upper body. The patient is prepared and draped, and surgery is started without incidence.

Two hours into the surgery, unanticipated difficulties arise with adhesions, and blood loss by that time is estimated at 1000 mL. A radial arterial catheter is inserted for the anticipated need of closer hemodynamic monitoring and blood draws. An 8F introducer is inserted into the right internal jugular vein, and all fluids are run through a fluid warmer. To this point, fluid replacement has consisted of 4 L of normal saline, 1000 mL of 5% albumin, and 2 U of packed RBCs. Blood gas analysis reveals pH 7.28, PCO_2 33 mmHg, PO_2 214 mmHg, bicarbonate 15.8 mEq/L, and base deficit 9.4 mEq/L.

Four hours into the surgery, the patient now has 3000 mL blood loss. Fluid replacement consists of 14 L of normal saline, 1500 mL of 5% albumin, 8 U of packed RBCs, and 2 U of fresh frozen plasma.

Additional Laboratory Findings: pH 7.14, PCO_2 36 mmHg, PO_2 156 mmHg, bicarbonate 14.3 mEq/L, base deficit 14.5 mEq/L. Sodium 144 mEq/L, potassium 3.3 mEq/L, chloride 128 mEq/L, lactate 0.8 mEq/L, anion gap of 3.

Questions: What impact may the choice of crystalloid have on acid-base status?
Do colloids have any advantages over crystalloids?
Review the different colloid solutions available, including content and side effects.

What impact may the choice of crystalloid have on acid-base status? The normal saline used worsened the acid-base status of the patient. A better fluid replacement regimen would consist of a combination of physiologically balanced crystalloids and colloids, such as lactated Ringer's solution and Hextend, with the appropriate blood products.

The proper choice of fluid to restore intravascular volume and maintain cellular perfusion continues to be debated. Matters of controversy and interest include the significance of acid-base disturbances resulting from excessive saline administration, the benefits of crystalloids compared with colloids, and the metabolic derangements associated with the particular colloid administered.

Do colloids have any advantages over crystalloids? Important considerations when comparing crystalloids include their composition and volumes of distribution. Investigations by Healy et al,[3] Scheingraber et al,[5] and Waters and Bernstein[8] all showed higher mortality with lower pH, increased base deficit, and higher chloride concentrations in resuscitations using normal saline compared with more physiologically balanced solutions such as lactated Ringer's, Plasma-Lyte, and Normosol. Wilcox[1] showed in greyhound kidneys that an increased chloride load causes renal vasoconstriction (related most likely to release of adenosine, prostaglandin E_1, or thromboxane), resulting in decreased glomerular filtration rate and renal blood flow. In humans, hyperchloremia likewise has been shown to decrease urine output.

The degree to which intravascular volume is increased by a given volume of fluid administered is a second consideration. Plasma volume expansion (PVE), based on Starling equilibrium, is equal to the volume infused $\times$ the plasma volume (PV) $\div$ volume of distribution (Vd) for that particular fluid. Normal saline and lactated Ringer's solution contain equal amounts of sodium and have equal volumes of distribution (which is the extracellular volume) and expand the plasma volume by about 21%. Dextrose in free water has a volume of distribution of total body water and a PVE of only 7% of the volume infused. Drobin and Hahn[4] studied PVE, applying a two volume fluid space kinetic model, and found that the degree of intravascular space expansion with lactated acetate was a function of time. Although initial plasma volume was 50% to 60% of the amount infused, the expansion decreased within 20 minutes to about 21% of the total fluid administered.

The purported advantage of colloids over crystalloids is their ability to remain in the intravascular space in higher concentrations for longer peri-ods. Commonly administered colloids include hetastarch, albumin, gelatins, and dextran.

Review the different colloid solutions available, including content and side effects. There are two commercially available hetastarch preparations. Hespan contains 6% hetastarch diluted in 0.9% sodium chloride, whereas Hextend contains 6% hetastarch in a balanced electrolyte solution similar to lactated Ringer's solution. Hespan and Hextend are similar in 24-hour plasma volume expansion: 38% remains intravascular, 23% diffuses into the interstitium, and the remainder is renally excreted. Amylopectin is the basic starch molecule in Hetastarch, which in the body is degraded rapidly to α-amylase, rendering amylase measurements invalid for several days after administration. Molecular weights vary from 70,000 to 800,000 kD in the various commercially prepared hetastarch products. The size of the molecules equates with their ability to remain intravascular and osmotically effective and is referred to as **polydispersity.** The larger the molecule, the longer it will remain intravascular, but these larger molecules also are reduced in number, decreasing the amount of their volume expansion. Hyperchloremic metabolic acidosis and decreased urine output have been noted after administration of starch products constituted with 0.9% normal saline when compared with more physiologically balanced formulations.

Serum albumin exerts 75% to 80% of the normal colloid osmotic pressure needed for fluid homeostasis. Albumin has been used for resuscitation of burn and other trauma patients; in patients in other shock states, with acute respiratory distress syndrome, undergoing hemodialysis, with acute nephrosis, with hyperbilirubinemia, with acute liver failure, after liver transplantation, with ascites, and with sequestration of protein-rich fluids in acute peritonitis, pancreatitis, and mediastinitis; and in neonates. Albumin rarely is first-line therapy for maintenance of intravascular volume. Albumin is administered as part of intracranial pressure therapy in head-injured patients to maintain colloid osmotic pressure and microcirculatory competence. Several metaanalyses examined the effect of albumin (and other colloids and hypertonic solutions) on mortality, with inconsistent results. Although some of these analyses had similar results, the authors arrived at different conclusions. Further well-designed and controlled studies are needed to define the benefit of albumin administration in the various subsets of patients previously mentioned. Some of the albumin preparations are 0.9% normal saline; others are more physiologically balanced, which lowers the incidence of developing hyperchloremic metabolic acidosis.

Albumin 5% has similar PVE to the starches but is more expensive. Each gram of circulating albumin binds an average of 18 mL of plasma water, expanding the intravascular space approximately 450 mL with the administration of 25 g (either 100 mL of 25% or 500 mL of 5%). Infused albumin leaks out of the intravascular space at a rate of about 5% per hour but is highly dependent on capillary leakage, which has been shown to be much higher in the critically ill. The average size of the albumin molecule is 65 kD. Similar to crystalloids and the starches, the carrier of albumin varies.

Dextran 40 and dextran 70 are carbohydrate-based colloids of 40 kD and 70 kD. The dextrans are similar in price to starches but have an intravascular retention of only 20% to 30% after 90 minutes. Gelatins are formed by the hydrolysis of bovine collagen and, similar to the dextrans, are packaged in normal saline. Of infused gelatin, 80% leaks to the extravascular space after 90 minutes. Gelatins are the most common colloid administered in the United Kingdom but have not been approved for use in the United States. All the colloids have the potential for anaphylactic and anaphylactoid reactions, dextran being the worse. Dextran hapten can be administered before dextran to reduce the anaphylactic potential.

Coagulation disturbances, including decreased von Willebrand factor and factor VIII, and decreased platelet function, and thromboelastographic abnormalities have been noted after colloid administration. Starches of sizes <130,000 kD may have a smaller impact on factor VIII and platelet glycoprotein concentrations. Hextend seems to have fewer effects on coagulation profile, as assessed by thromboelastography, compared with Hespan. Gan and et al[2] showed less blood loss, less calcium supplementation, and fewer blood products transfused when hetastarch was given in a balanced solution, rather than in 0.9% normal saline. Balanced hetastarch preparations have coagulation profiles similar to albumin, but studies comparing these two solutions have not been reported.

The Present Patient

In the present patient, it would be reasonable to start the case with lactated Ringer's solution. When blood loss dictates the use of >4 L of replacement fluid, it would be reasonable to start supplementing with a physiologically balanced colloid. As blood loss continues, blood products should be given based on hemodynamics, acid-base status, and measured hematologic and coagulation parameters.

Clinical Pearls

1. Large infusions of normal saline cause hyperchloremic metabolic acidosis, decreased renal blood flow, and reduced urine output. This acidosis also confounds interpretation of blood gases and acid-base status. Physiologically balanced solutions, such as Ringer's lactate, Normosol, and Plasma-Lyte, are preferred for crystalloid resuscitation.

2. Advantages of crystalloids include cost, efficacy, and preservation of renal function. The large volumes of crystalloids that may be necessary at times also increase soft tissue and pulmonary edema, however, often significantly.

3. For any given volume administration, colloids are more effective than crystalloids in expanding intravascular volume. Colloids also remain intravascular for longer periods relative to crystalloids. However, glomerular filtration rate is supported less with colloids, however, compared with crystalloids, and coagulation disturbances are noted after larger infusions of hydroxyethyl starch and dextran. Colloids are more expensive.

4. The main difference between the hetastarch products is their carrier. Hetastarch diluted in physiologically balanced solutions results in fewer coagulation disturbances, better urine output, and less hyperchloremic metabolic acidosis when compared with hetastarch in a normal saline carrier. It also may be given in greater quantities without adverse effects on coagulation.

5. The effect of albumin administration on mortality is disputed. Because of the smaller size of the albumin molecule, it may be lost from the intravascular space more easily than larger colloid molecules. Coagulation and patient-specific concerns offset the slightly higher cost of albumin.

6. The University HealthSystem Consortium[7] recommends crystalloids as the initial resuscitation fluid of choice. Nonprotein colloids are considered second line for ongoing hemorrhagic losses when 4 L of crystalloid has been given. When these nonprotein starches and dextrans are contraindicated, as in previous hypersensitivity, bleeding disorders, risk for intracranial hemorrhage, and oliguric renal failure, albumin should be used. Diminished oxygen carrying capability or bleeding disorders should prompt the use of blood products as part of fluid replacement.

REFERENCES

1. Wilcox CS: Renal haemodynamics during hyperchloremia in anaesthetized dog: Effects of captopril. J Physiol 406:27–34, 1988.
2. Gan TJ, Bennett-Guerrero E, Phillips-Bute B, et al: Hextend, a physiologically balanced plasma expander for large volume use in major surgery: A randomized phase III clinical trial. Hextend Study Group. Anesth Analg 88:992–998, 1998.
3. Healey MA, Davis RE, Liu FC, et al: Lactated Ringer's is superior to normal saline in a model of massive hemorrhage and resuscitation. J Trauma 45:894–899, 1998.
4. Drobin D, Hahn RG: Volume kinetics of Ringer's solution in hypovolemic volunteers. Anesthesiology 90:81–91, 1999.
5. Scheingraber S, Rehm M, Sehmisch C, et al: Rapid saline infusion produces hyperchloremic acidosis in patients undergoing gynecologic surgery. Anesthesiology 90:1247–1249, 1999.
6. Martin G, Wakeling H, El-Moalem H: Hextend has better coagulation profile than Hespan and Lactated Ringer's. Anesthesiology 93:A-508, 2000.
7. University HealthSystem Consortium: Technology assessment: Albumin, nonprotein colloid, and crystalloid solutions. May 2000.
8. Waters JH, Bernstein CA: Dilutional acidosis following hetastarch or albumin in healthy volunteers. Anesthesiology 93:1184–1188, 2000.
9. Cook D, Guyatt G: Colloid use for fluid resuscitation: Evidence and spin (editorial). Ann Intern Med 135:205–208, 2001.
10. Franz A, Bräunlich P, Gamsjäger T, et al: The effects of hydroxyethyl starches of varying molecular weights on platelet function. Anesth Analg 92:1402–1407, 2001.
11. Wilkes M, Navickis R: Patient survival after human albumin administration, a meta-analysis of randomized, controlled trials. Ann Intern Med 135:149–164, 2001.
12. Wilkes NJ, Woolf R, Mutch M, et al: The effects of balanced versus saline-based hetastarch and crystalloid solutions on acid-base and electrolyte status and gastric mucosal perfusion in elderly surgical patients. Anesth Analg 93:811–816, 2001.

Gordon H. Morewood, MD

PATIENT 30

A 65-year-old woman with abrupt intraoperative cardiac decompensation

A 65-year-old woman presents for total abdominal hysterectomy and bilateral salpingo-oopherectomy. She initially is referred for consultation with a gynecologist because of complaints of "bloating" and a palpable right-sided mass on pelvic examination. Ultrasonography revealed a 5-cm right ovarian mass, and the patient was scheduled for surgical staging and potentially curative resection of a presumed malignancy.

The patient's past medical history is remarkable for chronic, poorly controlled hypertension, hyperlipidemia, and borderline diabetes (diet controlled). She has smoked a pack of cigarettes a day for 40 years. She has no known allergies to medications and currently is treated with amlodipine, 10 mg orally daily; atorvastatin, 10 mg orally daily; and hydrochlorothiazide, 50 mg orally daily. She does not participate regularly in any significant physical activity but does walk 1 mile to the park occasionally with her grandson. She is able to carry the laundry from her basement to the upstairs bedroom (two flights of stairs) without stopping or experiencing excessive shortness of breath. She denies any symptoms suggestive of coronary artery disease.

Physical Examination: Pulse 67, blood pressure 165/90. General appearance: Patient is 5 feet 4 inches tall and weighs 184 lb. She is edentulous but her airway is otherwise unremarkable. Auscultation of heart and lungs: normal.

Laboratory Findings: All tests within normal limits. Hct 39%. ECG: (12-lead) changes suggestive of left ventricular hypertrophy, but otherwise unremarkable. Echocardiogram: severe concentric hypertrophy with normal left ventricular systolic function and mild mitral regurgitation. No regional wall motion abnormalities present. The report notes that the quality of the images obtained was limited by the patient's body habitus.

Operative Course: After discussing the expected perioperative course with the patient, she is taken to the operating room. A 16-G peripheral intravenous catheter is inserted, and an epidural catheter is placed via the T8–9 interspace for postoperative analgesia. General anesthesia is induced with fentanyl, propofol, and vecuronium. Transient but significant hypotension (60/40 mmHg) occurs shortly after tracheal intubation but responds promptly to a phenylephrine bolus and 500 mL of normal saline. The epidural catheter is bolused with 10 mL of 0.125% bupivacaine, and a bupivacaine infusion is started at 10 mL/h. Anesthesia is maintained with nitrous oxide and isoflurane. The anesthetic proceeds uneventfully for the first 90 minutes of the surgical procedure. At that point, the blood pressure falls abruptly from 115/60 to 65/40 mmHg. Her heart rate is 90 beats/min at that time. The hypotension responds transiently to phenylephrine, but repeated boluses are required. Total blood loss at that point is estimated to be 600 mL, and the patient has received 2500 mL of normal saline in replacement. An arterial catheter is placed, which confirms the noninvasive measurement. No ECG changes are seen in either lead II or V on the monitor. A pulmonary artery catheter is placed, and the following measurements are obtained: central venous pressure 12 mmHg, pulmonary arterial pressure 65/32 mmHg, cardiac output 2.8 L/min, cardiac index 1.5 L/min/m². The patient is started on infusions of nitroglycerin and epinephrine without improvement in the hemodynamics.

An intraoperative transesophageal echocardiogram (TEE) is performed. On the basis of the TEE findings, the nitroglycerin, epinephrine, and epidural infusions are stopped. A phenylephrine infusion is started, 5 mg of metoprolol is given IV, and a 500-mL bolus of hetastarch is given. The hemodynamics gradually improve. On completion of the surgical procedure, the patient is transferred to the intensive care unit, at which time her heart rate is 65 beats/min, blood pressure is 140/72 mmHg, pulmonary arterial pressure is 34/18 mmHg, and her cardiac output is 4.6 L/min. She is extubated 2 hours postoperatively.

Questions: What is the diagnosis?
Should further preoperative workup have been done, given the data available?
What is the role of intraoperative echocardiography under these conditions?
What factors likely contributed to the onset of intraoperative hemodynamic instability?

What is the diagnosis? Dynamic left ventricular outflow tract (LVOT) obstruction.

Should further preoperative workup have been done, given the data available? The preoperative assessment of patients at risk for cardiac morbidity during the perioperative period has received attention from anesthesiologists and cardiologists. In the present case, the patient had several known risk factors for coronary atherosclerosis. Nonetheless, she had no history of coronary disease, and moderate exertion did not elicit symptoms of myocardial ischemia. The planned surgical procedure carried only a moderate risk of cardiovascular morbidity. Under these conditions, most authors would not recommend further investigation of the patient's cardiac status. In such patients, the potential morbidity associated with further testing (false-positive stress tests, delay of surgery, catheterization) is likely equal to, or greater than, any potential benefit. The preoperative cardiovascular assessment of the patient described was appropriate.

When significant hemodynamic instability occurred intraoperatively, a stepwise approach was taken to diagnosis and management. When the hypotension became persistent, an arterial catheter was placed to confirm the noninvasive measurement. After confirmation of the hypotension, a pulmonary artery catheter was placed to determine cardiac filling pressures and cardiac output. The values given by the pulmonary artery catheter (high filling pressures and low cardiac output) seemed compatible with myocardial ischemia and resulting left ventricular dysfunction. Although no ischemic changes were present on the ECG, medical therapy was instituted with a venodilator and inotrope without improvement.

What is the role of intraoperative echocardiography under these conditions? According to practice guidelines published by the American Society of Anesthesiology and the Society of Cardiovascular Anesthesiologists,[5] "the emergent use of perioperative TEE to determine the cause of acute, persistent, and life-threatening hemodynamic disturbances in which ventricular function and its determinants are uncertain and have not responded to treatment is a category I indication." A TEE was performed when the appropriate therapies failed and apparent contradictions were present in the clinical presentation.

What factors likely contributed to the onset of intraoperative hemodynamic instability? Dynamic LVOT obstruction occurs when left ventricular geometry and intracavitary blood flow cause prolapse of the anterior mitral valve leaflet into the LVOT during systole (see Figure). Normally, during ventricular contraction, the mitral valve leaflets are pushed toward the left atrium by the rising pressure within the left ventricle. When the mitral valve is closed and the aortic valve is open, blood flows through the conical LVOT and reaches a maximum velocity as it passes through the aortic valve annulus. Severe hypertrophy of the interventricular septum may cause narrowing of the LVOT, however, such that maximum blood flow velocity occurs well below the aortic annulus. The pliable anterior mitral valve leaflet comprises one wall of the LVOT and can be pulled in toward the interventricular septum under such conditions secondary to a Venturi-like effect. As the mitral leaflet moves toward the septum during systole, the obstruction to blood flow increases and so does the pressure gradient between the left ventricle and the aorta. Movement of the anterior mitral valve leaflet also disrupts its relationship to the posterior mitral valve leaflet, resulting in acute (often severe) mitral regurgitation. The net clinical effect of the LVOT obstruction and the mitral regurgitation is systemic hypotension and pulmonary hypertension.

The *dynamic* nature of the LVOT obstruction manifests when changes in ventricular geometry occur. Any alteration in cardiac function that decreases left ventricular end-diastolic volume brings the anterior mitral valve leaflet closer to the septum and increases the obstruction (e.g., decreased preload, tachycardia). Conditions associated with increased blood flow velocity through the LVOT also may worsen the displacement of the mitral valve leaflet (e.g., states of increased inotropy, decreased afterload).

Dynamic outflow tract obstruction has been classically associated with the genetically determined disease hypertrophic obstructive cardiomyopathy. It now is recognized however, that hypertrophy of the interventricular septum resulting from other causes (such as concentric hypertrophy associated with systemic hypertension) also may result in the described pathophysiology. This concept is particularly relevant to anesthesiologists. Many of the expected cardiovascular responses to anesthesia and surgery may provoke dynamic LVOT obstruction in patients with an anatomic predisposition.

The Present Patient

The present patient's severe concentric hypertrophy provided the required substrate for a dynamic LVOT obstruction. Although she was asymptomatic in her daily life, the decreased preload (isoflurane, bleeding, third-space losses) and decreased afterload (isoflurane, sympathectomy

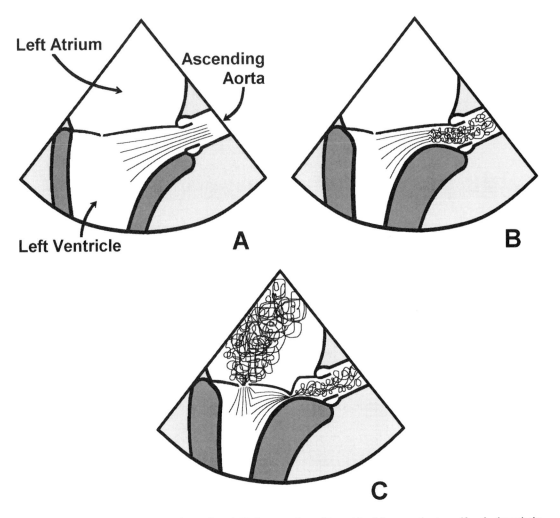

The pathogenesis of dynamic LVOT obstruction. *A,* Under normal conditions, blood flow accelerates uniformly through the LVOT and reaches peak velocity at the level of the aortic valve. *B,* In patients with thickening of the interventricular septum, peak flow velocity may occur well below the aortic valve and result in turbulent flow beyond the most narrow point in the LVOT. *C,* Subsequent changes in the loading conditions or the inotropic state of the heart may result in the anterior mitral valve leaflet being drawn into the LVOT, resulting in acute severe obstruction and mitral regurgitation.

from the epidural) that occurred during the surgical procedure ultimately resulted in an outflow tract obstruction. The initial therapy for myocardial ischemia (nitroglycerin, epinephrine) only exacerbated the underlying pathophysiology. When the correct diagnosis was made, increasing afterload with a pure α_1-agonist, decreasing heart rate and contractility with a β-blocker, and improving preload with moderate volumes of colloid relieved the LVOT obstruction.

Better control of this patient's systemic hypertension might allow regression of her left ventricular hypertrophy over the long-term and eliminate her predisposition to dynamic LVOT obstruction. Provocative maneuvers during transthoracic echocardiography (Valsalva, nitroglycerin) can help illustrate the degree to which she is susceptible to dynamic obstruction of her LVOT. Had her pathology been known preoperatively, appropriate management would have included β-blockade, adequate hydration beginning before induction, and avoidance of the sympathectomy and decreased afterload associated with epidural local anesthetics.

Clinical Pearls

1. Severe intraoperative hemodynamic disturbances not responding appropriately to therapy are one of the best indications for intraoperative TEE.

2. Hypertrophy of the interventricular septum from any cause may provide the anatomic substrate for a dynamic LVOT obstruction.

3. The cardiovascular changes associated with general and neuraxial anesthesia may provoke a dynamic LVOT obstruction.

4. Dynamic LVOT obstruction may mimic acute myocardial ischemia with left ventricular failure and cannot be differentiated from ischemia based on pulmonary artery catheter data alone.

5. Patients prone to dynamic LVOT obstruction should be kept "slow and full" during the perioperative period. Hypotension should be treated with a pure α_1-agonist.

REFERENCES

1. Bulkley BH, Fortuin NJ: Systolic anterior motion of the mitral valve without asymmetric septal hypertrophy. Chest 69:694–696, 1976.
2. Maron BJ, Epstein SE, Bonow RO, et al: Obstructive hypertrophic cardiomyopathy associated with minimal left ventricular hypertrophy. Am J Cardiol 53:377–379, 1984.
3. Pellikka PA, Oh JK, Bailey KR, et al: Dynamic intraventricular obstruction during dobutamine stress echocardiography. Circulation 46:1429–1432, 1992.
4. Armstrong WF, Marcovitz PA: Dynamic left ventricular outflow tract obstruction as a complication of acute myocardial infarction. Am Heart J 131:827–830, 1996.
5. Practice guidelines for perioperative transesophageal echocardiography. A report by the American Society of Anesthesiologists and the Society of Cardiovascular Anesthesiologists Task Force on Transesophageal Echocardiography. Anesthesiology 84:986–1006, 1996.
6. Mangano DT: Assessment of the patient with cardiac disease: An anesthesiologist's paradigm. Anesthesiology 91:1521–1526, 1999.
7. Eagle KA, Berger PB, Calkins H, et al: ACC/AHA guideline update for perioperative cardiovascular evaluation for noncardiac surgery update: Executive summary. A report of the American College of Cardiology/American Heart Association Task Force on Practice Guidelines (Committee to Update the 1996 Guidelines on Perioperative Cardiovascular Evaluation for Noncardiac Surgery). J Am Coll Cardiol 39:542–553, 2002.
8. Morewood GH, Weiss SJ: Intra-aortic balloon pump associated with dynamic left ventricular outflow tract obstruction following valve replacement for aortic stenosis. J Am Soc Echocardiogr 13:229–231, 2002.
9. Murtha W, Guenther C: Dynamic left ventricular outflow tract obstruction complicating bilateral lung transplantation. Anesth Analg 94:558–559, 2002.

Rodger E. Barnette, MD, FCCM

PATIENT 31

A 39-year-old woman with multisystem organ failure and no advance directives

A 39-year-old woman with a history of hypertension, diabetes mellitus, hypothyroidism, and morbid obesity (127 kg) is admitted in congestive heart failure. Workup reveals a severe idiopathic cardiomyopathy. A left ventricular assist device (LVAD) is implanted as a bridge to cardiac transplantation. Postoperatively, her condition stabilizes sufficiently to allow transfer to floor care. Two weeks later, sepsis and evidence of a right cerebral vascular accident necessitate readmission to the intensive care unit, where she requires mechanical ventilation, invasive monitoring, and administration of broad-spectrum antibiotics. Surgical exploration of the chest and abdomen is undertaken twice in an attempt to drain and treat an infected LVAD drive-line site. The sepsis is refractory to aggressive therapy, and the patient develops acute renal failure.

Neuropsychologic evaluation reveals that, although the patient responds to voice and intermittently follows simple commands, she is not capable of understanding complex questions or issues. There is a dense left hemiplegia. Despite tracheotomy and repeated weaning attempts, she continues to require ventilatory support. The LVAD continues to function adequately but is chronically infected. Removal of the LVAD is not considered clinically feasible. The patient is removed from the cardiac transplant list because of ongoing infection and significant multiorgan system dysfunction.

The intensive care unit physician responsible for the patient's care believes that further medical intervention would be futile. The patient does not have a living will, however, and had not conferred durable power of attorney for health care on a family member or friend.

Questions: Summarize the events leading up to the Self-Determination Act of 1990.

What responsibilities do physicians and hospitals have in ensuring patients have advance directives?

Describe advance directives for health care and how they assist in end-of-life decisions.

What resources do health care providers have when faced with patients who do not have advance directives?

Summarize the events leading up to the Self-Determination Act of 1990. In 1983 a 24-year-old woman named Nancy Cruzan was involved in a motor vehicle accident. Although resuscitated at the scene, her injuries were substantial and included a profound hypoxic encephalopathy. After 5 years in a persistent vegetative state, the family asked for withdraw of nourishment and hydration. This request was refused by the state hospital caring for Cruzan, and the family went to court. Although the Cruzan family's request was granted by the trial court, the decision was immediately appealed by the state of Missouri.

The Missouri Supreme Court overturned the lower court, stating there was no "clear and convincing evidence" that Cruzan would wish to have life support withdrawn. The Missouri Supreme Court believed that the family's quality-of-life arguments did not carry as much weight as the state's interest in the sanctity of human life. The case was appealed to the U.S. Supreme Court, where a majority of the court upheld the Missouri Supreme Court's decision. The U.S. Supreme Court stated: "The choice between life and death is . . . deeply personal. . . . Missouri may legitimately seek to safeguard the personal element of this choice through the imposition of heightened evidentiary requirements." Testimony by Cruzan's friends eventually led to "clear and convincing evidence" of her wishes, and care was withdrawn. That same year, and as a direct result of the Cruzan case, Missouri Senator Danforth sponsored the bill that became *The Self-Determination Act of 1990.*

What responsibilities do physicians and hospitals have in ensuring patients have advance directives? The Self-Determination Act is the major legal force that structures patient autonomy in regard to end-of-life issues. The law states:

1. Hospitals must provide written information at the time of admission that makes clear to patients their right to accept or refuse therapy and their right to create advance directives.
2. Health care providers must document in the patient's current medical record whether an individual has executed an advance directive.
3. Providers are not to condition care, or otherwise discriminate against the patient, based on the presence or absence of an advance directive.
4. States must develop state law regarding advance directives, and health care institutions must ensure compliance with these state laws.

Describe advance directives for health care and how they assist in end-of-life decisions. Implementation of the Self-Determination Act led to a variety of policies designed to strengthen patient autonomy and to prevent a reenactment of the Cruzan case. There are four basic types of advance directives: do-not-resuscitate (DNR) orders, living wills, durable power of attorney for health care, and, perhaps most important, verbal statements made when competent.

DNR orders allow patients or patients' advocates to structure the extent of heroic care. Most hospitals now have several levels of DNR status. At the hospital in the present case, the levels include withholding resuscitation in the face of an otherwise lethal event (DNR level I), DNR/do not add additional therapy (DNR level II), and DNR/withdraw life support (DNR level III). Most hospitals also address, through their individual internal policies, how DNR status is to be managed perioperatively if and when a patient with a DNR order requires a surgical procedure. This is necessary because a patient undergoing surgery and the administration of anesthesia may experience cardiovascular and airway perturbations that are not a direct result of the primary disease process. Temporary changes in DNR status should be clarified with the patient, the patient's family, and all physicians involved in the care of the patient before surgery.

Living wills are legal documents that specify the extent to which a patient is willing to accept artificial life support and resuscitation efforts. The living will takes effect only when the patient is incompetent, faces imminent death, or is otherwise considered terminal.

The durable power of attorney for health care is also a legal document. It gives a specified surrogate the power to make all decisions regarding health care. Similar to the living will, it takes effect when patients are incompetent to make their own decisions or face impending death.

Several studies have documented that advance directives are dramatically underused. For that reason, verbal statements made by patients while competent are often the only available indications of their views on these issues. In the present case, the family's testimony regarding what the patient had stated previously regarding her preference for end-of-life care, was crucial.

What resources do health care providers have when faced with patients who do not have advance directives? Even with The Self-Determination Act, difficulties and conflicts in end-of-life decision making are frequent. Many patients do not avail themselves of advance directives, and many physicians are uncomfortable raising this topic.

Another problem is the meaning of the term **medical futility.** Despite years of discussion among authorities, there is still no consensus definition. The attempt to define this term failed because the assumption that a specific definition existed that could be applied in all cases was flawed. **Medical futility** is a value-laden term—a term that acquires content from one's belief system or philosophy of life rather than from precise, empirically determined data.

Because there may be significant differences of opinion between physicians and patients or their proxies regarding values and goals of therapy, resolution by process-centered algorithms has been advocated. Process-centered algorithms attempt to resolve conflict through a series of sequential steps. These steps consist of consensus building through the use of outcome data and value judgments, joint decision making, consultants' expert opinions, involvement of ethics committees, and possibly transfer of care to another hospital or physician. Although some of these process-based algorithms advocate unilateral withdraw of care if resolution of conflict is not possible, the legal ramifications of such an action are unknown. Communication and negotiation are key skills when using these algorithms. Early involvement of the hospital's ethics committee is an important strategy and is usually a worthwhile option when faced with an end-of-life dilemma.

Advance directives are legal tools that are available to all patients. Through them the courts have generally upheld the patients' right to refuse therapy and have attempted to provide a mechanism for resolving many end-of-life conflicts. The right of patients to demand therapy and the right of physicians unilaterally to withdraw therapy considered medically futile persist as areas of difficulty.

The Present Patient

A series of family meetings was held concerning the present patient. Consultation was obtained with the ethics committee. Treatment was considered to be medically futile by all physicians caring for this patient. The family stated, based on previous discussions with the patient, that she would not have wanted to continue living given her condition. A decision was made by the family and physicians to make the patient DNR level III (do not resuscitate and withdraw support). The patient died shortly thereafter.

Clinical Pearls

1. Advance directives are concrete mechanisms with which patients may exercise autonomy in end-of-life decisions. They are underused.

2. Medical futility is a value-laden term; it does not have a precise, empirically determined definition.

3. The courts have generally upheld patients' and their surrogates' rights to refuse therapy. The rights of patients to demand therapy and of physicians unilaterally to withdraw therapy are not well established.

4. Medical ethics committees offer information and an objective third party. Early involvement of the ethics committee in end-of-life dilemmas is usually advantageous.

5. Process-based approaches are new and hold promise, but they are largely untested and may end up in the court system.

6. Perioperative DNR policies may differ among hospitals. Physicians should become familiar with their institutions' policies.

REFERENCES

1. *Cruzan v Director, Missouri Department of Health,* 497 US 261 (1990). Available at http://supct.law.cornell.edu/supct/html/88-1503.ZS.html.
2. Patient Self-Determination Act of 1990. 42 U.S.C. 1395.
3. Halevy A, Brody B: A multi-institutional collaborative policy on medical futility. JAMA 276:571–574, 1996.
4. Council on Ethical and Judicial Affairs, American Medical Association: Medical futility in end-of-life care. JAMA 281:937–941, 1999.
5. Freeborne N, Lynn J, Desbiens NA: Perspectives and reviews of support findings: Insights about dying from the SUPPORT project. J Am Geriatr Soc 48:1–13, 2000.
6. Helft P, Siegler M, Lantos J: The rise and fall of the futility movement. N Engl J Med 343:293–296, 2000.
7. Singer P, Barker G, Bowman KW, et al: Hospital policy on appropriate use of life-sustaining treatment. Crit Care Med 29:187–191, 2001.

Scott A. Schartel, DO

PATIENT 32

A 48-year-old woman with failure to separate from cardiopulmonary bypass

A 48-year-old woman is brought to the operating room for coronary artery bypass graft surgery. She was admitted to the hospital 2 days before surgery following 16 hours of intermittent chest pain. Initial ECG showed 2-mm horizontal ST segment depression in leads V1-V5. Her symptoms and ECG improved after treatment with intravenous nitroglycerin and heparin. Serial cardiac enzyme assays were elevated, and a diagnosis of non–Q wave myocardial infarction was made. Cardiac catheterization showed 80% stenosis of the left main coronary artery, 75% stenosis of the left anterior descending artery, 90% stenosis of the circumflex artery, and 50% stenosis of the right coronary artery. An echocardiogram showed normal valve function, normal right ventricular function, and a left ventricular ejection fraction of 40%. There was moderately severe hypokinesis of the anterior wall and the intraventricular septum.

Additional medical history includes hypertension; hypercholesterolemia; and diabetes mellitus type 2, controlled with diet. She smoked cigarettes until 6 months before admission. Medications on the day of surgery included intravenous infusions of heparin and nitroglycerin and oral metoprolol.

Operative Course: The patient is brought to the operating room where a left radial intraarterial catheter, right internal jugular pulmonary artery catheter, and a 16-G right arm intravenous catheter are placed before induction of anesthesia. Anesthesia is induced with sufentanil and lorazepam. Pancuronium bromide is administered to facilitate tracheal intubation. After induction of anesthesia, a transesophageal echocardiogram probe is placed without difficulty. The TEE examination is unchanged from the preoperative examination. Near completion of the internal mammary artery dissection, it is noted that ST segment elevation in lead V5 has increased from 0.5 mm to 3 mm. The surgeon is notified, heparin is administered (300 U/kg), and the nitroglycerin infusion is increased. Aortic and venous cannulae are placed, and cardiopulmonary bypass (CPB) is initiated. The aorta is cross-clamped, and cold blood cardioplegia is administered. The patient is cooled to 32°C. Three bypass grafts are constructed: Left internal mammary artery to the left anterior descending artery, reversed saphenous vein from aorta to circumflex artery, and reversed saphenous vein from aorta to right coronary artery.

After release of the aortic cross-clamp (total time 125 minutes), ventricular fibrillation develops. Defibrillation with 20 J results in sinus rhythm. The patient is rewarmed to a bladder temperature of 36.5°C. Infusions of epinephrine (4 μg/min) and milrinone (50 μg/kg loading dose followed by 0.5 μg/kg/minute) are begun. CPB is weaned slowly, then terminated. After separation from CPB, heart rate is 95 beats/min, mean arterial pressure is 46 mmHg, pulmonary arterial pressure is 54/28 mmHg with pulmonary capillary wedge pressure of 26 mmHg, right atrial pressure is 16 mmHg, and cardiac index is 1.6 L/min/m². TEE shows akinesis of the anterior and septal walls and hypokinesis of the lateral wall with ventricular distention. Two minutes after separation from CPB, mean arterial pressure is 40 mm Hg, pulmonary arterial pressure is 58/32 mmHg, and cardiac index is 1.3 L/min/m². CPB is reinstituted.

Questions: What is the diagnosis?
Describe the causes of failure to wean from CPB?
What can be done to facilitate separation from CPB on the next attempt?
Discuss the role of mechanical circulatory assist devices.

What is the diagnosis? Post-CPB pump failure resulting from the combined effect of pre-CPB myocardial ischemia and additional ischemic injury during aortic cross-clamping.

Describe the causes of failure to wean from CPB. Failure to separate from CPB can be caused by mechanical and pathophysologic factors.[5] Myocardial dysfunction, either global or regional, is a principal cause for failure to wean from CPB and may be related to preexisting cardiac dysfunction or ischemic injury. Ischemic injury may result from inadequate myocardial preservation during the period of aortic cross-clamping, from technical problems with coronary artery bypass grafts, or from coronary artery embolic events (air or debris). Heart rate and rhythm disturbances are another cause and may be related to electrolyte abnormalities, ischemic injury, or conduction system abnormalities. Tachyarrhythmias or bradyarrhythmias interfere with adequate cardiac output. Hyperkalemia, hypocalcemia, and metabolic acidosis also may contribute to inadequate cardiac function post-CPB. Mechanical causes that lead to inadequate cardiac filling or emptying may interfere with successful separation. These include cannula-related problems, external compression, or outflow obstruction (e.g., undiagnosed stenotic valve, dynamic subvalvular outflow tract obstruction, malfunction of prosthetic valve). Marked vasodilation, occult blood loss, and technical problems with drug delivery also must be considered.

What can be done to facilitate separation from CPB on the next attempt? The first step in achieving successful separation from CPB requires correction of metabolic abnormalities and establishing an acceptable cardiac rhythm and rate. Epicardial atrial and ventricular pacing can be used when spontaneous cardiac rhythm does not return or when the intrinsic rate is too slow. If pacing is required, atrioventricular pacing is preferred to take advantage of atrial augmentation to ventricular preload.

Inotropic support is the next step in treatment of failure to separate from CPB. A β-receptor agonist and a cardiac phosphodiesterase inhibitor are acceptable first choices. Consideration of the direct effects and side effects of the various agents and the specific patient's hemodynamic derangements allows the rational selection of an appropriate initial inotrope. If a second agent is required, an agent from a different class with a different mechanism of action might achieve synergy.

Discuss the role of mechanical circulatory assist devices. If the response to inotropic drugs is still inadequate to achieve separation from CPB, mechanical circulatory support is considered. Choices include intra-aortic balloon counterpulsation or a ventricular assist device (VAD).

Intra-aortic balloon pump (IABP) counterpulsation usually is the first choice for mechanical circulatory assist. Most commonly the IABP is placed through a femoral artery into the descending thoracic aorta. In patients with lower extremity peripheral vascular disease, the IABP can be placed by a transthoracic approach. In the transthoracic approach, the IAPB is introduced into the ascending aorta and passed distally into position in the descending thoracic aorta.

The IABP is timed so that the balloon will inflate with the onset of diastole and deflate just before the onset of systole. Inflation of the IABP augments diastolic blood pressure, which can lead to an increase in coronary artery flow. IABP deflation decreases systemic vascular resistance, resulting in increases in cardiac output in the range of 0.5 to 0.8 L/min.[1,2]

If IABP counterpulsation provides inadequate support or if the magnitude of the ventricular dysfunction is beyond the capabilities of IABP support, VAD support can be used. Two short-term VAD options include use of a centrifugal pump or the Abiomed BVS 5000 VAD (Abiomed Cardiovascular, Inc, Danvers, MA).

A centrifugal pump, such as is employed commonly during CPB, can be used to provide left or right ventricular assist; two devices can be placed if biventricular support is necessary. For left VAD support, the pump is configured with an inflow cannula in the left atrium and an outflow cannula in the ascending aorta. For right VAD support, cannulae are placed in the right atrium and pulmonary artery. Centrifugal pumps provide nonpulsatile flow and require systemic anticoagulation. Considerable experience exists for using centrifugal pumps for this purpose; however, the devices are not approved by the Food and Drug Administration for this indication. A perfusionist must be in attendance throughout the duration of VAD support.

The Abiomed BVS 5000 Bi-Ventricular Support System[3,4] is a pneumatically powered, pulsatile VAD. (see Figure). It is approved by the Food and Drug Administration for the treatment of ventricular failure after cardiac surgery. The device has a dual-chamber design with an upper collecting chamber (atrium analog) and a lower pumping chamber (ventricular analog). The system has two trileaflet unidirectional valves, one between the upper and lower chambers and the other between the lower chamber and the outflow tubing. The blood chambers are contained within a hard plastic shell. The pumping action is caused

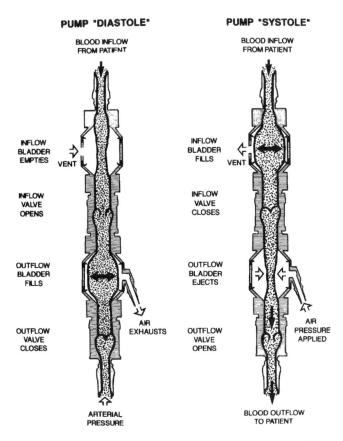

PUMP "DIASTOLE"

BLOOD INFLOW
FROM PATIENT

INFLOW
BLADDER
EMPTIES   VENT

INFLOW
VALVE
OPENS

OUTFLOW
BLADDER
FILLS

OUTFLOW   AIR
VALVE   EXHAUSTS
CLOSES

ARTERIAL
PRESSURE

PUMP "SYSTOLE"

BLOOD INFLOW
FROM PATIENT

INFLOW
BLADDER
FILLS   VENT

INFLOW
VALVE
CLOSES

OUTFLOW
BLADDER
EJECTS

OUTFLOW   AIR
VALVE   PRESSURE
OPENS   APPLIED

BLOOD OUTFLOW
TO PATIENT

Abiomed BVS 5000 Pump (Abiomed Cardiovascular, Inc, Danvers, MA).

by introducing compressed air into the hard plastic shell surrounding the lower blood chamber. A control module monitors the filling of the lower chamber with blood, and when it senses that the chamber is full, it pressurizes the shell outside the chamber, causing the chamber to empty. The blood chambers have a capacity of 100 mL and typically generate a stroke volume of 70 to 80 mL with flow rates up to 5 L/min.

The cannulae are passed through subcostal stab wounds into the thorax. The cannulae have external polyester sleeves that are positioned in the subcutaneous tissue to aid in hemostasis and to decrease the risk of infection. When used as a left VAD, the inflow cannula is placed into the left atrium, and the outflow cannula is connected to the ascending aorta with an end-to-side anastomosis. Right ventricular assist is achieved by placing the inflow cannula into the right atrium and the outflow cannula into the pulmonary artery. A single control module can control two VADs and provide biventricular support (see Figure).

The Abiomed BVS requires systemic anticoagulation to prevent clot formation within the VAD circuit. The manufacturer recommends that anti-

coagulation begin within 24 hours of implantation. A continuous infusion of heparin is begun when surgical bleeding is under control and titrated to achieve a target activated coagulation time between 180 and 200 seconds. Ventricular assist support is continued until independent ventricular function has recovered. The device must be removed in the operating room. The Abiomed BVS is designed to provide support for days to several weeks. If ventricular function does not recover sufficiently in this period, conversion to a long-term VAD or heart transplantation is necessary.

Complications with the Abiomed BVS system include bleeding, thromboembolism, central nervous system embolism, renal failure, infection, and hemolysis. In two reviews of the use of the Abiomed, VAD weaning from assist occurred in the patients studied in 49%, with 31% surviving to discharge,[8] and in 66%, with 42% surviving to discharge.[7]

Experience with the use of VAD support for postcardiotomy ventricular failure showed that such devices should be used early. Samuels et al[6] showed a lower incidence of multisystem failure, improved device weaning, and improved dis-

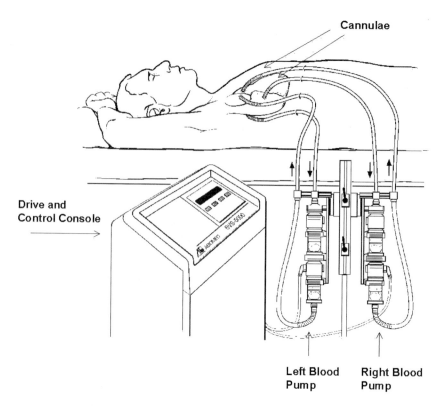

Cannulae

Drive and
Control Console

Left Blood
Pump

Right Blood
Pump

The Abiomed BVS 5000 configured for biventricular support.

charge rates when VAD therapy was initiated within the first 3 hours of failed weaning.

The Present Patient

The present patient was unable to be weaned from CPB with inotropic and IABP support. Separation from CPB succeeded after the placement of an Abiomed left VAD. The chest was closed, and the patient was transferred to the intensive care unit. Left VAD support was continued for 7 days. On postoperative day 1, the IABP was removed. Two days later, the patient was weaned from mechanical ventilation. TEE on postopera-tive day 7 showed improved left ventricular function. The patient was returned to the operating room, general anesthesia was administered, and the chest was reopened. After institution of infusions of epinephrine (2 μg/min) and milrinone (0.4 μg/kg/min), the left VAD support was decreased slowly, then discontinued. The cannulae were removed, and the chest was closed after ensuring hemostasis. On TEE, the overall left ventricular ejection fraction was 55%. The patient was weaned from mechanical ventilation on post-VAD day 1 and discharged from the intensive care unit on post-VAD day 2.

Clinical Pearls

1. In patients who fail to wean from CPB, a careful search should be done for all reversible and treatable causes, including electrolyte abnormalities, rhythmn disturbances, and mechanical issues.

2. Rational selection of inotropic agents in patients with postcardiotomy ventricular failure should match the direct effects and side effects of the drugs with the patient's hemodynamic abnormalities.

3. For patients who cannot wean from CPB, IABP counterpulsation is a good first step for mechanical support.

4. In patients who do not wean from CPB after instituting reasonable doses of two or more inotropic agents, VAD support should be considered. VAD therapy should be used early. Prolonged attempts to correct post-cardiotomy shock before VAD placement increase the incidence of multisystem organ failure and poor outcome.

5. The Abiomed VAD system is a good choice for short-term VAD support. It requires systemic anticoagulation.

REFERENCES

1. Dunkman WB, Leinbach RC, Buckely MJ, et al: Clinical and hemodynamic results of intraaortic balloon pumping in surgery for cardiogenic shock. Circulation 46:465–477, 1972.
2. Scheidt S, Wilner G, Mueller H, et al: Intra-aortic balloon counterpulsation in cardiogenic shock: Report of a co-operative clinical trial. N Engl J Med 288:979–984, 1973.
3. Abiomed BVS 5000 Bi-Ventricular Support System Training Manual. Danvers MA, Abiomed Cardiovascular, Inc, 1994.
4. Abiomed BVS 5000 Bi-ventricular Support System: Guide to Patient Management. Danvers MA, Abiomed Cardiovascular, Inc, 1994.
5. Michelsen LG, Shanewise JS: Discontinuation of cardiopulmonary bypass. In Mora CT, Gutyon RA, Finlayson DC, Rigatti RL (eds): Cardiopulmonary Bypass: Principles and Techniques of Extracorporeal Circulation. New York, Springer-Verlag, 1995, pp 289–292.
6. Samuels LE, Kaurman MS, Thomas MP, et al: Pharmacological criteria for ventricular assist device insertion following postcardiotomy shock: Experience with the Abiomed BVS system. J Card Surg. 14:288–293, 1999.
7. Dekkers RJ, Fitzgerald DJ, Couper GS: Five-year clinical experience with Abiomed BVS 5000 as a ventricular assist device for cardiac failure. Perfusion 16:13–8, 2001.
8. Samuels LE, Homes EC, Thomas MP, et al: Management of acute cardiac failure with mechanical assist: Experience with the Abiomed BVS 5000. Ann Thorac Surg 71(3 suppl):S67–72, 2001.

David M. Polaner, MD, FAAP

PATIENT 33

A 22-month-old with postoperative respiratory complications

A 22-month-old girl is scheduled for tonsillectomy and adenoidectomy because of obstructed breathing during sleep. She has had an upper respiratory illness (URI) for the past 4 days, with mild cough and mucopurulent rhinitis but no respiratory distress. She does not have a history of reactive airway disease. She has been eating and drinking normally. The child was born at 33 weeks' gestation, received exogenous surfactant at birth, and had no subsequent problems of prematurity other than an oxygen requirement for the first week of life.

Physical Examination: Heart rate 106, respirations 22, oxygen saturation in room air 97%. Lungs: upper airway rhonchi, but no rales, wheezes, or asymmetry of breath sounds. Normal external airway; no murmurs are audible.

Laboratory Findings: Polysomnogram showed repeated episodes of desaturation to <80% during deep sleep coincident with upper airway obstruction. No central apnea detected. No other laboratory data available.

Hospital Course: The patient receives oral premedication with midazolam, 0.5 mg/kg, and acetaminophen, 15 mg/kg. Anesthesia was induced with sevoflurane in nitrous oxide and oxygen. She was intubated deep, but developed laryngospasm during the initial attempt at laryngoscopy, which was broken with continuous positive airway pressure (CPAP). Anesthesia was maintained with halothane and a total of 2.5 μg/kg of fentanyl administered in incremental doses. The operation lasted 30 minutes. She was extubated awake at the end of the procedure but had pronounced coughing, which lasted for more than 5 minutes. During this time, oxygen saturation fell to 75% despite the administration of 100% oxygen by facemask from the anesthesia circuit with 5 cm H_2O of CPAP. A chest radiograph was normal. She continued to require oxygen in the postanesthesia care unit for >2 hours to maintain oxygen saturations >85%.

Questions: What is the most likely cause of the oxygen desaturation?
What are the surgical and anesthetic factors that increase the risk of postoperative respiratory complications in children with URIs?
When should a case be postponed?
What are the patient-related factors that increase risk?
What may be done to decrease the risk of complications?

What is the cause of the oxygen desaturation?
Recent acute viral illness.

What are the surgical and anesthetic factors that increase the risk of postoperative complications in children with URIs? Viral respiratory illnesses are common in children presenting for elective surgery and create a dilemma for the anesthesiologist in deciding whether to proceed with surgery. The average child contracts six to eight viral respiratory illnesses a year, and children in day care have even more. Judging which children pose an increased risk of developing respiratory complications and should have their surgery postponed is a difficult decision that must be based on limited data. Studies have determined that there are increased risks associated with certain patient, surgical, and anesthetic factors that can guide the clinician in making a decision.

Children with viral URI are at increased risk for intraoperative and postoperative respiratory complications after anesthesia. This risk is present not only while they have an active URI, but also during recovery and for 8 weeks after resolution of the acute illness, owing to persistent airway hyperresponsiveness.

Airway irritability or bronchoreactivity increases during viral respiratory illness. These increases are more profound if the patient has an underlying history of reactive airways disease (e.g., asthma, bronchopulmonary dysplasia) but occur even in otherwise normal subjects. The reactivity can occur in the lower respiratory tract even if the primary symptoms seem to be confined to the upper tract. Several mechanisms probably are involved in producing airway reactivity. Vagal hyperreactivity, caused by the effects of virus on inhibitory M2 muscarinic receptors in the airways, has been identified as one significant mechanism. Increases in tachykinins, leukotrienes, and other cytokines have been implicated as important mediators of airway inflammation and irritation in URI. Viral infections also have been reported to reduce the ability to degrade these mediators, prolonging their action and increasing their concentration.

A hypersecretory response commonly occurs in the airways of children with viral respiratory illness. This response is a product of the inflammatory reactions to viral infection in mucus-producing cells and to edema of the airway and sloughing of debris resulting from injury to the respiratory epithelium. These secretions may be more viscid than normal and plug the bronchioles, leading to areas of microatelectasis or, in severe cases, to subsegmental or segmental atelectasis. This may be part of the cause of the frequent need

for supplemental oxygen in the immediate postoperative period in these children. Alternatively, investigators found that inflammation of the lung in sheep induced by viral illness increased oxygen consumption, increasing shunt.

When should a case be postponed? The presence of significant fever ($>38.5°C$), toxicity, or substantial airway congestion or the detection of hypoxemia, wheezing, or airway obstruction would lead most anesthesiologists and surgeons to cancel an elective surgical procedure. The child with a mild-to-moderate URI presents the diagnostic dilemma. Certain characteristics of a URI have been associated with increased risk of respiratory complications, including copious sputum production, severe nasal congestion, severe cough, the presence of wheezing or bronchospastic symptoms, and snoring. There are no diagnostic tests (e.g., lymphocyte count, differential, sedimentation rate) with any predictive value to assess the fitness of a child with URI for anesthesia. A chest radiograph is worth obtaining only if there are focal findings on physical examination. Peak expiratory flow rate, although not studied specifically in this situation, is a useful indicator of control in asthmatics and may be helpful in the subset of children with a history of reactive airways disease. One of the best discriminators, according to several investigators, is the impression of the parents as to the severity of the child's illness.

What are the patient-related factors that increase risk? Any child with a chronic respiratory disease, such as asthma or reactive airway disease, or bronchopulmonary dysplasia (chronic lung disease owing to prematurity), is at increased risk of respiratory complications with a URI. A history of prematurity is a risk factor even in a child without a history of reactive airway disease when well and even when the child is several years old. The age at which prematurity no longer is a risk is unclear. The more severe the underlying condition, and the more severe the alteration from baseline, the more thought that must be given to postponement and aggressive treatment.

Parental smoking and other chronic exposure to second-hand tobacco smoke have been identified as a risk factor for increased respiratory complications in several studies even in the absence of URI. Passive smoking with a coexisting URI has been shown to increase risk further.

The child with sickle cell disease is at increased risk for developing acute chest syndrome after anesthesia and surgery, but the presence of a URI may cause additive risks. The early symptoms of chest syndrome may be difficult to distinguish from a cold. Heightened consideration should be given to cancellation in these children.

Children with congenital heart disease, especially children with increased pulmonary blood flow or pulmonary hypertension, are at considerably increased risk and must be evaluated with special care. Consultation with the child's pediatric cardiologist may be helpful.

What may be done to decrease the risk of complications? Certain surgical and anesthetic procedures are more likely to result in respiratory complications in children with URIs. Instrumentation of the airway has been shown repeatedly to be a major factor in precipitating respiratory problems. Endotracheal intubation produces an 11-fold increase in the incidence of problems. The laryngeal mask is less stimulating to the airway and produced fewer complications, and a conventional mask fewer still, in two studies. Surgery of the airway, especially bronchoscopy, but also tonsillectomy and adenoidectomy, increases risk. Although studies with large numbers of patients are lacking, operations that predispose to intraoperative or postoperative respiratory insufficiency, such as pectus excavatum repair, thoracotomy, and upper abdominal procedures, are likely to carry increased risk. Tympanostomy and myringotomy tube placement may carry a decreased risk — one well-controlled study showed more rapid resolution of URI in this selected population. It is not clear if this rapid resolution was due to the operation itself or to the antiviral activity of halothane, which has been shown in *in vitro* studies.

The principal complications in children with URI are bronchospasm, laryngospasm, hypoxemia, breath holding and cough, and increased secretions. The incidence of laryngospasm is more than doubled in children with URI. Many children with URI have mild-to-moderate degrees of oxygen desaturation in the postanesthesia care unit, although virtually all simply require supplemental oxygen for a longer period than healthy children (an additional 1 to 2 hours) before normoxia in ambient air returns. Respiratory failure is a rare but reported complication and may represent either an exacerbation of an unrecognized pneumonia, critical airway plugging resulting in severe shunt, or the unusual patient who has an exaggerated irritability of the airways and pulmonary vasculature. An extremely rare (but reported) complication is a child who has unrecognized postviral cardiomyopathy and develops dysrhythmias and cardiovascular collapse on induction.

The magnitude of risk is a big remaining question. A more recent large prospective controlled study (1078 patients) suggested that although complications are increased in children with intercurrent and recent mild URI, the severity of these complications usually is either mild or manageable, and morbidity is minimal. With careful screening and selection and the judicious choice of anesthetic technique and perioperative management, most of these children can undergo anesthesia and surgery with good outcomes. There is a small but real risk of more serious complications, however, including respiratory failure, and the potential risks must be discussed realistically with the parents when obtaining consent. The anesthesiologist must be prepared to deal with bronchospasm and laryngospasm, and the postanesthesia care unit staff must anticipate that some of these children may require a longer than average stay. Patients in the highest risk categories should be considered for postponement.

The Present Patient

After 4 hours of oxygen supplementation and treatment with nebulized ipratroprium bromide, the patient was able to sustain oxygen saturation of 97% in ambient air. During episodes of coughing, her oxygen saturation would fall to 88-90%, but returned to greater than 95% within a minute of stopping coughing. She was observed overnight in the hospital, where oxygen saturation remained >93% during sleep, and minimal airway obstruction was observed. She was discharged home the next afternoon in stable condition.

Clinical Pearls

1. Airway reactivity should be treated aggressively in susceptible patients in the preoperative period. If proceeding in a child with asthma, the clinician should consider the use of preoperative bronchodilators. A short course of preoperative steroids (24 hours) should be used if possible. Asthma is an inflammatory disease of the airways, not simply bronchospasm. Asthmatics must use all of their medications preoperatively. Children who were premature may respond well to ipratroprium bromide.

2. Airway stimulation should be minimized. The use of a mask or laryngeal mask, if feasible, is preferable to an endotracheal tube. If intubation is necessary, an adequate depth of anesthesia must be reached before laryngoscopy and intubation (may need to be deeper than usual). Deep extubation, which eliminates the need to have a light patient with a tube in place, should be strongly considered. Topicalization of the airway might be considered (be careful of local anesthetic toxicity). The use of regional anesthesia in conjunction with general anesthesia may facilitate the use a laryngeal mask with spontaneous ventilation instead of intubation for some operations.

3. Airway irritants should be avoided. Isoflurane and desflurane are considerably more irritating to the airways than halothane or sevoflurane. Isoflurane maintenance increases the risks of respiratory complications and emergence delirium in these patients.

4. If surgery is cancelled, the clinician should allow adequate time for recovery. There is little to be gained by waiting until the overt symptoms of the cold go away without waiting until resolution of the airway irritability (minimum of 4 weeks). A procedure should not be rescheduled before 4 weeks. If the case cannot be postponed that long, symptoms should be treated aggressively, and the surgery should proceed.

REFERENCES

1. Empey DW, Laitinen LA, Jacobs L: Mechanisms of bronchial hyperreactivity in normal subjects after upper respiratory infections. Am Rev Respir Dis 113:131–139, 1976.
2. Tait AR, Knight PR: The effects of general anesthesia on upper respiratory tract infections in children. Anesthesiology 67:930–935, 1987.
3. Tait AR, Knight PR: Intraoperative respiratory complications in patients with upper respiratory tract infections. Can J Anaesth 34:300–303, 1987.
4. Cohen MM, Cameron CB: Should you cancel the operation when a child has an upper respiratory tract infection? Anesth Analg 72:282–288, 1991.
5. Rolf N, Cote CJ: Frequency and severity of desaturation events during general anesthesia in children with and without upper respiratory infections. J Clin Anesth 4:200–203, 1992.
6. Williams OA, Hills R, Goddard JM: Pulmonary collapse during anaesthesia in children with respiratory tract symptoms. Anaesthesia 47:411–413, 1992.
7. Rieger A, Schroter G, Philippi W, et al: A comparison of sevoflurane with halothane in outpatient adenotomy in children with mild upper respiratory tract infections. J Clin Anesth 8:188–197, 1996.
8. Schreiner MS, O'Hara I, Markakis DA, Politis GD: Do children who experience laryngospasm have an increased risk of upper respiratory tract infection? Anesthesiology 85:475–480, 1996.
9. Borland L: Sinusitus in children. In Borland L (ed): Airway Management in Pediatric Anesthesia. Philadelphia, Lippincott-Raven, 1997.
10. Nandwani N, Raphael JH, Langton JA: Effect of an upper respiratory tract infection on upper airway reactivity. Br J Anaesth 78:352–355, 1997.
11. Tait AR, Pandit UA, Voepel-Lewis T, et al: Use of the laryngeal mask airway in children with upper respiratory tract infections: A comparison with endotracheal intubation. Anesth Analg 86:706–711, 1998.
12. Tait AR, Malviya S, Voepel-Lewis T, et al: Risk factors for perioperative adverse respiratory events in children with upper respiratory tract infections. Anesthesiology 95:299–306, 2001.

Elaine Broad, MD, and Anthony Lee, MD

PATIENT 34

A 68-year-old man with colon cancer scheduled for right hemicolectomy

A 68-year-old man with colon cancer is scheduled for a right hemicolectomy. He has a 35-pack-year smoking history, hypertension, gastroesophageal reflux disease, and chronic obstructive pulmonary disease (COPD). He has excessive daytime somnolence and is undergoing a sleep study for evaluation. He has been hospitalized three times in the last year for what he describes as *COPD exacerbations*. He had acute paralytic poliomyelitis in 1952 and recovered well with no clinical deficits but has noticed of late unexplained progressive atrophy and decreased strength of his right calf. He reports no anesthetic complications during prior surgeries. Current medications include 1 aspirin daily, lisinopril, hydrochlorothiazide, omeprazole, and an albuterol inhaler as needed. His is able to walk approximately 3 to 4 blocks without shortness of breath but is limited by arthritis.

Physical Examination: Pulse 82, respirations 20, blood pressure 178/82 mmHg, pulse oximetry 92% on room air, afebrile. General appearance: Well-appearing 80-kg man. Chest: Clear to auscultation with no wheezes, rales, or ronchi. Thoracic kyphosis present. Cardiac: normal S_1 and S_2 without murmurs. Airway: unremarkable.

Laboratory Findings: Hct 52%. Electrolytes, renal function, glucose, prothrombin time, partial thromboplastin time, and liver function tests all within normal limits. ECG: normal sinus rhythm.

Hospital Course: A thoracic epidural catheter placement was attempted to manage postoperative pain, but placement was unsuccessful secondary to kyphosis of the thoracic spine. During attempted epidural placement, the patient was given midazolam, 3 mg, and fentanyl, 100 μg, and he became somnolent, he developed snoring respirations, and his oxygen saturation decreased to 84%. He aroused with stimulation, the airway was supported with a chin lift, and oxygen was administered at 4 L/min by nasal cannula, resulting in improvement in oxygen saturation.

The patient received a general anesthetic induction, and intubation was nonincidental. He had a grade II airway, visible with direct laryngoscopy, and an 8.0 endotracheal tube was passed atraumatically through the vocal cords on the first attempt. A right radial arterial line was inserted, as was an additional large-bore peripheral intravenous catheter. The patient received 1500 mL of colloid and 3000 mL of crystalloid during the procedure; total blood loss was 500 mL, and urine output was adequate. At case conclusion, the patient was found to have one twitch with nerve stimulation and was reversed with neostigmine, 5 mg, and glycopyrrolate, 0.8 mg. The patient was breathing spontaneously and generating tidal volumes of 3 mL/kg; respirations were 25/min. Fentanyl was titrated to respiratory rate, and the patient was extubated when he could follow commands and showed a vigorous grip. Before extubation, thick secretions were suctioned from the pharynx and endotracheal tube. The patient was transferred to the postanesthesia care unit, but despite aggressive oxygen therapy via nonrebreather mask, he was dyspneic and could not maintain oxygen saturations around 90%. He subsequently was reintubated.

Questions: What is the cause of the patient's perioperative anesthetic complication?
What are the criteria for diagnosing this condition?
Discuss special considerations for patients with a history of APPM scheduled for surgery.
What are the specific perioperative respiratory concerns?

What is the cause of the patient's perioperative anesthetic complications? Postpolio syndrome.

What are the criteria for diagnosing postpolio syndrome (PPS)? There are an estimated 250,000 to 300,000 individuals in the United States alone who developed acute paralytic poliomyelitis (APPM) in the epidemic of 1940–1950. These individuals have deficits from their polio episode ranging from minimal symptoms to severe neuromuscular disability. All of these patients pose anesthetic challenges and must be approached in an individualized fashion.

Many patients have secondarily developed progressive muscular weakness and fatigue in skeletal and bulbar musculature. The symptoms of PPS usually develop 25 to 35 years after APPM. Initially described by Mulder in 1972, characteristics of PPS include:

1. A confirmed prior episode of acute poliomyelitis with residual motor neuron loss. This loss may not be clinically evident and may require close neurologic examination and electromyography.
2. A period >15 years of neurologic and functional stability after recovery from the initial acute illness.
3. Report of gradual onset of new muscle weakness, abnormal muscle fatigue, muscular atrophy, or generalized fatigue.
4. Exclusion of other conditions that could cause similar manifestations.

Although the mechanism of PPS is unknown, it is hypothesized that there is excessive metabolic stress on the remaining, unaffected neurons. Longterm follow-up of polio patients showed that there is about a 1% decrease in strength per year attributable to slow disintegration of the terminals of the individual axons.

Discuss special considerations for patients with a history of APPM scheduled for sugery. Of particular concern to the anesthesiologist are patients in whom bulbar muscle weakness develops. These patients suffer from pharyngeal muscle weakness, dysphagia, chronic aspiration, and laryngeal dysfunction secondary to unilateral or bilateral vocal cord paralysis. A traumatic intubation could lead to devastating consequences in these patients, and their induction and intubation plan should be approached conservatively.

About a quarter of patients with PPS have sleep apnea, and sleep disturbances in a patient with a history of APPM must be evaluated with this in mind. Central sleep apnea may be secondary to dysfunction of brainstem neurons; obstructive sleep apnea may be due to oropharyngeal muscle weakness. These patients also may hypoventilate secondary to intercostal and diaphragmatic weakness. Untreated sleep apnea can lead to hypoxemia, hypercarbia, polycythemia, pulmonary hypertension, and right heart failure. Patients with a history of APPM and COPD exacerbations should have PPS with bulbar involvement suspected.

Besides symptoms attributable to the initial attack of APPM, when interviewing these patients, it is appropriate to inquire about swallowing or voice difficulties, fatigue, muscle atrophy, cold intolerance, and joint pain (suggesting loss of muscular stabilization to joints). Patients with PPS also may have developed significant vertebral curvatures. Polio patients with scoliosis regularly have a more significant degree of pulmonary functional impairment compared with other scoliotic patients. Pulmonary function tests in PPS patients often show a combined mixed and obstructive pattern of disease and are difficult to interpret.

What are specific perioperative respiratory concerns? Important perioperative concerns in patients with PPS include prevention of aspiration and vocal cord damage associated with airway management, particularly in patients with known preexisting vocal cord dysfunction. Succinylcholine may be ill advised in patients with residual motor impairment from APPM because hyperkalemia may result. Patients in whom succinylcholine is used are likely to experience intense muscle pain postoperatively and should be forewarned. Patients with a history of PPS may be sensitive to nondepolarizing muscle relaxants to the degree that doses may need to be halved, and neuromuscular monitoring is essential. The postoperative period is of particular concern because laryngeal dysfunction and vocal cord dysfunction may lead to airway obstruction and respiratory insufficiency, requiring urgent reintubation. Strict extubation criteria should be met before extubation, although this does not guarantee an uncomplicated postextubation course.

The Present Patient

The present patient remained intubated overnight. He underwent standard weaning protocols the next day and was extubated without difficulty.

Clinical Pearls

1. Patients with PPS may have vocal cord dysfunction, chronic aspiration, and pulmonary hypertension and be an anesthetic challenge preoperatively, intraoperatively, and postoperatively.

2. Postoperative recovery of patients with PPS may be complicated by ventilatory failure secondary to neuromuscular weakness, inability to generate effective coughs, thoracic deformity, dysphagia, or obstructive apnea. These patients may need to be reintubated.

3. Dysphagia can occur in patients with a history of APPM but without a history of bulbar involvement and may increase the risk of aspiration significantly.

4. Patients with a history of APPM reporting frequent unexplained pulmonary infections warrant a complete swallowing study to rule out dysphagia and chronic aspiration.

5. Patients with PPS may be sensitive to nondepolarizing relaxants; these medications should be titrated based on neuromuscular monitoring. Patients with significant motor impairment may develop hyperkalemia after succinylcholine administration.

REFERENCES

1. Janda A, Urschutz L: Postoperative respiratory insufficiency in patients after poliomyelitis. Anaesthetist 28:249, 1979.
2. Gyermek L: Increased potency of nondepolarizing relaxants after poliomyelitis. J Clin Pharmacol 1990:170–173, 1990.
3. Dalakas MC: The post-polio syndrome as an evolved clinical entity: Definition and clinical description. Ann N Y Acad Sci 753:68–80, 1995.
4. Macario A, Mackey S, Terris D: Bilateral vocal cord paralysis after radical cystectomy in a patient with a history of bulbar polio. Anesth Analg 85:1171–1172, 1997.
5. Jubelt B, Agre J: Characteristics and management of postpolio syndrome. JAMA 284: 412–414, 2000.
6. Lin MC, Liaw MY, Chen WJ, et al: Pulmonary function and spinal characteristics: Their relationships in persons with idiopathic and postpoliomyelitic scoliosis. Arch Phys Med Rehabil 82:335–341, 2000.
7. Mahgoub A, Cohen R, Rossoff L: Weakness, daytime somnolence, cough, and respiratory distress in a 77 year old man with a history of childhood polio. Chest 120:659–661, 2001.
8. Shaoxiong L, Modell J: Anesthetic management for patients with postpolio syndrome receiving electroconvulsive therapy. Anesthesiology 95:799–801, 2001.

Ken Swank, MD

PATIENT 35

A 54-year-old trauma patient with cardiovascular collapse

A 54-year-old woman presents to the operating room for washout and external fixation of an isolated open right tibial fracture sustained during an auto-pedestrian accident. The patient was admitted to the emergency department (ED) in mild shock, which rapidly responded to resuscitation with 2 L of IV isotonic crystalloid. A right internal jugular triple-lumen catheter was placed, and the patient remained hemodynamically stable through the balance of her 3-hour ED course.

Physical Examination: Pulse 84, respirations 16, blood pressure, 100/50 mmHg, arterial oxygen saturation 98% on 2 L oxygen by nasal cannula, central venous pressure 10. General appearance: Patient in minimal distress secondary to right lower extremity pain.

Laboratory Findings: Blood work unremarkable except for Hct 38.2% decreasing to 33%. Chest radiograph and abdominal ultrasound: no positive findings. Right lower extremity angiogram: no vascular injury. Right femoral arterial angiography sheath left in place.

Operative Course: Routine monitors are placed. The patient's 16G peripheral IV catheter is connected to a pressurized-heated fluid infusion system. Right femoral arterial blood pressure is monitored throughout the procedure. General endotracheal anesthesia is induced without difficulty in rapid sequence fashion, and an uneventful balanced general anesthetic is administered using desflurane, 60% nitrous oxide in oxygen, and fentanyl. The patient receives positive-pressure ventilation. Resuscitation continues during surgery guided by vital signs, central venous pressure, urine output, and serial arterial blood gas and hematocrit determinations and consists of 3 L of lactated Ringer's solution and 2 U of packed RBCs given for a hematocrit of 24%. Estimated blood loss during the procedure is 400 mL. The patient's metabolic status is improving as judged by decreasing base deficit (-3 mmol/L from -8 mmol/L), and the procedure is drawing to a close. Precipitously, acute severe cardiovascular deterioration ensues. Over seconds, the systolic blood pressure falls to 40 mmHg, a sinus tachycardia of 100 beats/min develops, end-tidal carbon dioxide decreases from 33 mmHg to 14 mmHg. The central venous pressure remains unchanged at 12 mmHg. Ventilatory parameters including peak airway pressure remain unchanged.

Questions: What is the diagnosis?
What immediate steps should be taken to resuscitate the patient?
Form a differential diagnosis.
How would you narrow the differential diagnosis?
Describe the pathophysiology of this condition.
Review other consequences of this condition.
In what other situations might this condition be a concern?
Describe the effect of (N_2O) in this setting.
Besides fluid and cardiotonic therapy, what other maneuvers might be of benefit after this acute episode?

What is the diagnosis? Iatrogenic venous air embolism.

What immediate steps should be taken to resuscitate the patient? Regardless of the exact diagnosis, prompt aggressive intervention is necessary. The clinician should immediately increase inspired oxygen concentration to 100%, turn off the volatile anesthetic, auscultate the chest and verify adequate ventilation, increase fluid resuscitation, consider administration of potent cardiotonic medications such as epinephrine, advise the surgeons, and call for assistance.

Form a differential diagnosis. Possible causes of acute intraoperative cardiovascular collapse, especially in a recently traumatized patient, include cardiac tamponade or tension pneumothorax. Myocardial infarction, anaphylaxis, hemolytic transfusion reaction, hypovolemia, severe anemia, and medications are other possibilities. An embolism of some type (e.g., thrombus, fat, air, foreign body) can produce sudden and dramatic cardiovascular collapse, and fat embolization is a well-described complication of long bone fractures.

How would you narrow the differential diagnosis? A central catheter was started in the ED, and the patient was maintained on 60% nitrous oxide (N_2O), which may accelerate development of a tension pneumothorax. Auscultation of the chest showed equal breath sounds, trachea was midline, and neck vein distention was absent. Although tension pneumothorax may be present despite seemingly normal breath sounds, before the precipitous event, tachycardia and hypoxemia had been absent, and these are two early signs of tension pneumothorax. Had tension pneumothorax continued to be a concern, inserting needles into the hemithoraces would have been accompanied by a rush of air out of the affected compartment, and vital signs likely would have stabilized. Because this was a case of isolated extremity trauma, pericardial tamponade was thought unlikely. Heart sounds were distinct, although an unusual murmur was discerned. Electrocardiographic abnormalities likely, although not invariably, would accompany myocardial ischemia or infarction. A transfusion or other anaphylactic reaction would have been accompanied by wheezing and perhaps cutaneous erythema, both of which were absent. No medications had been given recently. Intravascular volume status and anemia were issues continuously addressed throughout the case. Although sometimes the amount of occult blood loss is surprising, it usually presents in a gradual fashion, in contrast to this patient's event.

In this patient, it was quickly noted that the pressurized infusion system was empty of fluid, and an unknown quantity of air had been infused into the patient. The heart murmur detected earlier was believed to be the **mill wheel murmur** associated with an air embolus. Resuscitative measures as previously discussed were initiated, and epinephrine, 50 μcg was given after the IV line was fluid primed. At this point, the heart rate was 140 beats/min, and the blood pressure was 50/20 mmHg.

Describe the pathophysiology of VAE. VAE leads to precipitous cardiovascular impairment and has a mortality rate of approximately 30%. Bolus air LD_{50} volumes in humans are estimated to be 200 to 300 mL. Successful treatment requires rapid recognition. VAE may occur in two distinct ways. The first is when a large volume of air reaches the venous system as a bolus. This bolus moves to the right atrium and ventricle and immediately interferes with the normal functioning of the tricuspid and pulmonic valves, resulting in a *vapor lock* of the right heart, drastically reducing the forward flow. This severe decrease in cardiac output is accompanied by hypotension, tachycardia or bradycardia, decreased pulmonary arterial pressure, and perhaps increased central venous pressure.

The second way VAE may occur is by a slow entraining of air over a longer period of time—an *air infusion*. This type of VAE is associated more often with procedures such as sitting craniotomy. The pathophysiologic consequences are different from the large air bolus in that the small air bubbles pass through the right side of the heart and lodge in the pulmonary circulation. This results in progressive pulmonary embolization, creating increasing mechanical obstruction to pulmonary flow. Depending on the air infusion rate, signs of VAE may be delayed. Eventually, cardiovascular decompensation occurs as a result of progressive right ventricular overload. In contrast to what is observed with a large air bolus, pulmonary arterial and central venous pressures gradually increase in concert with gradual reductions in cardiac output. Dose-dependent hemodynamic effects begin in dogs at infusion rates of 0.5 mL air/kg/min with severe cardiovascular impairment occurring at rates >1.5 mL air/kg/min.

Review other consequences of VAE. Other consequences of VAE include paradoxical systemic embolization and adult respiratory distress syndrome (ARDS). Approximately 25% of normal patients have a patent foramen ovale, which in the setting of VAE may allow air to pass from the right to left atrium and from there into the systemic circulation. The worst complications involving paradoxical emboli are cerebral and myocardial infarction. In the setting of paradoxical embolization, there is some evidence that treatment with hyperbaric oxygen, which reduces bubble size, is beneficial. Initial work with artificial oxygen carriers, such as perfluorocarbon emulsions, shows some promise in hastening air bubble resorption and reducing ischemia distally.

Although air bubbles within the pulmonary vasculature are reabsorbed over 15 to 30 minutes, they directly irritate the endothelium, resulting in the release of inflammatory mediators. ARDS has been noted after VAE and may be secondary to release of these toxic compounds. Treatment of ARDS is usually supportive.

In what other situations might VAE be a concern? VAE can occur in many different settings. It has been reported during a host of different operative procedures, but sitting posterior fossa craniotomy is the most common. The incidence of VAE in this situation is reported to be 45% to 55%, which warrants the use of increased monitoring for VAE, such as precordial Doppler and consideration of placement of a right atrial large-bore multiorifice catheter for air aspiration. VAE can occur during central catheter placement and withdrawal or through a catheter that is improperly capped or defective. Placing the patient in Trendelenburg position before catheter placement or withdrawal can minimize VAE in these instances.

Iatrogenic VAE can occur with any type of pressurized IV infusion system. Commercially available rapid infusion systems include built-in air traps to prevent inadvertent infusion of air. These should not be relied on. VAE can be prevented completely during the use of these systems simply by removing the air from the IV fluids being infused before being placed in the infusor.

Describe the effect of N_2O on VAE. Because the severity of VAE depends on volume of air infused, the consequences of VAE occurring in the presence of N_2O are greater, and N_2O should be promptly discontinued. N_2O is much more soluble in blood than nitrogen (blood—gas partition coefficients of 0.46 and 0.013 respectively, which causes N_2O moves into air-filled body spaces 34 times faster than the nitrogen can leave. N_2O also expands the volume of blood-borne air bubbles dramatically; bubble volume can double in the presence of 50% N_2O.

Besides fluid and cardiotonic therapy, what other maneuvers might be of benefit after acute VAE? Placing the patient in a left lateral decubitus, head-down position (Durant's position) is attractive in theory because air would accumulate at the right ventricular apex and away from the outflow tract. Studies in dogs showed resuscitation outcome may be independent of position. Closed chest cardiac massage was shown to hasten the exit of air from the right ventricle and may be as effective as Durant positioning. Aspiration of air from the right atrium may be effective, provided that the proper catheter is already in place *and* in the correct position. The utility of this modality is much greater when air embolization is considered likely and is anticipated, such as for sitting craniotomies. The best catheter for this purpose is a large-bore multiorifice catheter positioned with its tip just distal to the superior vena cava–right atrial junction. Aspiration of other types of catheters, such as triple-lumen or pulmonary artery catheters, is ineffective. Because of its limited efficacy, placement of a multiorifice catheter in the acute setting should not supersede other treatments.

The use of positive end-expiratory pressure (PEEP) to treat VAE is controversial. Its efficacy in reducing the amount of air entering the blood seems limited, and removal of PEEP can increase right-to-left interatrial shunting, increasing the risk of paradoxical emboli. By impeding venous return, PEEP could worsen already impaired cardiac output.

The Present Patient

In the present patient, the N_2O was immediately turned off, and elimination increased with high-flow oxygen. The distal 16 G lumen of the triple-lumen catheter was aspirated without obtaining any air. Additional fluids and another 50 μg of epinephrine were given. The patient was turned to left lateral decubitus head-down position without effect. The patient was returned to supine position in preparation for closed chest cardiac massage, at which point the hemodynamic situation rapidly improved and within minutes had returned to baseline. The mill wheel murmur was no longer present. No paradoxical embolization or ARDS occurred as a result of this episode.

Clinical Pearls

1. VAE can lead to acute cardiovascular collapse and has significant mortality. A high index of suspicion is necessary for prompt identification and treatment.

2. Prevention is the best treatment for iatrogenic VAE. When using pressurized infusion systems, all air always should be removed from IV fluid bags before use. Trendelenburg position should be used when placing or removing central venous catheters.

3. In situations in which the risk of VAE is high, as in sitting craniotomy, increased monitoring for VAE, such as precordial Doppler ultrasound, should be used. Prior placement of a large-bore multiorifice catheter positioned for effective air removal should be considered. N_2O should not be used in these settings.

4. Treatments for VAE include identifying and eliminating the source of venous air, discontinuing N_2O if in use, aspiration of venous air if an appropriately positioned catheter is already in place, standard cardiopulmonary resuscitative measures, and position change to the left lateral head-down position.

5. Paradoxical systemic embolization may occur leading to long-term sequelae even after successful acute treatment. Hyperbaric oxygen therapy may be of benefit in this situation by reducing bubble size.

REFERENCES

1. Munson E: Effect of nitrous oxide on the pulmonary circulation during venous air embolism. Anesth Analg 50:785–793, 1971.
2. Adornato DC: Pathophysiology of intravenous air embolism in dogs. Anesthesiology 49:120–127, 1978.
3. Orebaugh S: Venous air embolism: Clinical and experimental considerations. Crit Care Med 20:1169–1177, 1992.
4. Black S: Venous air embolism. In Zornow MH, Prough DS (eds): Problems in Anesthesia. Philadelphia, Lippincott-Raven, 1997, pp 113–124.

Brian J. Hopkins, MD

PATIENT 36

A 54-year-old man undergoing left hemicolectomy

A 54-year-old man is scheduled for left hemicolectomy after a near-obstructing mass is found during colonoscopy. The patient has a history of well-controlled hypertension for which he takes atenolol and is otherwise healthy.

Physical Examination: General appearance: a healthy-appearing thin man. Temperature normal; pulse 62; respirations 14; blood pressure 142/88; SpO_2 98% on room air. Airway and cardiopulmonary examinations unremarkable.

The patient was brought to the operating room after insertion of a 16G intravenous catheter. The standard monitors were applied to the patient as he was preoxygenated. After administration of midazolam 2 mg and fentanyl 100 µg intravenously, the patient was induced with propofol 160 mg, paralyzed with rocuronium 50 mg, and intubated.

The surgery and postanesthetic recovery proceeded without incident. On postoperative day 3, the patient becomes febrile, tachypneic, tachycardic, and hypotensive and is transferred to the surgical intensive care unit, where fluid resuscitation is begun. Despite fluid therapy, the patient remains hypotensive and tachycardic. Radial artery and pulmonary arterial catheters are inserted.

Laboratory Findings: Pulmonary arterial pressure 35/17 mmHg; pulmonary arterial occlusion pressure 15 mmHg; cardiac index 4.3 L/min/m^2; systemic vascular resistance 450 dyne $\cdot$ sec $\cdot$ cm^{-5}.

Norepinephrine is administered at 0.1 µg/kg/min and titrated upward to maintain a mean arterial pressure of 70 to 80 mmHg. Blood cultures are sent, and the patient is started on empirical antibiotics. Over the next 24 hours, the patient's extremities are noted to be mottled and cool; serum lactate concentrations are increasing, urine output is decreased, and the patient's creatinine is increased to 1.6 mg/dL from a baseline value of 0.7 mg/dL.

Questions: What is the diagnosis?
What are the characteristics of endotoxic or septic shock?
What are major side effects associated with use of catecholamines in septic shock?
What beneficial effects have been reported with the use of vasopressin in the treatment of septic shock?
What are vasopressin's cellular mechanisms of action?

What is the diagnosis? Septic shock.

What are the characteristics of endotoxic or septic shock? Endotoxic shock is a syndrome of cardiovascular collapse and multiple organ failure in response to overwhelming infection. The central characteristic of septic shock is systemic vasodilation secondary to disordered vasoconstrictor and vasodilator processes. Excessive vasodilation is due to excess generation of nitric oxide and vasodilatory prostaglandins and activation of adenosine triphosphate (ATP)–sensitive potassium channels in vascular smooth muscle cells. Abnormalities in vasoconstrictor mechanisms have been less well examined, but vascular smooth muscle is poorly responsive to norepinephrine in the setting of septic shock.

What are major side effects associated with use of catecholamines in septic shock? Vasopressor catecholamines, such as norepinephrine, epinephrine, and dopamine, have been traditional treatments for severe hypotension in septic shock. These patients may develop adrenergic hyposensitivity, however, resulting in loss of catecholamine pressor effects leading to refractory hypotension. Catecholamine administration also carries with it significant toxicity. Norepinephrine increases tissue oxygen demand, decreases renal and mesenteric blood flow, increases pulmonary vascular resistance, and may produce tachyarrhythmias.

What beneficial effects have been reported with the use of vasopressin in the treatment of septic shock? Several studies showed beneficial effects when vasopressin was used in patients with septic shock. Arginine vasopressin is an endogenous peptide hormone secreted by the neurohypophysis in response to an increase in serum osmolality or a decrease in plasma volume. Vasopressin administration increases systemic vascular resistance and mean arterial blood pressure and usually is accompanied by a decrease in heart rate and mean pulmonary arterial pressure. Vasopressin is devoid of direct inotropic effects but improves myocardial perfusion, enhancing myocardial performance, and may have selective coronary vasodilatory effects. As opposed to norepinephrine and epinephrine, afferent renal arterioles are not vasoconstricted during vasopressin use, maintaining glomerular filtration, creatinine clearance, and urine output. Vasopressin does vasoconstrict efferent renal arterioles, a beneficial effect. Administration of vasopressin often results in significant reductions in norepinephrine infusion rates. Vasopressin also produces cerebral vasodilation.

What are vasopressin's cellular mechanisms of action? Proposed cellular mechanisms for vasopressin's effects include the following: (1) Stimulation of vascular smooth muscle V_1-receptors by vasopressin increases cytoplasmic ionized calcium; (2) blockage of activated ATP/potassium channels within the muscle cell membrane facilitates myocyte depolarization and vasoconstriction; (3) vasopressin attenuates endotoxin and interleukin-1β–stimulated generation of nitric oxide and its second messenger, cyclic guanosine monophosphate, inhibiting excessive arteriolar vasodilation; and (4) during endotoxemia, vasopressin enhances adrenergic responsiveness through stimulation of smooth muscle V_1-receptors.

The Present Patient

The patient was started on a vasopressin infusion of 0.04 U/min and simultaneously was weaned from norepinephrine while maintaining satisfactory perfusion pressures. The patient's urine output increased significantly, and serum creatinine decreased to 0.9 mg/dL. Blood cultures were positive for *Enterococcus faecalis,* and the patient was treated with the appropriate antibiotics. When the sepsis resolved, he was weaned successfully from the vasopressin infusion and subsequently transferred to the surgical ward. The patient was discharged home on postoperative day 9.

Clinical Pearls

1. Catecholamine-resistant hypotension is a severe and often fatal complication in patients with septic shock and severe multiple organ dysfunction syndrome.

2. Catecholamine infusions are used in this setting to maintain important organ infusion. Catecholamine use has several potential adverse effects, however, including increased tissue oxygen demand, decreased renal and mesenteric blood flow, increased pulmonary vascular resistance, and arrhythmias.

3. Vasopressin may be an important adjunct in the treatment of patients with septic shock because it causes vasodilation of cerebral, coronary, and pulmonary vasculature, while maintaining renal and mesenteric perfusion.

REFERENCES

1. Landry DW, Levin HR, Gallant EM, et al: Vasopressin deficiency contributes to the vasodilation of septic shock. Circulation 95:1122–1125, 1997.
2. Landry DW, Levin HR, Gallant EM, et al: Vasopressin pressor hypersensitivity in vasodilatory septic shock. Crit Care Med 25:1279–1282, 1997.
3. Malay MB, Ashton RC, Landry DW, et al: Low-dose vasopressin in the treatment of vasodilatory septic shock. J Trauma 47:699–703, 1999.
4. Dunser MW, Mayr AJ, Ulmer H, et al: The effects of vasopressin on systemic hemodynamics in catecholamine-resistant and postcardiotomy shock: A retrospective analysis. Anesth Analg 93:7–13, 2001.
5. Patel BH, Chittock DR, Russell JA, et al: Beneficial effects of short-term vasopressin infusion during severe septic shock. Anesthesiology 96:576–582, 2002.

Kristin Woodward, MD

PATIENT 37

A 5-year-old girl manifesting difficulty with oral opening during anesthetic induction

A 5-year-old girl is scheduled for bilateral ureteral reimplants secondary to vesicoureteral reflux. Her past medical history is significant for repeated hospital admissions because of recurrent pyelonephritis. She is otherwise healthy, is active, and has never had surgery. She is adopted.

Physical Examination: General appearance: shy-appearing, well-developed girl who cries when clinician enters the room. Weight 18 kg; height 105 cm. Temperature 37.1°C; Pulse 114; respirations 22; blood pressure 95/64; oxygen saturation 98% in room air. General physical examination, including HEENT and airway examination: unremarkable.

Laboratory Findings: Electrolytes and renal panel normal; hematocrit 43%.
The patient is given midazolam 0.5 mg/kg orally and brought to the operating room without difficulty. Inhalation induction is begun with progressively increasing sevoflurane concentrations while the monitors are placed. The child develops airway obstruction as the plane of anesthesia deepens, and assisting by mask ventilation proves difficult. Attempts to open the child's mouth to insert an oral airway prove almost impossible.

Questions: What is the cause of the child's airway obstruction?
Should the case continue or be cancelled?
Describe the underlying pathology in malignant hyperthermia (MH).
Review disease processes with an association with masseter muscle rigidity (MMR) and MH.
How should an operating room be prepared for a patient at risk?
What is the mechanism of action of dantrolene?
How should MH be recognized and treated?
What drugs are known to be safe and unsafe in MH-prone populations?
How should families of susceptible individuals be screened for MH?
What resources are available for patients with MH?

What is the cause of the child's airway obstruction? The diagnosis is masseter muscle rigidity (MMR).

As this child's airway obstructs and attempts to establish a patent airway prove difficult, it may not be immediately clear what is the cause. The child may have significant temporomandibular articular dysfunction or distinct anatomic abnormalities, but these likely would have been apparent on physical examination. Myopathies may have limited jaw motion as part of their complex, but this child has a healthy history. A concerning possibility is MMR. Also known as *trismus-masseter spasm,* MMR is jaw muscle rigidity associated with limb muscle flaccidity after the use of succinylcholine. Of pediatric anesthetic regimens including succinylcholine and inhalation agents, 1% may have associated MMR. Initially described by van der Spek, the mechanism is believed to be slow tonic masseter muscle fibers responding to depolarizing muscle relaxants with contracture. A spectrum in the severity of jaw tightness exists; somewhere within this spectrum lies the boundary above which the MH population exists. An exaggerated degree of jaw tightness has been called *jaws of steel,* and this degree might be described as exaggerated, prolonged, and tight. Patients who have MMR after succinylcholine use may have a 50% chance of developing MH. If MMR is associated with generalized muscular rigidity, the association with MH is absolute.

Should the case continue or be cancelled? This child developed MMR during an inhalation induction, not after receiving succinylcholine, increasing the child's likelihood of subsequently developing MH. The volatile anesthetic should be turned off, 100% oxygen should be administered, and the child should be treated expectantly for MH.

Had the child received succinylcholine and an inhalation agent, the decision to continue would be more circumstantial. The degree of jaw tightness is useful in deciding whether or not to proceed with the case. With jaws of steel, the procedure should be halted, particularly if the degree of spasm lasts for several minutes, and the patient should be monitored for further development of signs of MH. If there is a slight degree of tightness, the anesthesiologist, with a heightened awareness for developing MH, may continue using a nontriggering anesthetic, monitoring appropriately. The patient should be monitored for a rise in end-tidal carbon dioxide, increasing temperature, and tachycardia not otherwise explainable. Any patient showing these features should have potassium and creatine kinase checked and blood gas analysis for metabolic and respiratory acidosis. The urgency of the surgical procedure and personal or family history suggesting MH susceptibility may influence the decision to continue. Authorities recommend patients experiencing significant MMR undergo testing for MH.

Describe the underlying pathology in MH. MH is an autosomal dominant disorder with variable penetrance and is an ordinarily subclinical myopathy characterized by the inability of the sarcoplasmic reticulum to reuptake calcium, leading to an uncontrolled increase in muscle metabolism. The underlying defect is a mutation leading to an abnormal ryanodine receptor. This receptor is integral in maintaining acceptable intracellular calcium concentrations during the cycle of excitation coupling and relaxation. The defect results in failure to sequester calcium within the sarcoplasmic reticulum during muscular relaxation. Pathologic increases in intracellular calcium result in unbridled excitation (rigidity), increased aerobic and anaerobic metabolism, increased oxygen consumption, and increased heat production.

Review disease processes with an association with MMR and MH. Patients at risk for MMR and progression to MH include patients with a previous or family history of MH, central core disease, King-Denborough syndrome, Duchenne's muscular dysrophy and related muscular dystrophies, and myopathies. Disorders with a *possible* association with MH include sudden infant death syndrome, Smith-Lemi-Opitz syndrome, Charcot-Marie-Tooth syndrome, heatstroke, and mitochondrial cytopathies. In these patients, MH precautions always should be instituted, and a nontriggering anesthetic technique routinely should be used.

How should an operating room be prepared for a patient at risk? Concerning the anesthesia machine, anesthetic vaporizers must be removed, soda lime must be replaced, and fresh gas should purge a new disposable circuit disposable at a flow of 10 L/min for at least 10 minutes. Verifying absence of volatile anesthetics with an expired gas analyzer is helpful. Dantrolene, dextrose, and sodium bicarbonate should be available for intravenous administration. A method to cool a hot patient is recommended. Should a hypermetabolic event ensue, the anesthesiologist would need assistance to perform all necessary interventions.

What is the mechanism of action of dantrolene? Although the mechanism has not been characterized definitively, dantrolene reduces calcium release from the sarcoplasmic reticulum. It relaxes but does not totally paralyze skeletal muscle. Dantrolene is useful for preventing and treating MH episodes.

How should MH be recognized and treated?
The early signs of MH, unless the process is fulminant, are nonspecific and include tachycardia, tachypnea in spontaneously breathing patients, sweating, unstable blood pressure, cyanosis, skin mottling, increasing temperature, muscular rigidity, and arrhythmias.

Patients developing MH should have triggering agents discontinued and receive dantrolene 2 mg/kg every 5 minutes up to 10 mg/kg. Sodium bicarbonate 2 to 4 mEq/kg should be administered. Hyperthermia should be treated aggressively with cooling blankets and iced fluids; cooling to 38°C to 39°C is suggested to avoid hypothermic overshoot. Urine output should be monitored, and urine should be examined for myoglobin because rhabdomyolysis and acute tubular necrosis are features of MH. Blood gases, electrolytes, renal and hepatic function, coagulation profile, hemoglobin, and serum glucose should be studied. Arrhythmias may require treatment.

What drugs are known to be safe and unsafe in MH-prone populations?
The following table lists safe and unsafe drugs.

Unsafe Drugs	Safe Drugs
Volatile anesthetics	Amide anesthetics
Desflurane	Barbiturates
Enflurane	Calcium
Halothane	Dantrolene
Isoflurane	Ester anesthetics
Sevoflurane	Etomidate
	Ketamine
Muscle relaxants	Nitrous oxide
Succinylcholine	Nondepolarizing
	neuromuscular agents
	Opiates
	Propofol

How should families of susceptible individuals be screened for MH?
Measurement of creatine kinase is a basic screening tool. Creatine kinase elevation in a relative of a patient who had an MH episode suggests MH susceptibility. A finding of a normal creatine kinase on numerous occasions does not definitively establish MH nonsusceptability, however. A muscle biopsy and contracture study are necessary to characterize the individual further. Contracture responses also may be positive in individuals with other myopathies that bear no direct relationship to MH. In patients with concerning family histories, the best practice is to administer a nontriggering anesthetic and monitor the patient closely.

What resources are available for patients with MH?
The Malignant Hyperthermia Association of the United States (MHAUS) provides education for affected families. There is a 24-hour phone line for emergencies and a website, www.mhaus.org. Patients should be referred to this organization as soon as the diagnosis is suspected. The professional subsidiary of MHAUS is the North American MH Registry.

The Present Patient
The patient was treated as if she were developing MH. Volatile anesthesia was discontinued, and she was ventilated with 100% oxygen. She was given dantrolene 2 mg/kg, which was repeated every 5 minutes to a total of 6 mg/kg. The MMR improved after the third dose of dantrolene. She did not show further signs or symptoms of MH.

Clinical Pearls

1. MMR is common, particularly in pediatric patients immediately after the use of succinylcholine. The degree of rigidity is some indication of the likelihood that the patient may go on to develop MH. The degree of rigidity, urgency of the case, and patient and family history should dictate whether the anesthetic is continued.

2. Jaws of steel should be treated as MH syndrome. The anesthetic should be halted, and the patient should be monitored for signs and symptoms of MH. MH may develop postoperatively. Tachypnea is an early sign in spontaneously breathing patients.

3. In patients with a family history of poorly characterized anesthetic complications or perioperative death, it may be wise to administer regional anesthesia or a general anesthetic with nontriggering agents.

4. MH requires aggressive therapy. Many tasks are required, and one provider cannot reasonably achieve them all in a short time frame: Call for help!

REFERENCES

1. van der Spek AFL, Reynolds PI, Fang WB, et al: Changes in resistance to mouth opening induced by depolarizing and non-depolarizing neuromuscular relaxants. Br J Anaesth 64:21, 1990.
2. Albrecht A, Wedel DJ, Gronert GA, et al: Masseter muscle rigidity and non-depolarizing neuromuscular blocking agents. Mayo Clin Proc 72:329, 1997.
3. Gronert GA, Antognini JF, Pessah: Malignant hyperthermia. In: Miller RD (ed): Anesthesiology, 5th ed. New York, Churchill Livingstone, 2000, pp 1033–1052.
4. Rosenberg H: Testing for malignant hyperthermia. Anesthesiology 96:1, 2002.

Ron Valdivieso, MD

PATIENT 38

A 70-year-old man with respiratory depression

A 70-year-old man is scheduled to undergo a radical cystectomy for bladder cancer. He is otherwise healthy except for a long-standing history of sleep apnea, for which he uses a continuous positive airway pressure mask. He denies any allergies and uses only multivitamins and over-the-counter nonsteroidal antiinflammatory drugs on a regular basis.

Physical Examination: Unremarkable, including airway examination.

Laboratory Findings: Serum chemistries, hematology, and coagulation profiles normal. Resting ECG, sinus rhythm at a rate of 74 with normal axis and occasional premature atrial contractions. No ST segment abnormalities appreciated.

The patient consents to a combined regional and general anesthetic. Before induction, he receives intrathecal preservative-free morphine 1 mg through a 27G spinal needle at the L3–4 interspace. An epidural catheter is inserted and secured with 4 cm in the epidural space, and a test dosing is unremarkable. General anesthesia is induced, the patient is endotracheally intubated, and the balanced general anesthetic proceeds without incident. At the conclusion of an uncomplicated surgery, the patient emerges from anesthesia, is extubated, and is transferred to postanesthetic care in good condition. The remainder of postoperative day 0 is unremarkable, and the patient has no pain complaints.

On postoperative day 1, the patient starts complaining of increasing pain, especially while trying to ambulate. An epidural infusion of morphine 100 µg/mL in 0.0625% bupivacaine is started at 10 mL/h. A few hours later, he requests a "sleeping pill," and lorazepam 0.5 mg is administered orally.

During night rounds, the urology resident is unable to awaken the patient. His respiratory rate is 6 breaths/min, and his pulse oximeter reads 82% saturation on 3 L of oxygen via nasal cannula.

Questions: What do you think is the cause of the patient's presentation?
What are the different opioid receptors and their effects?
What is the relationship between µ receptors and respiratory depression?
Describe predisposing factors for respiratory depression after the use of neuraxial opioids
Is there a difference between opioids in their ability to cause respiratory depression after neuraxial administration?
Review the usual opioid doses for spinal and epidural administration.
Describe the treatment of a patient who has opioid-induced respiratory depression.

What do you think is the cause of the patient's presentation? Respiratory depression secondary to excessive epidural morphine, exacerbated by administration of benzodiazepines.

What are the different opioid receptors and their effects? Although opioids have been used for millennia, the locus of analgesic effects was not identified until the late 1960s. Yaksh and Rudy identified receptors within the dorsal horn of the spinal cord that, when bound with opioids, afforded excellent analgesia without producing many of the untoward side effects normally associated with the use of systemic preparations. Opioid receptors also are found in other areas of the central nervous system, including periaqueductal gray matter, locus caeruleus, and nuclei within the medulla, notably the nucleus raphes magnus, nucleus tractus solitarius, and nucleus ambiguus. These loci not only are responsible for the analgesic effect of opioids, but also, depending on the specific receptor that is activated, mediate the side effects that commonly arise from the use of these medications. There are at least three different types of opioid receptors, μ, κ, and δ, although there is conflicting evidence suggesting the existence of two other receptors (σ and ϵ). μ receptors are responsible for the analgesic effect and for pruritus, urinary retention, biliary spasm, and respiratory depression. Clinical and experimental studies showed a dose-related depression of ventilatory drive (responsiveness to carbon dioxide) and respiratory frequency. These are μ receptor–mediated events because reversal of these effects is noted after administration of the pure μ receptor antagonist, naloxone. κ receptors mediate the sedative effects of opioids and may be involved in respiratory depression, whereas δ receptors are associated with nausea and vomiting.

What is the relationship between μ receptors and respiratory depression? The principal opioid receptor responsible for analgesia and respiratory depression is the μ receptor. The are two types of μ receptors, μ_1 and μ_2. μ_1 has great affinity for opioids and is the major receptor responsible for analgesia. Activation of this receptor by morphine seems to stimulate ventilation. μ_2 receptors have a low affinity for opioids and depress ventilation. Because of the low affinity of the μ_2 receptor, smaller doses of opioids are bound preferentially to the high-affinity μ_1 receptors, and respiratory depression is relatively unlikely to occur. As opioid doses increase, however, and the high-affinity receptors are occupied, drug is available to occupy μ_2 receptors, and respiratory depression is more likely to occur. Opioid-induced respiratory depression has been noted after all forms of administration, including oral, intramuscular, intravenous, transdermal, mucosal, and neuraxial routes, and is noted especially in opioid-naive patients.

Multiple studies showed neuraxial opioids to provide better postoperative analgesia and patient satisfaction than systemic opioid therapy. The likelihood of respiratory depression and other side effects is least after neuraxial administration because the opioid doses required to achieve adequate analgesia are the least when given by this route. Nonetheless, there seems to be considerable trepidation among some health care providers to allow general use of neuraxial opioids after surgical or obstetric procedures. Perhaps this fear is due to the delayed nature of respiratory depression when opioids are so administered.

Describe predisposing factors for respiratory depression after the use of neuraxial opioids. The first approved opioid for intrathecal use was morphine. Intrathecal morphine was administered for multiple indications, including relieving cancer pain refractory to opioid therapy by other routes. The initial success with the use of neuraxial narcotics soon was followed by reports of severe respiratory depression. This situation could be explained partially by the fact that the initial patient population in whom spinal opioids were used was tolerant to opioids, and the doses that were reported as effective were extremely high. An extreme example, Saami reported using 20 mg of subarachnoid morphine in a hyperbaric solution without respiratory depression. A particular group of patients that seemed prone to respiratory depression were opioid-naive patients, particularly if other central nervous system depressants (benzodiazepines, neuroleptics, and opioids by other routes) were given concomitantly. Many of these reports of delayed respiratory depression mentioned doses of subarachnoid morphine that today are considered excessive, ranging from 3 to 5 mg. Other factors that may contribute to respiratory depression include dose, intrathecal as opposed to epidural administration, extremes of age, general poor health, concomitant administration of intravenous opioids or other central nervous system depressants, and respiratory disease, including sleep apnea.

In 1984, a large nationwide Swedish study found 19 cases of respiratory depression (defined as a respiratory rate <10 breaths/min) among 14,139 cases of *epidural* morphine administration, an incidence of 1:1,100 (0.09%). Four patients developed respiratory depression after 1,103 *intrathecal* morphine injections, an incidence of 1:275 (0.36%).

The doses used at that time were not significantly different from the ones in use today, (e.g., epidural morphine 4 mg and intrathecal morphine 0.2 to 0.8 mg). Most of the patients who experienced respiratory depression possessed multiple risk factors as described previously, were American Society of Anesthesiologists patient classes III and IV, had repeated doses of extradural opioids or general anesthesia, and may have received additional opioids by other routes. All cases of respiratory depression involved the use of morphine. Almost all of the respiratory events occurred within 12 hours of the last neuraxial injection of morphine. The authors concluded that surveillance for >12 hours seemed unnecessary, although there are a few cases in the literature of respiratory depression persisting for >24 hours.

Is there a difference between opioids in their ability to cause respiratory depression after neuraxial administration?   Morphine is hydrophilic, and owing to this morphine may not be bound up by lipid-rich tissues near the site of injection. It has the propensity to migrate rostrally to respiratory centers, and this is the proposed mechanism for morphine's delayed respiratory depression. Lipophilic drugs (e.g., as fentanyl and sufentanil) also produced respiratory depression after intrathecal injection, however, although in an immediate manner. Highly lipophilic opioids have a greater propensity to be absorbed systemically. It is well established that systemic levels of epidurally administered lipophilic opioids are no different when compared with the same drug administered intravenously. There is little difference in the potential for respiratory depression between equipotent doses of intravenous and epidural sufentanil or fentanyl.

Review the usual opioid doses for spinal and epidural administration.   Most institutions use either morphine or fentanyl as their neuraxial opioids. Concentrations usually range from 30 to 50 μg/mL for morphine and 2 to 10 μg/mL for fentanyl, with the concentration of bupivacaine ranging from 0.0625% to 0.125%, depending on the level at which the epidural catheter is inserted. After neuraxial opioids have been given, patients can be transferred to surgical wards, where proper training has been given to nursing and ancillary personal. Monitoring of respiratory rate and sedation scores should be recorded every hour for the first 2 hours the patient is on the floor, every 2 hours for the following 6 hours, and every 4 hours thereafter, until the infusion is discontinued. In the case of one-time administration of intrathecal opioids, the same parameters are monitored for 24 hours. When excessive sedation is noted, the anesthesia service should be contacted immediately and therapeutic measures instituted before further depression occurs.

Describe the treatment of a patient who has opioid-induced respiratory depression.   When encountering a patient experiencing respiratory depression, tailor the treatment to the magnitude of the symptoms. Somnolence and mild respiratory depression require a different response than apnea and cyanosis. Stimulate or support respiration to the extent necessary, maintain a patent airway, administer supplemental oxygen, and titrate opioid antagonists, keeping in mind that aggressive opioid reversal would render the patient in agony. Should pharmacologic reversal be chosen, the μ receptor antagonist naloxone can be administered in divided doses, followed by a continuous infusion if necessary. Usual initial bolus doses are in the range of 100 to 120 μg administered every few minutes until respiratory depression and excessive sedation are reversed. An infusion of naloxone may be initiated if believed necessary. A recommended starting point is 3 to 5 μg/kg/h, titrated to patient response. For sufentanil, antagonist doses are likely to be greater because of the opioid's high affinity for the μ receptor. If benzodiazepines have been given, flumazenil effectively reverses their sedative properties. The patient requires a closely monitored bed.

The Present Patient

When the respiratory depression was noted, the the patient's level of consciousness was vigorously increased. Oxygen saturation improved. The anesthesiologist on duty was called; the epidural infusion was stopped; nalaxone 100 μg was given twice over a 10-minute period with marked improvement in his condition; and the patient was transferred to the surgical intensive care unit, where a prophylactic continuous infusion of naloxone was started at 5 ug/kg/h.

The patient's mental and respiratory status improved overnight. He continued to have excellent pain relief even while receiving the naloxone infusion. He was transferred to the surgical ward that morning, and his epidural solution was changed to morphine 30 μg/mL in 0.1% bupivacaine at 8 mL/h. The epidural catheter was discontinued on the fourth postoperative day, and he was transitioned to oral opioids. The patient was discharged from the hospital without incident the next day.

Clinical Pearls

1. Opioids by any route may induce respiratory depression. There is a higher incidence of respiratory depression after intravenous opioid administration when compared with neuraxial opioid–related respiratory depression. The incidence of respiratory depression after neuraxial opioid administation is <1%.

2. Opioids administered by the neuraxial route provide superior analgesia. Use of intrathecal and epidural opioids should not be avoided out of concern for respiratory depression.

3. Certain scenarios potentiate the risk for respiratory depression after neuraxial opioids. Factors include opioid-naive patients, patients coadministered central nervous system depressants, extremes of age, poor general health, and respiratory diseases. Supplemental intravenous opioids also contribute to respiratory depression.

4. Patients can be monitored on routine nursing floors after neuraxial opioids have been given. Nurses and other personnel benefit from proper training and educational activities. Respiratory rate, oxygen saturation, and level of sedation should be monitored regularly although time intervals may increase in stepwise fashion.

5. Should respiratory depression be noted, the aggressiveness of therapy is tailored to the degree of symptoms.

REFENCES

1. Yaksh TL, Rudy TA: Studies on the direct spinal action of narcotics in the production of spinal analgesia in the rat. J Pharmacol Exp Ther 202:411, 1977.
2. Jones RDM, Jones JG: Intrathecal morphine: Naloxone reverses respiratory depression but not analgesia. B MJ 281:645–646, 1980.
3. Reiz S, Westberg M: Side effects of epidural morphine. Lancet 1:203–204, 1980.
4. Davies GK, Toulhurst-Cleaver CL, James TL: CNS depression from intrathecal morphine. Anesthesiology 52:280, 1980.
5. Reiz S, Ahlin J, Ahrenfeldt B, et al: Epidural morphine for postoperative pain relief. Acta Anaesth Scand 25:111–114, 1981.
6. Bromage P, Camporesi E, Durant P, et al: Rostral spread of morphine. Anesthesiology 56:431–436, 1982.
7. Odoom J, Sih IL: Respiratory depression after intrathecal morphine. Anesth Analg 61:70, 1982.
8. Rawal N, Wattwil M: Respiratory depression after epidural morphine—an experimental and clinical study. Anesth Analg 63:8–14, 1984.
9. Lamarche Y, Martin R, Reiher J, et al: The sleep apnoea syndrome and epidural morphine. Can Anaesth Soc J 33:231–233, 1986.
10. Rawal N, Arner S, Gustafsson LL, Allvin R: Present state of extradural and intrathecal opioid analgesia in Sweden: A national follow up survey. Br J Anaesth 59:791–799, 1987.
11. Cornish PB: Respiratory arrest after spinal anesthesia with lidocaine and fentanyl. Anesth Analg 84:1387–1388, 1997.
12. Fournier R, Gamulin Z, Van Gessel E: Respiratory depression after 5 μg of intrathecal sufentanil. Anesth Analg 87:1377–1378, 1998.
13. Dworzak H, Fuss F, Buttner T: Persisting respiratory depression following intrathecal administratation of morphine and simultaneous sedation with midazolam. Anaesthetist 48:639–641, 1999.

Kenneth M. Swank, MD

PATIENT 39

A 71-year-old man with acute onset of hypotension and tachycardia after percutaneous transluminal coronary angioplasty

A 71-year-old man presents with chest pain resulting from an acute anterior myocardial infarction. He had no other significant medical history. Initial treatment consisted of intravenous heparin and nitroglycerin, which failed to relieve the pain. He underwent emergent percutaneous transluminal coronary angioplasty, which successfully dilated two high-grade stenoses of the left anterior descending artery. The patient does well for several hours after the procedure but suddenly develops hypotension and tachycardia.

Physical Examination: SpO$_2$ 97% on 2-L nasal cannula. Heart rate 132; respirations 24; blood pressure 75/40 (radial arterial line) with pulsus paradoxus; General appearance: pale, confused. Neck examination: Jugular venous distention. Cardiac examination: rapid regular rhythm, tachycardia with distant heart sounds, no murmurs. Chest examination: lung fields clear. Extremities: Cool extremities with prolonged capillary refill.

Laboratory Findings: CBC, electrolytes, partial thromboplastin time: normal. ECG: sinus tachycardia. Chest radiograph: mildly enlarged globular-shaped heart with clear lung fields. Transthoracic echocardiogram: large pericardial effusion. Pulmonary artery pressure: 37/24 mmHg with an occlusion pressure of 18 mmHg; central venous pressure 22 mmHg.

Questions: What is the likely diagnosis?
Describe the pertinent anatomy and physiologic role of the pertinent structures.
What are the causes of acute deterioration?
Describe the pathophysiology of this condition.
What are the clinical manifestations?
How should this patient be optimized preoperatively?
Discuss the key issues affecting anesthetic management.

What is the likely diagnosis? Acute pericardial tamponade.

Describe the pertinent anatomy and physiologic role of the pertinent structures. The pericardium consists of two layers: the visceral pericardium, which is adherent to the epicardium, and the parietal pericardium, which is a tough, fibrous layer resistant to stretch in the acute setting. Normally, 15 to 25 mL of serous fluid is in the pericardial space. The physiologic roles of the pericardium are not clear, but it is thought that it limits cardiac size during acute volume overload, maintains optimal cardiac position and shape within the mediastinum, provides mechanical separation of the heart from other structures, augments cardiac diastolic filling, and plays a role in cardiac chamber interactions. At normal cardiac and pericardial fluid volumes, the pressure within the pericardial space is negative and is similar to the interpleural pressure at any given moment of the respiratory cycle. As the following Figure shows, the pericardium is compliant up to a certain volume, above which the compliance decreases markedly because of the indistensible nature of the parietal pericardium.

What are the causes of acute deterioration? Acute pericardial tamponade results from a sudden increase in intrapericardial pressure secondary to accumulation of fluid within the pericardium. In acute tamponade, the fluid is usually blood (hemopericardium), whereas in less acute tamponade situations, such as viral pericarditis, uremia, malignancy, and autoimmune diseases, the fluid is usually serous or serosanguineous. Causes of acute cardiac tamponade include penetrating and blunt chest trauma and aortic dissection. Iatrogenic causes include central venous catheter placement; cardiac surgery; pericardiocentesis; or any instrumentation of the heart such as catheterization, pacemaker lead placement, or transluminal angioplasty. Acute pericardial tamponade usually occurs within hours of the inciting event.

Describe the pathophysiology of this condition. The degree of hemodynamic impairment depends on the amount of fluid within the pericardium and the rapidity with which it accumulates. The increase in intrapericardial pressure impairs diastolic filling of all the cardiac chambers, with the thinner walled right atrium and right ventricle being the most affected. This impaired filling in turn leads to decreased stroke volume and cardiac output. Sympathetic reflexes initially maintain the blood pressure by increases in heart rate, inotropic state, central venous tone, and systemic vascular resistance. As intrapericardial pressure continues to increase, the pressures within all the cardiac chambers approach the intrapericardial pressure (equalization of pressures). At this point, compensatory mechanisms are exhausted, leading to decreased cardiac output, hypotension, and inadequate peripheral oxygen delivery. Myocardial oxygen balance, a particularly important consideration in the present patient with a recent myocardial infarction, is impaired severely by tamponade. Myocardial oxygen consumption is increased because of increased heart rate and inotropic state, whereas myocardial oxygen delivery is decreased by tachycardia, hypotension, and elevated left ventricular end-diastolic pressure.

What are the clinical manifestations? Acute pericardial tamponade classically manifests as hypotension, distended neck veins, and a quiet precordium and muffled heart sounds (Beck's triad). Patients are usually tachycardic and may complain of dyspnea or chest tightness. Pulsus paradoxus, a decrease in systolic blood pressure of ≥10 mmHg

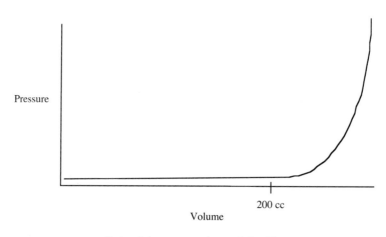

Pericardial pressure - volume relationship

during inspiration, is often present. Pulsus paradoxus may not be present in the face of severe hypotension, left ventricular dysfunction, atrial septal defect, or aortic valvular incompetence. There is usually no evidence of pulmonary edema, which differentiates tamponade from cardiogenic shock. The presence of tamponade not only elevates the central venous pressure, but also, by impairing ventricular filling, it diminishes or eliminates the y descent of the right atrial pressure waveform. The pericardial fluid collection may alter the ECG by decreasing QRS voltage or causing the appearance of electrical alternans, alternating high-voltage and low-voltage QRS complexes. The chest radiograph may show an enlarged cardiac silhouette, which in itself is not specific for tamponade unless the cardiac size is increased from that of previously obtained recent chest radiographs. These radiographs are often of limited use, however, in the diagnosis of tamponade because at least 250 mL of pericardial fluid must be present to enlarge the cardiac silhouette. Echocardiography is an excellent tool to diagnose tamponade. Not only can small amounts (15 mL) of pericardial fluid be visualized, but also it can provide information regarding impairment of diastolic filling and can guide percutaneous needle pericardiocentesis.

How should this patient be optimized preoperatively? Definitive treatment of acute pericardial tamponade consists of removal of accumulated pericardial fluid. Percutaneous subxiphoid pericardiocentesis is useful for temporary drainage and usually can be done rapidly. A small drainage catheter may be placed into the pericardial space to allow for more prolonged drainage. If the tamponade is due to trauma, however, pericardiocentesis is a temporary measure because surgical exploration is almost always necessary. Because of the nature of the pericardial pressure-volume relationship, the removal of even a small amount of fluid may result in significant hemodynamic improvement. For this reason, pericardiocentesis always should be considered before anesthetic induction for definitive surgical drainage. Other treatment consists of aggressive intravenous volume expansion and inotropic support.

Discuss the key issues affecting anesthetic management. Although many different anesthetic techniques may be used under these circumstances, minimizing negative anesthetic effects on an already impaired cardiovascular system is crucial. Subxiphoid and left anterior thoracotomy are the two most commonly used surgical approaches. Local anesthesia is useful for patients undergoing subxiphoid pericardiotomy and is the preferred approach in hypotensive patients. The dissociative anesthetic ketamine, administered intravenously in small divided doses, is useful for sedation and analgesia in this situation.

Ketamine also is a good choice for general anesthetic induction because it is more likely to maintain sympathetic tone, heart rate, and peripheral vascular resistance than other induction agents. General anesthesia adversely affects all of the compensatory mechanisms maintaining blood pressure during tamponade, and induction of anesthesia in this situation may result in extreme hypotension or cardiac arrest or both. In addition to the adverse effects of anesthetic drugs, positive-pressure ventilation further reduces venous return to the heart and can exacerbate any existing hypotension. For this reason, positive end-expiratory pressure should be avoided. Awake intubation with maintenance of spontaneous respiration may be useful in this situation to avoid the adverse effects of positive-pressure ventilation.

Because of the potential for dramatic hemodynamic deterioration on general anesthetic induction, the patient should be prepared and draped, and the surgeons should be ready to perform thoracotomy before induction. Preinduction arterial pressure monitoring is essential. In a patient with significant prior cardiac disease, pulmonary arterial pressure monitoring is a consideration to aid in assessment and manipulation of intravascular volume and selection and dosing of inotropic drugs. Because central venous pressure and pulmonary arterial occlusion pressure equalize with the intrapericardial pressure in severe tamponade, however, the utility of this information may be limited. Maximizing preload before induction is important, as is the immediate availability of inotropic drugs and other resuscitation equipment, including a cardiac defibrillator.

The Present Patient

The diagnosis of acute pericardial tamponade was verified by transthoracic echocardiography shortly after the onset of the hypotension. Pericardial fluid was present and was impairing right atrial filling. Systolic cardiac function seemed normal except for mild hypokinesis of the anterior left ventricle. After several unsuccessful attempts at percutaneous, echocardiographically guided pericardiocentesis, an emergent pericardial window was planned. Intravenous fluid expansion was the initial treatment for the hypotension. Dopamine 10 µg/kg/min was added for inotropic support before arrival in the operating room. A radial arterial catheter was already in place. Before induction, a large-bore peripheral IV catheter was placed, and the patient was positioned, prepared, and draped. Ketamine 1 mg/kg and succinylcholine were administered in rapid-sequence fashion to induce general anesthesia. After intubation of the trachea, intermittent small doses of ketamine (10 to 20 mg) and fentanyl 1 μg/kg were used for anesthetic maintenance until a subxiphoid pericardial window relieved the patient's hemopericardium, with immediate dramatic hemodynamic improvement. At this point, isoflurane safely replaced ketamine as the anesthetic agent. The patient was transferred to the intensive care unit in stable condition with a pericardial drain in place. Pericardial drainage was minimal postoperatively. The patient was discharged home 10 days postoperatively.

Clinical Pearls

1. The rapid accumulation of fluid within the pericardium can cause dramatic hemodynamic compromise by limiting cardiac filling, resulting in cardiac tamponade. Acute cardiac tamponade caused by blood within the pericardium can occur secondary to penetrating or blunt chest trauma and iatrogenic causes.

2. Cardiac tamponade decreases cardiac output, resulting in shock. Hallmarks of tamponade include shock with jugular venous distention, pulsus paradoxus (a >10 mmHg decrease in systolic blood pressure during inspiration), and no evidence of pulmonary edema.

3. Drainage of the pericardial fluid (even small volumes) results in improvement and is the primary treatment. Fluid administration to maximize preload and inotropic support are temporizing therapies.

4. Surgical drainage via pericardial window is often necessary. Percutaneous pericardiocentesis should be done to improve the hemodynamic status before anesthetic induction. Local anesthesia with judicious sedation is the preferred technique. If general anesthesia is required, extreme care must be taken to minimize the negative hemodynamic effects of anesthetic drugs and positive-pressure ventilation. Because of the high expected degree of hemodynamic instability in these situations, arterial pressure monitoring is essential.

REFERENCES

1. Lake CL: Anesthesia and pericardial disease. Anesth Analg 62:431–443, 1983.
2. Spodick DH: Pericarditis, pericardial effusion, cardiac tamponade, and constriction. Crit Care Clin 5:455–476, 1989.
3. White JB, Macklin S, Studley JG, et al: Cardiac tamponade: A review of diagnosis and anaesthetic and surgical management illustrated by three case reports. Ann R Coll Surg Engl 20:386–390, 1988.
4. Reddy PS, Curtiss EI: Cardiac tamponade. Cardiol Clin 8:627–637, 1990.

Anthony Lee, MD

PATIENT 40

A 55-year-old woman develops a dysrhythmia

A 55-year-old woman presents for an appendectomy. She is otherwise healthy. Her only complaints are left lower quadrant pain and nausea, for which she received 1.25 mg of droperidol IV in the emergency department. The patient states she ate a cheeseburger 2 hours ago. Recently she developed a sore throat, for which her primary care physician prescribed erythromycin, and she has been taking this for 6 days. The patient denies any history of palpitations, coronary artery disease, syncope, or irregular heart rhythms. An uncomplicated open reduction and internal fixation of the right ankle was done 3 years previously under spinal anesthesia.

Physical Examination: Temperature 38.9°C; heart rate 95; respirations 20/min; blood pressure 123/71; and oxygen saturation of 96%. Abdominal examination: decreased bowel sounds and left lower quadrant pain with rebound tenderness.

Laboratory Findings: Electrolytes: all normal except for a magnesium level of 1.2 mEq/L (normal range 1.3 to 1.9 mEq/L). ECG: sinus rhythm at 71 beats/min with Q-T interval of 0.54 second (normal <0.45 second) and Q-T dispersion of 66 msec (normal range 20 to 50 msec). A 1-mm U wave is seen in lead V2. Previous ECG from 6 months prior does not show these changes.

General endotracheal anesthesia is initiated without complications with thiopental, fentanyl, and succinylcholine. While the patient's abdomen is being prepared, precordial lead V shows elongation of the Q-T interval to 0.6 second and a bradycardia of 35 beats/min with a blood pressure of 100/50 mmHg. Before any intervention is taken, the patient's rhythm changes to what is shown below.

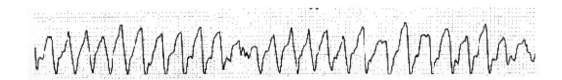

Questions: Diagnose the rhythm disturbance.
What are the causes of this rhythm disturbance?
What ECG changes favor the development of this dysrhythmia?
Which of this patient's medications predispose to the development of this dysrhythmia?
What other medications have been implicated in the development of this dysrhythmia?
Discuss the electrolyte abnormalities that play a role in the pathogenesis of this dysrhythmia.
What is the treatment?
Are there congenital causes for Q-T prolongation, and how is their treatment different from that for acquired Q-T syndromes?
Does epidural or spinal anesthesia carry less risk in people with a prolonged Q-T interval?

Diagnose the rhythm disturbance. Torsades de pointes.

What are the causes of this rhythm disturbance? Torsades de pointes is a polymorphic ventricular tachycardia that shows a peculiar ECG pattern characterized by a continuous twisting in QRS axis around an imaginary baseline. Torsades de pointes most likely is caused by early after-depolarizations, which are depolarizations of the transmembrane voltage occurring during the plateau phase (phase 2) or early rapid depolarization phase (phase 3) of the Purkinje fiber or ventricular muscle action potentials. Decreasing net outward potassium current or increasing net inward sodium or calcium current during phase 2 delays depolarization and causes Q-T prolongation. An increased Q-T interval is a risk factor for torsades de pointes, but for a gross index of electrical instability, a better estimate of dysrhythmia susceptibility may be represented by the dispersion of depolarization. Dispersion of repolarization can be assessed on ECG by comparing the duration of Q-T interval in all 12 leads. The way to quantify this is to compare the difference between the longest and the shortest Q-T intervals. The larger the variability in Q-T interval between leads, the more disperse the activation of the myocardium, and the more likely torsades de pointes is to develop. The development of these ECG changes depends on several factors. Certain medications and electrolyte abnormalities are synergistic in the development of torsades de pointes.

What ECG changes favor the development of this dysrhythmia? Favorable conditions include bradycardia, Q-T elongation (specifically dispersion of elongated Q-T intervals), and prominent U waves.

Which of this patient's medications predispose to the development of this dysrhythmia? This patient received droperidol in the emergency department and had been taking erythromycin for 6 days. Butyrophenones such a droperidol and haloperidol produce Q-T elongation and afterde-polarizations, which are thought to be part of the underlying mechanism for torsades de pointes. Macrolide antibiotics such as erythromycin block depolarizing potassium currents and exhibit similar effects of class I antiarrhythmic agents.

What other medications have been implicated in the development of this dysrhythmia? Class I antiarrhythmic agents, such as quinidine, disopyramide, and procainamide, predispose patients to torsades de pointes. Prevalence of tor-sades de pointes in quinidine-treated patients has been estimated to range from 1.5% to 8%. These drugs block sodium channels and prolong the Q-T interval. Vasopressin and tricyclic antidepressants also have been implicated.

Several anesthetic agents predispose patients to the development of torsades de pointes. Thiopental has been shown to elongate the Q-T interval more than propofol. Succinylcholine prolongs the Q-T interval by stimulating simultaneously parasympathetic and sympathetic ganglia, resulting in imbalanced cardiac innervation. Precurarization has been shown to prevent this effect. Volatile anesthetics, particularly halothane, but also isoflurane and sevoflurane, may prolong Q-T intervals and predispose patients to torsades de pointes secondary to alterations in calcium and potassium channel currents in the myocardium. Other agents that may be synergistic in causing torsades de pointes include large doses of opioids, β-blockade, or insufficient anticholinergic dosing after muscle relaxant reversal. Any medication that produces bradycardia can predispose to torsades de pointes.

Discuss the electrolyte abnormalities that play a role in the pathogenesis of this dysrhythmia. Hypokalemia, hypomagnesemia, and hypocalcemia have been implicated in the development of torsades de pointes. Hypocalcemia prolongs repolarization, whereas hypokalemia and hypomagnesemia prolong the Q-T interval and produce prominent U waves.

What is the treatment? Initial treatment is to discontinue any offending agents. Electrolyte disturbances, including hypokalemia, hypomagnesemia, and hypocalcemia, are corrected. Magnesium sulfate 2 to 3 g IV may terminate and prevent recurrence of drug-induced torsades de pointes. If magnesium treatment is ineffective, cardiac pacing should be initiated. Pacing at a rate of 90 to 100 beats/min shortens the action potential, preventing early afterdepolarizations.

Are there congenital causes for Q-T prolongation, and how is their treatment different from that for acquired Q-T syndromes? Two congenital conditions, Romano-Ward syndrome and Jervell and Lange-Nielsen syndrome, are associated with torsades de pointes. These patients have episodes of torsades de pointes that result in syncope and sudden cardiac death. In contrast to patients with acquired prolonged Q-T syndromes, torsades de pointes episodes in patients with congenital prolonged Q-T syndromes are treated with β-blockers. Patients with congenital prolonged Q-T syndromes are at risk of torsades de pointes with sympathetic stimulation because they fail to shorten appropriately the Q-T interval with sympathetic stimulation. When these patients are refractory to β-blockade, left cardiac sympathetic denervation may be considered. This intervention involves the ablation of the lower part of the left stellate ganglion and the first four or five thoracic ganglia.

Does epidural or spinal anesthesia carry less risk in people with a prolonged Q-T interval? In patients with an acquired prolonged Q-T interval, epidural or spinal anesthesia may result in bradycardia from sympathetic blockade or vagal predominance. Bradycardia or vagal predominance predisposes patients to further Q-T interval elongation, which places them at further risk for the development of torsades de pointes. The way to combat this problem is to volume load patients and limit the height of sympathetic block. In patients with congenital prolonged Q-T syndrome, epidural or spinal anesthesia is beneficial. As noted earlier, these patients are at risk of torsades de pointes with sympathetic stimulation because they fail to shorten appropriately the Q-T interval with sympathetic stimulation. With high thoracic sympathetic block, these patients are protected against adrenergic stimulation.

The Present Patient

The anesthesiologist treated the patient with 1 g of magnesium sulfate in two boluses over 4 minutes for a total of 2 g. The patient's torsades de pointes subsided 5 minutes after onset, and the procedure was completed with no complications.

Clinical Pearls

1. The most significant risk factor for the development of torsades de pointes is Q-T interval prolongation.

2. Often, Q-T interval prolongation evolving into torsades de pointes is caused by the synergistic interaction of medications, electrolyte abnormalities, and sympathetic blockade. Medications implicated include macrolide antibiotics, butyrophenones such as droperidol and haloperidol, vasopressin, tricyclic antidepressants, induction agents, volatile anesthetics, and succinylcholine. Electrolyte abnormalities implicated are hypomagnesemia, hypokalemia, and hypocalcemia.

3. Initial treatment of torsades de pointes is magnesium sulfate 2 to 3 g IV. This treatment is effective in treating and suppressing recurrence of drug-induced torsades de pointes. In patients who are refractory to this treatment, cardiac pacing is recommended.

REFERENCES

1. Tzivoni D, Banal S, Shuger C, et al: Treatment of torsades de pointes with magnesium sulfate. Circulation 7:392–397, 1988.
2. Schmeling W, Warltier D: Prolongation of the QT interval by enflurane, isoflurane, and halothane in humans. Anesth Analg 72:137–144, 1991.
3. Schwartz J, Locati, H, Moss J: Cardiac sympathetic denervation in the therapy of the congenital long QT syndrome: A worldwide report. Circulation 84:503–511, 1991.
4. Wilt J, Minnema M, Johnson F, et al: Torsades de pointes allocated with the use of intravenous haloperidol. Ann Intern Med 119:391–394, 1993.
5. Napolitano C, Priori S, Scwartz J, et al: Torsades de pointes mechanisms and management. Drugs 47:51–65, 1994.
6. Faigel D, Metz, D, Kockman M, et al: Torsades de pointes complicating the treatment of bleeding esophageal varices: Association with neuroleptics, vasopressin, and electrolyte Imbalance. Am J Gastroenterol 90:822–824, 1995.
7. Kazuo A, Takada K, Yoshiya I, et al: Intraoperative torsades de pointes ventricular tachycardia and ventricular fibrillation during sevoflurane anesthesia. Anesth Analg 86:701–702, 1998.
8. Lustik S, Eichelberger J, Chibber A, et al: Torsades de pointes during orthoptic liver transplantation. Anesth Analg 87:300–303, 1998.

Mark H. Chandler, MD
Howard J. Miller, MD

PATIENT 41

A 38-year-old woman with postintubation stridor

A 38-year-old, 79-kg woman presents for total abdominal hysterectomy under general anesthesia. Past medical history is significant for intermittent use of tobacco and a remote history of asthma. She has no known drug allergies, and her medications include a multivitamin and an albuterol metered-dose inhaler, which she uses only 1 to 2 times per year. Past surgical history is significant only for an appendectomy, under general anesthesia, without complication.

Physical Examination: Vital signs unremarkable. Patient was quite anxious about upcoming surgical procedure. No wheezing detected on auscultation of the chest.

The patient underwent a general anesthetic. After induction with propofol and demonstration of easy mask ventilation, fentanyl and vecuronium were administered. The patient was intubated easily with a 7.0 endotracheal tube and maintained on oxygen, isoflurane, vecuronium, and fentanyl. The surgery concluded uneventfully, and the patient's neuromuscular blockade was reversed with neostigmine and glycopyrrolate. When the patient was awake and responsive and able to sustain a 5-second head lift, she was suctioned, extubated, and transported to the postanesthesia care unit (PACU) on 4 L/min of oxygen per nasal cannula without incident. After 15 minutes in the PACU, the patient is noted to be extremely anxious and uncooperative, is stridorous, and is pointing to her larynx.

Questions: What form of stridor has been noted in recently intubated patients with psychiatric disease and perioperative anxiety?

What is the differential diagnosis of stridor after general endotracheal anesthesia?

Review the natural history of this unusual form of postoperative stridor.

This form of stridor has a unique treatment. What is the treatment, and why is it effective?

Describe a stepwise treatment algorithm for a stridorous patient.

What form of stridor has been noted in recently intubated patients with psychiatric disease and perioperative anxiety? Paradoxical vocal cord motion (PVCM).

What is the differential diagnosis of stridor after general endotracheal anesthesia? Immediately after extubation, the differential diagnosis for stridor includes laryngospasm, laryngeal or pulmonary edema, residual neuromuscular blockade, oversedation, foreign-body aspiration, and vocal cord dysfunction.

Review the natural history of this unusual form of postoperative stridor. PVCM is a relatively rare syndrome that is known by many other names, including episodic paroxysmal laryngospasm, paradoxical vocal fold movement/adduction, pyschogenic stridor, functional stridor, hysterical stridor, Munchausen stridor, emotional laryngeal wheezing, and spasmodic croup. Rogers and Stell first described two cases of PVCM in 1978, but the syndrome probably has been seen for years in recovery rooms and other settings masquerading as acute airway obstruction or acute bronchospasm. When an episode of PCVM begins, the patient often presents with choking, stridor, and wheezing on inhalation (rather than on exhalation, distinguishing it from asthma). Often the patient points to the larynx as the site of the problem. Given the frequency of PVCM in the recovery room, it seems that mechanical vocal cord stimulation, such as that from intubation and extubation, may trigger this disorder. Frequently, PVCM presents in the emergency department, where it commonly is misdiagnosed as an acute exacerbation of asthma. There seems to be a pyschogenic component to PVCM, and in some patients, PVCM may represent a formal conversion reaction.

Although a comprehensive study of PVCM patients has not been undertaken, an emerging pattern from various case reports is apparent. These patients share the following qualities: Most are female, <40 years old, and with a history of respiratory complaints (chiefly asthma) and psychiatric stress–related conditions. Some authors also observed that many PVCM patients have jobs in the health care industry. It is important to consider this syndrome in any stridorous patient; although PVCM is a diagnosis of exclusion, and any such patient is likely to receive some form of nebulized therapy, episodes of reintubation might be avoided with accurate diagnosis.

The pathophysiology of PVCM is unclear. The vocal cords paradoxically adduct on inspiration, causing either a partial or complete obstruction of the airway at the glottis. Patients with PVCM have shown extrathoracic airflow obstruction during inspiration on a spirometric flow volume loop. With a fiberscope, Collett evaluated the glottic area and pulmonary resistance in patients with PVCM during normal breathing, stridorous episodes, and passive breathing and found glottic narrowing and increased pulmonary resistance only during active stridorous inspiration. In a pattern pathognomonic for PVCM, the anterior two thirds of the vocal cords adduct during inspiration, leaving a diamond-shaped glottic chink or gap in the posterior one third of the cords. Collett speculated that PVCM is due to a *phase reversal* between the activity of inspiratory neurons and that of laryngeal motor neurons. What exactly triggers this phase reversal is unclear.

This form of stridor has a unique treatment. What is the treatment, and why is it effective? Benzodiazepines have proved to be an effective treatment for PVCM, reinforcing the belief that there is a psychogenic component to the disorder; however, benzodiazepines in this setting may have more than one action. Benzodiazepines attenuate the Kratschmer reflex, a protective reflex evoked by chemical or mechanical stimulation of the larynx and hypopharynx, resulting in temporary closure of the vocal cords. Centrally acting benzodiazepines may help treat PVCM not only by sedating an anxious patient, but also by attenuating this reflex.

Describe a stepwise treatment algorithm for a stridorous patient. The treatment begins with an assessment of adequate airway patency and oxygenation and ventilation. If oxygenation and ventilation are not adequate, stepwise treatment, including selective nebulized therapy, continuous positive airway pressure, bag-and-mask ventilation with 100% oxygen, administering small doses of succinylcholine in an effort to relax the vocal cords, and intubation of the trachea or surgical airway, must proceed. As always, the degree of intervention is a function of the gravity of the situation. If the patient is in minimal respiratory distress and cooperative, and the diagnosis of PVCM is thought likely, the patient should be reassured; some authors suggest panting, sniffing, and breath holding may be beneficial. Inhaled corticosteroids are not recommended because they only further irritate the airway. Pathognomonic findings on fiberscopic laryngoscopy confirm the diagnosis of PVCM. When diagnosed, sedation should be administered in an attempt to relieve symptoms.

The Present Patient

The patient first was thought to have had either an acute exacerbation of her asthma or postextubation laryngospasm. Despite the fact that this patient was agitated and tachypneic, oxygen saturations were satisfactory. Auscultation determined that the patient was moving air and not wheezing, and the patient was able to phonate. There was a small, intermittent element of paradoxical movement of the chest, suggesting a degree of upper airway obstruction. Nebulized racemic epinephrine failed to improve the stridor. Because of the atypical clinical picture, an ENT surgeon was consulted to perform flexible fiberscopic laryngoscopy, and PVCM was identified. The patient was verbally reassured, and her condition improved almost immediately after administering midazolam 2 mg. After her symptoms resolved, the patient revealed she had been under an intense amount of emotional strain over the prior weeks and that she had been particularly anxious about this surgery. She experienced no further episodes of stridor in the PACU and was discharged from the hospital 2 days later without further incident.

Clinical Pearls

1. The first step in dealing with acute airway obstruction is to ensure adequate oxygenation and ventilation by whatever means necessary.

2. After ensuring an adequate airway, more common and worrisome causes of postoperative stridor are ruled out, including residual neuromuscular blockade, oversedation, foreign-body aspiration, bronchospasm, or pulmonary or laryngeal edema.

3. Although rare, PVCM must be considered after other causes of stridor are ruled out, especially in a patient with a history of respiratory complaints or psychiatric disorders, to prevent unnecessary and sometimes harmful interventions.

4. Benzodiazepines are the drug of choice for PVCM because of their anxiolysis and their attenuation of airway reflexes.

REFERENCES

1. Rogers JH, Stell PM: Paradoxical movement of the vocal cords as a cause of stridor. J Laryngol Otol 92:157–158, 1978
2. Collett PW, Brancatisano T, Engel LA: Spasmodic croup in the adult. Am Rev Respir Dis 127:500–504, 1983.
3. Hammer G, Schwinn D, Wollman H: Postoperative complications due to paradoxical vocal cord motion. Anesthesiology 66:686–687, 1987.
4. Michelson LG, Vanderspek AF: An unexpected functional cause of upper airway obstruction. Anaesthesia 43:1028–1030, 1988.
5. Arndt GA, Voth BR: Paradoxical vocal cord motion in the recovery room: A masquerader of pulmonary dysfunction. Can J Anesth 43:1249–1251, 1996.
6. Robert KW, Crnkovic A, Steiniger J: Post-anesthesia paradoxical vocal cord motion successfully treated with midazolam. Anesthesiology 89:517–519, 1998.
7. Wynnchencko TM: Paradoxical vocal cord adduction. Anesthesiology 93:894–895, 2000.
8. Gallivan GJ: Paradoxical vocal cord movement. Chest 119:1619, 2001.

Rita Agarwal, MD

PATIENT 42

A 26-month-old boy with a choking episode followed by wheezing

The parents of a 26-month-old boy witnessed the child putting peanuts in his mouth just before a choking episode. The child developed difficulty breathing precipitated by a severe coughing and choking episode. He is otherwise healthy.

Physical Examination: General appearance: a well-nourished boy sitting up in bed with labored breathing. Weight 14 kg. Heart rate 130; respirations 50; blood pressure 90/60; oxygen saturation 90% on room air. The child is not cyanotic at examination. Audible wheezes heard over the right upper lobe. Substernal retractions apparent.

Laboratory Findings: Chest radiograph shows hyperinflation of the right lung.

Questions: What is the likely cause of this child's presentation and radiographic appearance?
In what age group does this problem occur most frequently?
What are the major preoperative anesthetic concerns?
Is it reasonable to administer premedication to the patient?
During anesthesia, is controlled or spontaneous ventilation preferred in these patients?
Review the options for anesthesia. If the child had eaten just before presentation, how would that affect anesthetic management?

What is the likely cause of this child's presentation and radiographic appearance? The child has aspirated a peanut into the right pulmonary tree. Such a child usually presents after a sudden episode of coughing or choking while eating or playing with a small object; subsequent wheezing, coughing, gagging, or stridor in this situation is diagnostic of foreign-body aspiration (FBA). The more difficult cases to diagnose are those in which aspiration is not witnessed or is unrecognized and unsuspected. In these situations, the child may present with persistent wheezing, persistent or recurrent pneumonia, lung abscess, focal bronchiectasis, or hemoptysis. If the material is in the subglottic space, complaints may include stridor, recurrent or persistent croup, and voice changes. On physical examination, new-onset wheezing or stridor may be heard. Often, there are asymmetric breath sounds. The physical examination also may be normal, however.

Chest radiography can be helpful in aiding diagnosis and determining the location of the foreign body. Because most objects are radiolucent, inspiratory and expiratory films are obtained in the posteroanterior and lateral positions and show evidence of air trapping or hyperinflation.

In what age group does this problem occur most frequently? FBA is most common in infants 1 to 3 years old, although it can occur at any age. Children are more prone to FBA because of their decreased ability to chew and their tendency to talk, run, or laugh while consuming a variety of objects. The most common objects aspirated are small food items (e.g., peanuts, other nuts, raisins) or improperly chewed foods (e.g., grapes, pieces of meat, hot dog). These may be large enough to cause tracheal obstruction and asphyxiation. Nonfood items that are small enough to pass into the trachea include pieces of balloons, pills, buttons, pieces of plastic or toys, safety pins, or coins. FBA is the cause of death in >300 children per year in the United States. Most foreign bodies lodge in right main bronchus, bronchus intermedius, or right lower lobe bronchus. The left main bronchus is smaller than the right main bronchus and slightly angled. In the supine child, material usually enters the right main bronchus, but then falls into the orifice of the right upper lobe, which is dependent in the supine position. The left main bronchus and its lobes are not immune from FBA, however.

What are the major preoperative anesthetic concerns? Preoperative evaluation includes assessment of respiratory distress, including the presence of retractions, increased work of breathing, decreased oxygen saturation, and tachypnea. The location of the foreign body and probability of tracheal obstruction should be discussed with the surgeon. Recent intake of food significantly affects the anesthetic plan.

Is it reasonable to administer premedication to the patient? If the child has significant anxiety, the appropriateness of administering a premedication should be considered. Several studies showed an increase in postoperative anxiety in patients who had significant preoperative anxiety. Of patients with preoperative anxiety, 60% develop maladaptive behaviors for 2 weeks after surgery (Kain et al, Kotiniemi et al). These include new-onset enuresis, apathy, withdrawal, sleep disturbances, and nightmares. Most of these changes resolved after 2 weeks. Kain et al found a decreased incidence of such behavior in children who received oral midazolam preoperatively. Midazolam has been shown, however, to prolong emergence and recovery (although not discharge from the hospital) in short procedures. Parental presence in the operating room during induction may help decrease patient anxiety, particularly in children >4 years old and with calm parents. Premedication with oral midazolam may be superior to the combination of premedication and parental presence. Decisions regarding premedication, timing of surgery and induction techniques depend on the urgency of the situation.

During anesthesia, is controlled or spontaneous ventilation preferred in these patients? Spontaneous and controlled ventilation have been shown to be safe and effective for maintenance, and both have their proponents. There is less turbulent flow, improved alveolar ventilation, better ventilation-perfusion matching, and less air trapping in spontaneously breathing patients. It is easier to ventilate through the bronchoscope, and there is less chance of dislodging the foreign body in a spontaneously breathing patient. The airway is preserved and ventilation maintained better during manipulation. There is a higher incidence of patient movement, hypercarbia, and prolonged emergence, however. Patients may require conversion to controlled ventilation. The advantages of controlled ventilation include less patient movement, less hypercarbia, and more rapid emergence. The disadvantages are that high peak inspiratory pressures may be required to ventilate the patient adequately, air trapping can be significant, and ventilation must be coordinated with the surgeon.

Review the options for anesthesia. If the child had eaten just before presentation, how would that affect anesthetic management? Airway emergencies can be life-threatening in children. The rapidity with which a child's condition can deteriorate is frightening. There is probably no other situation in which it is as crucial to have the surgeons, nurses, and anesthesia care providers function as a team. Space, airways, and often equipment are shared.

In the patient with a full stomach, with respiratory distress, and who requires spontaneous respiration, communication with the entire team is mandatory. All equipment should be present, ready, and *functional,* IV induction probably is most appropriate, although some report sevoflurane induction with cricoid pressure. The surgeon should put the bronchoscope in as soon as patient is anesthetized and while cricoid pressure is being maintained.

A multitude of anesthetic techniques can be used for maintenance. If the surgeon requires spontaneous respiration because of fear that controlled ventilation will move the foreign body, the inhalation agents halothane or sevoflurane may work better because of evidence that they might have decreased airway reactivity (Kai et al, Pappas et al).

Emergence can occur with or without the patient intubated; however, if the patient had a full stomach before the procedure, he or she should be intubated at the conclusion of bronchoscopy and extubated awake. Foreign body removal is successful in 95% to 98% of patients. A few require repeat bronchoscopy to remove completely all the foreign material. Occasionally, fluoroscopy aids in locating the object, and rarely thoracotomy is required.

The Present Patient

The child was extremely anxious, crying, and clinging to his mother. By the time he arrived in the operating room, it had been 6 hours since his last oral intake (which consisted of the peanuts). He did not have an IV catheter, although several attempts had been made in the emergency department. Midazolam 0.5 mg/kg was administered orally, and the patient calmly was taken from his parents to the operating room. The radiographs suggested a right-sided foreign body. The patient was anesthetized using oxygen, nitrous oxide, and sevoflurane. Spontaneous ventilation was maintained. The vocal cords were visualized by the anesthesiologist and sprayed with 1 mL of 2% lidocaine. Maintenance was with sevoflurane and 0.3-μg/kg boluses of fentanyl to help decrease airway reactivity. Total fentanyl administered was 1.5 μg/kg. The surgery was uneventful with easy retrieval of the peanut.

Clinical Pearls

1. FBA presents most commonly in 1- to 3-year-olds but can occur at any age.
2. Most foreign bodies lodge on the right side because the left bronchus is smaller and slightly angled.
3. An inspiratory and expiratory chest radiograph may help with diagnosis because evidence of air trapping, atelectasis, or hyperinflation on one side can identify the presence and location of a foreign body.
4. The presence of respiratory distress dictates the urgency of the situation.
5. Either controlled or spontaneous ventilation can be used.
6. Object removal is successful 95% of the time.

REFERENCES

1. Kotiniemi LH, Ryhanen PT, Moilanen IK: Behavioral changes in children following day-case surgery: A 4-week follow-up of 551 children. Anaesthesia 52:970–976, 1997.
2. Kai T, Bremerich DH, Jones KA, et al: Drug specific effects of volatile anesthetics on Ca^{2+} sensitization in airway smooth muscle. Anesth Analg 87:425–429, 1998.
3. Kain ZN, Wang SM, Mayes LC, et al: Distress during the induction of anesthesia and postoperative behavioral outcomes. Anesth Analg 88:1042–1047, 1999.
4. Kain ZN, Mayes LC, Wang SM, et al: Postoperative behavioral outcomes in children: Effects of sedative premedication. Anesthesiology 90:758–765, 1999.
5. Kain ZN, Mayes LC, Wang SM, et al: Parental presence and a sedative premedicant for children undergoing surgery: A hierarchical study. Anesthesiology 92:939–946, 2000.
6. Litman RS, Ponnuri J, Tragan I: Anesthesia for tracheal or bronchial foreign body removal: An analysis of ninety four cases. Anesth Analg 91:1389–1391, 2000.
7. McCann MA, Kain ZN: The management of preoperative anxiety in children: An update. Anesth Analg 93:98–105, 2001.
8. Pappas AL, Sukhani R, Lurie J, et al: Severity of airway hyperreactivity associated with laryngeal mask airway removal: Correlation with volatile anesthetic choices. J Clin Anesth 13:498–503, 2001.

Gordon H. Morewood, MD

PATIENT 43

A 79-year-old man with a hip fracture and a heart murmur

A 79-year-old man presents for a unipolar hip replacement after a subcapital fracture of the right hip. He reports that he slipped on a wet bathroom floor that morning after his shower. He is adamant that the accident occurred when he lost his footing and that he had no symptoms of dizziness, weakness, chest pain, or palpitations before falling. He has bruises on his right forearm and over his right zygomatic arch, but a thorough assessment in the emergency department revealed no significant associated injuries.

The patient's past medical history is remarkable for hypothyroidism and chronic, well-controlled hypertension. His medications include aspirin 325 mg orally daily, thyroxine 200 μg orally daily, and ramipril 5 mg orally daily. He has no known allergies to medications and quit smoking 15 years ago. He was last hospitalized 10 years ago for a laparoscopic cholecystectomy; his recovery from that procedure was uneventful. He reports that he is regularly active and considers himself to be physically fit. He works in his garden several times a week and mows his own lawn. He plays golf once a week during the summer and walks nine holes pulling his clubs on a cart. He has never suffered chest pain during physical activity and does not become short of breath except after prolonged exertion.

Physical Examination: General appearance: a tall, thin man who appears roughly his stated age. Height 6 feet 2 inches, weight 180 lb. Pulse 72; blood pressure 140/80. Auscultation of chest: clear air entry throughout both lung fields and a harsh systolic murmur that is heard easily on either side of the sternum in the second intercostal space and radiates to both carotids.

Laboratory Findings: Serum electrolytes, BUN, creatinine, prothrombin time, and partial thromboplastin time: all normal. Hematocrit 39%; platelet count 166×10^9/L. ECG: changes suggestive of left ventricular hypertrophy but no other abnormality.

The patient is only mildly uncomfortable and is eager to chat. He states that a close associate recently had an elective hip replacement that was done under a spinal anesthetic. The patient's friend reportedly chose this technique after being told of the "significant benefits of spinal anesthesia for hip surgery patients." The patient does not want to "be put out" and believes that a general anesthetic would "be more risky anyways, right, Doc?"

Questions: What is the diagnosis?

What is the significance of an asymptomatic heart murmur detected preoperatively?

Discuss concerns associated with the patient's valvular lesion.

What are the benefits of neuraxial anesthetic techniques for lower limb arthroplasty?

Does the patient's daily use of aspirin affect the risks associated with neuraxial techniques?

What is the diagnosis? Asymptomatic aortic stenosis.

What is the significance of an asymptomatic heart murmur detected preoperatively? An accurate patient history is the most important aspect of any preoperative evaluation. In the present case, the patient's excellent general health and exercise tolerance suggest a low risk of perioperative morbidity. Nonetheless, key abnormalities on physical examination or laboratory evaluation must not be overlooked, even in seemingly healthy patients.

A heart murmur may have several implications for perioperative care. Certain valvular abnormalities may require antibiotic prophylaxis against endocarditis when surgical procedures are planned that will penetrate the urogenital, gastrointestinal, or respiratory mucosa. The hemodynamic effects of the lesion causing the murmur may alter the patient's expected physiologic responses to general or regional anesthetic techniques. Many cardiac abnormalities that cause audible murmurs eventually may result in impaired myocardial function because of chronic pressure or volume overload. The resulting ventricular dysfunction may accentuate further abnormal responses to the administration of anesthetics.

A conservative approach is justified when a patient's preanesthetic evaluation reveals a murmur. In many patients, the abnormality will have been detected and investigated previously. In most such cases, a review of the records documenting the cardiac abnormality in addition to the anesthesiologist's assessment of the patient's current tolerance for physical activity should be adequate to guide perioperative care. For patients in whom the murmur is a new finding, an echocardiographic assessment should be done before surgery.

In the present case, preoperative echocardiography revealed calcific aortic stenosis. The mean transvalvular gradient was 50 mmHg, the calculated valve area was 1.1 cm², and the stenosis was graded as *moderate to severe* (see Table).

Hemodynamic Assessment of Aortic Stenosis

Grade	Valve Area (cm²)	Mean Gradient (mmHg)
Mild	> 1.5	< 20
Moderate	1.0–1.5	20–50
Severe	< 1.0	> 50

Discuss concerns associated with the patient's valvular lesion. Aortic stenosis is a disease of chronic progressive obstruction to left ventricular emptying. As obstruction to flow through the aortic valve worsens, the systolic pressure within the left ventricle rises. This rise results in an increase in the mechanical stress experienced by the myocytes in the ventricular wall, as described by the law of Laplace. Over time, the ventricular myocytes increase in size, and the total wall thickness of the ventricle increases to compensate for this rising mechanical stress. Concentric left ventricular hypertrophy is an adaptive mechanism to reduce wall stress and myocardial oxygen requirements in aortic stenosis. This adaptive mechanism also often results in significantly enhanced sensitivity to loading conditions. As left ventricular wall thickness increases, compliance decreases, and left ventricular end-diastolic pressure must rise to maintain diastolic filling and stroke volume. An incremental reduction in left ventricular filling pressure that would be of little consequence to most patients can result in an abrupt reduction in stroke volume and hypotension when a stenotic aortic valve is present. Concentric left ventricular hypertrophy in combination with elevated left ventricular end-diastolic pressures also leads to a reduction in diastolic coronary blood flow to the left ventricle, especially in the region of the subendocardium. Because cardiac output is relatively fixed in advanced aortic stenosis, blood pressure depends more directly on systemic vascular resistance. If vascular resistance falls, profound hypotension may result, leading to subendocardial ischemia (left ventricular intracavitary pressures remain high, even as perfusion pressure falls). If the left ventricle becomes ischemic, cardiac output begins to fall, aortic pressures decline further, and recovery quickly may become impossible. These mechanisms are at least partly responsible for the increased risk of sudden death in patients with severe obstruction to flow through the aortic valve.

Historically, severe aortic stenosis has been associated with a significantly increased mortality rate after noncardiac surgery. Small retrospective reviews in more recent years showed, however, that patients known to have this abnormality can undergo surgery safely using modern anesthetic and monitoring techniques. Practice guidelines published in cooperation by the American Heart Association and the American College of Cardiology do not recommend valve replacement for aortic stenosis until the development of symptoms. Even patients with severe aortic stenosis enjoy a relatively good long-term prognosis if they are asymptomatic, but these patients should be followed yearly to gauge the progression of their disease and to detect the onset of symptoms. It is reasonable for the present patient to proceed to surgery without intervention for aortic stenosis.

Does aortic stenosis require an alteration in anesthetic management? The answer is a firm *maybe*. Traditionally, neuraxial anesthetic techniques have been avoided in patients with aortic stenosis. This avoidance was due to a concern that the rapid onset of an extensive sympathetic blockade might result in cardiovascular collapse. General anesthesia also is associated commonly with a reduction in peripheral vascular resistance, however, resulting from a depression of sympathetic nervous system activity and from direct pharmacologic vasodilation of resistance arterioles. Significant blockade of the sympathetic nervous system is not inevitable when neuraxial techniques are employed for lower limb surgery. The last fibers of the sympathetic chain depart from the spinal cord at the L2 segment. A neuraxial technique that produces a somatic blockade to the upper lumbar or lower thoracic segments should not alter peripheral vascular resistance substantially but would provide adequate conditions for lower limb arthroplasty. Slow titration of intrathecal isobaric bupivacaine, intrathecal hypobaric tetracaine, or epidural bupivacaine or lidocaine could provide an adequate anesthetic state with hemodynamic stability comparable to a general anesthetic. No prospective data are available to compare directly neuraxial versus general anesthesia for patients with aortic stenosis. It is likely that the manner in which the anesthetic is administered is more important than the technique chosen.

What are the benefits of neuraxial anesthetic techniques for lower limb arthroplasty? If the risks do not favor one anesthetic technique over another in the present patient, neither do the benefits. Notwithstanding the patient's claim, there is little to suggest a neuraxial technique would decrease the perioperative morbidity associated with his surgery. Early studies suggested a decrease in perioperative blood loss and the incidence of deep venous thromboses when spinal anesthesia was used for lower limb arthroplasties. Subsequent investigations failed to support the notion of decreased blood loss with neuraxial techniques but did corroborate the finding that patients suffered fewer thrombotic complications postoperatively when a spinal anesthetic was employed. Data col-

lected in the current environment of aggressive pharmacologic prophylaxis for deep venous thromboses with either warfarin or low-molecular-weight heparin have not found a benefit for neuraxial techniques. The patient should be advised that no clear medical benefit can be expected from one anesthetic technique versus another.

Does the patient's daily use of aspirin affect the risks associated with neuraxial techniques? The issue of anticoagulation and neuraxial anesthesia justifiably provokes much concern among anesthesiologists. For the current patient, neither aspirin nor any of the nonsteroidal antiinflammatory drugs are believed to increase the risk of complications after spinal or epidural anesthesia. (See Patient 28 for a further discussion of anticoagulation and neuraxial anesthesia.)

The Present Patient

The patient required an echocardiogram to determine the cause of his murmur before surgery for his hip fracture. Intervention for the patient's valvular disease was not recommended before the orthopedic procedure. Aspirin was not considered a contraindication to regional anesthesia. After a discussion of the relevant risks and benefits, the patient wished to proceed with a spinal anesthetic.

In the operating room, a large-bore intravenous catheter was placed and a radial arterial catheter to facilitate beat-to-beat monitoring of blood pressure. The patient received 500 mL of 6% hydroxyethyl starch IV while the regional block was prepared. With the patient in the left lateral decubitus position and slight (approximately 10°) Trendelenburg position, a lumbar puncture was performed with a 17G Touhy needle via the L4–5 interspace (care was taken to align the bevel of the needle parallel to the long axis of the patient's spine and parallel to the dural fibers). A standard epidural catheter was threaded 3 cm into the intrathecal space and secured. A hypobaric solution of 0.1% tetracaine (20 mg of niphanoid tetracaine hydrochloride dissolved in 20 mL of preservative-free sterile water) was administered via the catheter in 2-mL increments, waiting roughly 5 minutes between each dose. After 6 mL (6 mg of tetracaine), the patient was unable to sense a vigorous pinch below the T11 dermatome on the right and the L2 dermatome on the left. The blood pressure had decreased gradually from 150/80 mmHg to 105/60 mmHg. A low-dose phenylephrine infusion was begun and titrated to maintain a minimal diastolic blood pressure of 65 mmHg (within

20% of the baseline value). Blood loss throughout the case was replaced with an equal volume of 6% hydroxyethyl starch, and the patient received 1,000 mL of IV crystalloid. On arrival to the recovery room, the patient's blood pressure was 124/70 mmHg, and no phenylephrine had been required for 30 minutes. The patient's hospital recovery was uncomplicated, and he was discharged to a rehabilitation program 3 days after surgery. Arrangements were made for yearly follow-up with a cardiologist, and the patient was instructed to return earlier if he experienced angina, unusual dyspnea, or presyncope.

Clinical Pearls

1. An accurate patient history is often the most important component of the preoperative workup and is always necessary for the interpretation of abnormal physical findings or test results.

2. Knowledge of a patient's valvular pathology may affect the choice of prophylactic antibiotics, the anesthetic approach, or the decision to proceed with noncardiac surgery. All patients with an undiagnosed murmur should undergo echocardiographic examination preoperatively except when such a delay potentially would result in a loss of life or limb.

3. Aortic stenosis does not require surgical intervention until the onset of symptoms, and noncardiac surgery may be done with due caution in active but asymptomatic patients with this diagnosis.

4. In patients with aortic stenosis undergoing noncardiac surgery, the overall anesthetic technique (general versus regional) is not as important as the choice of individual drugs and their dosages.

5. When pharmacologic prophylaxis for deep venous thrombosis is to be used after lower limb arthroplasty, there is no proven difference between general anesthesia and neuraxial anesthesia with regard to perioperative morbidity.

6. Aspirin and nonsteroidal antiinflammatory drugs are the only *anticoagulants* that do not require careful timing of administration when used in patients undergoing neuraxial anesthesia.

REFERENCES

1. Sculco TP, Ranawat C: The use of spinal anesthesia for total hip-replacement arthroplasty. J Bone Joint Surg 57:173–177, 1975.
2. Goldman L, Caldera DL, Nussbaum SR, et al: Multifactorial index of cardiac risk in noncardiac surgical procedures. N Engl J Med 297:845–850, 1977.
3. Modig J, Borg T, Karlstrom G, et al: Thromboembolism after total hip replacement—role of epidural and general anesthesia. Anesth Analg 62:174–180, 1983.
4. O'Keefe JH Jr, Shub C, Rettke SR: Risk of noncardiac surgical procedures in patients with aortic stenosis. Mayo Clin Proc 64:400–405, 1989.
5. Modig J: Influence of regional anesthesia, local anesthetics, and sympathicomimetics on the pathophysiology of deep vein thrombosis. Acta Chirurg Scand 550:119–124, 1989.
6. Sorenson RM, Pace NL: Anesthetic techniques during surgical repair of femoral neck fractures—a meta-analysis. Anesthesiology 77:1095–1104, 1992.
7. Collard CD, Eappen S, Lynch EP, et al: Continuous spinal anesthesia with invasive hemodynamic monitoring for surgical repair of the hip in two patients with severe aortic stenosis. Anesth Analg 81:195–198, 1995.
8. Favarel-Garrigues JF, Sztark F, Petitjean ME, et al: Hemodynamic effects of spinal anesthesia in the elderly—single dose versus titration through a catheter. Anesth Analg 82:312–316, 1996.
9. Brinker MR, Reuben JD, Mull JR, et al: Comparison of general and epidural anesthesia in patients undergoing primary unilateral total hip replacement. Orthopedics 20:109–115, 1997.
10. Bonow RO, Carabello B, deLeon AC, et al: ACC/AHA guidelines for the management of patients with valvular heart disease—a report of the American College of Cardiology/American Heart Association Task Force on Practice Guidelines (Committee on Management of Patients with Valvular Heart Disease). J Am Coll Cardiol 32:1486–1582, 1998.
11. Torsher LC, Shub C, Rettke SR, et al: Risk of patients with severe aortic stenosis undergoing noncardiac surgery. Am J Cardiol 81:448–452, 1998.
12. Anonymous: Recommendations for neuraxial anesthesia and anticoagulation. American Society of Regional Anesthesia, 1998. Available at www.asra.com/iteams_of_interest/consensus_statements/.

13. Koval KJ, Aharonoff GB, Rosenberg AD, et al: Hip fracture in the elderly—the effect of anesthetic technique. Orthopedics 22:31–34, 1999.
14. Gilbert TB, Hawkes WG, Hebel JR, et al: Spinal anesthesia versus general anesthesia for hip fracture repair—a longitudinal observation of 741 elderly patients during 2-year follow-up. Am J Orthop 29:25–35, 2000.
15. O'Hara DA, Duff A, Berlin JA, et al: The effect of anesthetic technique on postoperative outcomes in hip fracture repair. Anesthesiology 92:947–957, 2000.

Jason Krutsch, MD

PATIENT 44

A 69-year-old woman with difficulty inserting a pulmonary artery catheter

A 69-year-old woman is scheduled for three-vessel coronary artery bypass graft surgery. She has a history of coronary artery disease, type 2 diabetes mellitus, and hypertension. Previous anesthetics were without complication. Medications include lisinopril and isosorbide mononitrate.

Physical Examination: Afebrile; pulse 67; respirations 16; blood pressure 145/85; oxygen saturation 95% on room air. General appearance: moderately obese woman in no apparent distress. Cardiac, chest, abdomen, neurologic, and extremity examinations all unremarkable.

Laboratory Findings: Blood glucose 165 mg/dL. Remaining hematology, coagulation profiles, and chemistries: normal. ECG: normal sinus rhythm, left ventricular hypertrophy, and evidence of previous anterior-septal myocardial infarction. Transthoracic echocardiogram: normal with left ventricular ejection fraction of 55%. Chest radiograph: normal.

The patient underwent induction and intubation. A 9F percutaneous sheath was inserted into the right internal jugular vein without incident. Next, a balloon-tipped, flow-directed pulmonary artery catheter (PAC) is inserted through the introducer. The PAC is advanced to 30 cm, where a right ventricular waveform is obtained. The waveform remains unchanged despite catheter insertion to 50 cm. Subsequently the PAC can be withdrawn only to 25 cm; all further attempts to withdraw the catheter are met with marked resistance. Blood pressure, heart rate, and rhythm remain normal throughout this sequence of events.

Questions: What is the problem with the PAC?
How is the diagnosis made?
How is this complication removed?
What are the risks associated with this complication?
What are other complications of PAC?

What is the problem with the PAC? Knotted intracardiac PAC.

How is the diagnosis made? Fluoroscopy and chest radiographs reveal knotted PACs. In this case, a distinct knot was palpated in the right atrium after sternotomy.

How is this complication removed? There are several options. Knots have been reduced noninvasively under fluoroscopic guidance. When a knot is incomplete (i.e., loose), the problem often is overcome easily and the knot is reduced by manipulation of the catheter in the veins or cardiac chambers. Occasionally the PAC has to be directed into the vena cava or right atrium, where better maneuvering is possible. Alternatively, a semiflexible steel guidewire may be inserted and advanced to the catheter's tip. This option is not effective for complete knotting, however, and carries a theoretical hazard of perforating the catheter, blood vessel, or cardiac chamber. Fluoroscopically guided capture and extraction of knotted PACs using a goose-neck wire loop is another option; this involves cannulation of a large vein (i.e., femoral) with subsequent fluoroscopic guidance of a wire loop to the location of the knot. When captured, the knot may be reduced or incised and removed. In cases in which the catheter is completely knotted (i.e., tightly knotted), withdrawal of the catheter to a peripheral vein with surgical removal has been the rule. Sometimes a surgical procedure is necessary to remove a stubbornly knotted PAC.

What are the risks associated with this complication? Knotted PACs may become incorporated into intracardiac structures (i.e., valve leaflets, chordae tendinae); these structures can be damaged during attempted catheter extraction. Vascular structures also can be lacerated during removal attempts.

What are other complications of PACs? Potential complications from the placement and residence of PACs include arrhythmias, valvular injury, pulmonary artery perforation, pulmonary infarction, infection, and venous thrombosis.

The Present Patient

The PAC was removed after the patient was placed on cardiopulmonary bypass. The right atrium was incised, and the knotted distal portion of the catheter was removed. The proximal section of the PAC was removed through the introducer.

Clinical Pearls

1. Intracardiac knotting is a rare but dangerous complication of PACs.

2. A knotted PAC should be suspected in the settings of persistent right ventricular waveforms, failure to wedge the PAC, or when a PAC cannot be extracted; it can be confirmed using fluoroscopy or chest radiography.

3. Prompt diagnosis and management of knotted PACs are crucial because knots may be incorporated into intracardiac and vascular structures, and damage can occur secondary to forced removal.

REFERENCES

1. Baldi J, Jaco F, Benchinol A: Complete knotting of a catheter and a non-surgical method of removal. Chest 65:93–95, 1974.
2. Mond H: A technique for unknotting an intracardiac flow directed balloon catheter. Chest 67:731–732, 1975.
3. Bottiger B, Schmidt H, Bohrer H, et al: Non-surgical removal of knotted Swan-Ganz catheter. Anaesthetist 40:682–686, 1991.
4. Practice guidelines for pulmonary artery catheterization. American Society of Anesthesiologists Task Force on Pulmonary Artery Catheterization. Anesthesiology 78:380–394, 1993.
5. Ismail K, Deckmyn T, Vandermeersch E, et al: Non-surgical extraction of intracardiac double knotted pulmonary artery catheter. J Clin Anesth 10:160–162, 1998.

Cyrus Mirshab, MD

PATIENT 45

A 19-year-old man with postoperative respiratory insufficiency

A 19-year-old man presents for reconstruction of the right anterior cruciate ligament. He is American Society of Anesthesiologists class 1 with no medical problems and on no medications. He has had no prior anesthetics, and there is no family history of problems associated with anesthesia.

Physical Examination: Cardiac and respiratory examination unremarkable. Airway is Mallampati class I with full range of motion of the neck.

Laboratory Findings: All within normal limits.

IV general anesthetic induction and endotracheal intubation are accomplished using propofol 150 mg, midazolam 2 mg, fentanyl 250 μg, and rocuronium 40 mg. General anesthesia is maintained with desflurane 6% in 50% oxygen. The duration of the surgery was 90 minutes; blood loss was minimal, and 800 mL of lactated Ringer's solution was given intravenously. The patient had 5 seconds of sustained tetanus, so no reversal agents were administered.

Soon after extubation, the patient is agitated and displays respiratory difficulty shown by stridor, impressive rib retractions, and use of accessory muscles. Hemoglobin saturation as measured by pulse oximetry rapidly declines to 65% from the previous value of 98%. Positive-pressure ventilation by mask does not result in improved ventilation. Succinylcholine 20 mg is given intravenously. In contrast to the initial intubation attempt, visualization of the glottis is inadequate on this attempt, and further episodes of mask ventilation ensue. Although there is some chest expansion, oxygen saturation never improves beyond 90%. The patient is reintubated after an additional dose of succinylcholine (80 mg) is given.

He is transferred to postanesthetic care and connected to a mechanical ventilator. Positive end-expiratory pressure (PEEP) 8 cm H_2O and 100% fraction of inspired oxygen (FIO_2) are required to maintain an SpO_2 of 98%. Auscultation of the chest reveals bilateral rhonchi, and frothy serosanguineous fluid is suctioned from the endotracheal tube. The impairment in oxygenation persists, and PEEP is increased to 12 cm H_2O. Pulmonary secretions are hemorrhagic. A chest radiograph shows diffuse bilateral interstitial infiltrates with peribronchial cuffing associated with a normal heart size.

Questions: What was the precipitating event that led to the patient's clinical picture and radiographic appearance?

Are there any predisposing risk factors for this precipitating event?

Review the intrathoracic pressure changes during normal respiration and during inspiration against a closed glottis.

What forces determine fluid flux within the lungs?

Describe the net movement of fluid during inspiration against a closed glottis.

Is the fluid flux only a matter of pressure gradients or is it due to alveolar injury?

What are the clinical signs and presentation of the observed pulmonary insufficiency?

What is the appropriate treatment for this condition?

What was the precipitating event that led to the patient's clinical picture and radiographic appearance? The patient experienced laryngospasm after extubation. Attempts to inspire against a closed glottis generated significant negative intrathoracic pressures.

Are there any predisposing risk factors for this precipitating event? Laryngospasm is common in children after airway instrumentation, including oral suctioning and placement of an oral airway, during intubation attempts with inhalation induction, and especially during extubation. Barbiturates and volatile anesthetic agents also have been associated with laryngospasm. Pharyngeal blood, regurgitated gastric contents, pain, peritoneal traction, and anal dilation also may cause laryngospasm.

Review the intrathoracic pressure changes during normal respiration and during inspiration against a closed glottis. Relative to atmospheric pressure, the intrapleural pressure at the base of the lungs is normally -2.5 mmHg at the start of inspiration, decreasing to about -6.0 mmHg at end expiration. Air flows into the lungs as a result of this pressure differential. Strong inspiration can generate a negative intrapleural pressure of -30 mmHg. Should the glottis be closed, however, as during laryngospasm, generated negative pressure gradients increase substantially and may reach -100 mmHg in muscular individuals.

What forces determine fluid flux within the lungs? Alveolar-capillary hemodynamics are a function of the hydrostatic and oncotic properties within the pulmonary vessels and alveoli and determine net fluid movement. The equation is as follows:

$$\text{Fluid movement} = \kappa[(P_c + \pi_i) - (P_i + \pi_c)]$$

where κ is capillary filtration coefficient, P_c is capillary hydrostatic pressure, P_i is interstitial hydrostatic pressure, π_c is capillary colloid osmotic pressure, and π_i is interstitial colloid osmotic pressure.

The hydrostatic pressure gradient (P_c-P_i) is the difference between the hydrostatic pressures in the capillary and the interstitium. The osmotic pressure gradient (π_c-π_i) is the difference between the colloid osmotic pressures of the plasma and interstitial fluid. The capillary filtration coefficient, κ, is proportionate to the permeability of the tissue. Normally, there is a small net fluid flux out of the capillaries. Reuptake of this fluid is accomplished through lymphatic transport.

Describe the net movement of fluid during inspiration against a closed glottis. Significant negative intrathoracic pressure gradients, as might be generated when inspiring against a closed glottis, dramatically increase intrathoracic venous return, increasing capillary hydrostatic pressure, while decreasing the perivascular interstitial hydrostatic forces. The net result is an increase in the transcapillary pressure gradient from capillary to interstitium, resulting in transudation of fluid into the intersitial space and, if severe enough, into the alveoli. Increases in negative intrathoracic pressure also increase left ventricular afterload, decreasing left ventricular stroke volume. Additionally, increase in venous return impedes lymphatic drainage. Release of catecholamines in response to anxiety, hypoxia, and hypercapnia also increases capillary hydrostatic pressure as blood pressure and pulmonary blood volume increase, favoring the shift of fluid into the interstitium. This phenomenon has been termed *negative pressure pulmonary edema* (NPPE).

NPPE occurs generally after relief of upper airway obstruction. The obstruction may be acute or chronic. Laryngospasm and upper airway tumors are the most common causes. Other causes include supraglottitis, aspiration, foreign bodies, bronchospasm, strangulation, and airway trauma. NPPE also has been noted after surgery for tonsillar and adenoidal hypertrophy, goiter, and nasopharyngeal masses and in patients with obstructive sleep apnea. Obese patients and patients predisposed to airway management difficulties because of anatomic abnormalities also are at risk. The period of airway obstruction may be extremely brief; the onset of NPPE may be precipitous, on the order of minutes, or may occur over a few hours.

Is the fluid flux only a matter of pressure gradients, or is it due to alveolar injury? It has been a long-held belief that NPPE occurring after relief of airway obstruction was a result of the altered intrathoracic pressure relationships as has been described, and when normal pressure relationships are reestablished, the problem is self-limited and resolves. Negative pressure pulmonary hemorrhage after such episodes has been increasingly reported, however, suggesting that some degree of alveolar injury has occurred. Alveolar stretch may result in loss of alveolar-capillary integrity and result in capillary leak, alveolar edema, and hemorrhage. Alveolar damage has been shown in a rabbit model to occur after generated negative pressures of only -40 mmHg. The threshold for alveolar damage in humans is not known. The character of pulmonary fluid after negative pressure injury has been found to be near that of serum protein, suggesting there is loss of alveolar integrity and capillary leak. A pulmonary transudate has only 50% to 65% the protein content of serum. Pulmonary hemorrhage also may be due to bronchial vascular injury. Other factors that may contribute to alveolar-capillary damage include rapid pulmonary reexpansion and oxidant injury.

What are the clinical signs and presentation of the observed pulmonary insufficiency? Acutely, signs of partial or complete airway obstruction are noted, including patient agitation, dyspnea and tachypnea, tachycardia (or bradycardia as hypoxemia becomes extreme), stridorous breath sounds, paradoxical respiratory motion of the chest and abdomen (the chest retracts and the abdomen expands), and use of accessory muscles of respiration. Oxygen saturation declines, and cyanosis may be noted. Differential diagnosis includes aspiration, pulmonary edema from fluid overload, congestive heart failure, adult respiratory distress syndrome, and anaphylaxis.

After an airway has been reestablished, pulse oximetry values may be poor despite administration of increased inspired oxygen concentrations. An astute clinician may note that an SpO_2 of 100 while the patient is assisted with a nonrebreathing mask at 15 L/min reflects substantial impairment in oxygenation. Additionally, copious secretions or pink or bloody fluid aspirated from an endotracheal tube would lead one to consider this diagnosis.

What is the appropriate treatment for this condition? The goal of initial treatment is to reestablish airway patency. The patient should be assisted with mask ventilation with 100% oxygen. An attempt to coordinate assisted ventilation with the patient's respiratory attempts should be made. High airway pressures may force gas into the stomach, predisposing the patient to regurgitation, so some moderation must be exercised during assisted ventilation. Should this maneuver fail to result in satisfactory airway movement, succinylcholine 10 to 20 mg may relax the vocal cords without resulting in total skeletal muscle paralysis. If oxygen saturation does not improve, reintubation may be indicated. At this point, it would be prudent to ensure loss of patient recall, either with administration of an anesthetic induction agent, benzodiazepine, or the like. When the patient has been intubated, the issue becomes will the patient develop laryngospasm again at the second intubation attempt? If the initial episode of laryngospasm had occurred as the patient was emerging from anesthesia but still obtunded, the time many consider to be a vulnerable period for laryngospasm, a more circumspect approach to reextubation may avoid a secondary episode of airway obstruction.

The treatment for NPPE and negative pressure pulmonary hemorrhage is mostly supportive in nature, addressing oxygenation, ventilation, and maintenance of hemodynamic stability. The severity of the injury determines the extent of treatment required. Mild pulmonary edema resolves without significant intervention. Although diuretic therapy may be considered, the patient's volume status determines the wisdom of this intervention. Diuretic therapy may render some surgical patients hypovolemic, whereas what was necessary was "tincture of time." Further fluid restriction may be appropriate, however. In any intubated patient, continuous positive airway pressure or some level of PEEP may be beneficial. Patients who are experiencing pulmonary hemorrhage should be treated with lung-protective strategies to prevent further alveolar injury. To accomplish this, smaller tidal volumes, higher respiratory rates, and PEEP are instituted. Rarely a pulmonary artery catheter may aid management. Severe pulmonary hemorrhage may require transfusion. Patients having procedures originally planned as outpatient are a concerning group because the process may continue to worsen after discharge. These patients should have at a minimum a protracted period of observation before discharge; admission and observation might be the best strategy.

The Present Patient

The patient persisted in having hemoptysis. Inspired oxygen concentration was increased to 100%, and PEEP was increased to 15 cm H_2O. Dopamine 5 µg/kg/min was initiated to support blood pressure. A radial arterial catheter was inserted for continuous monitoring and blood draws. Because the patient stabilized on the initial dose of dopamine, pulmonary arterial catheterization was not undertaken. The patient's hematocrit decreased to 22%, he was transfused 2 U of packed RBCs. During the following 24 hours, the patient's condition improved remarkably as hemoptysis resolved. He was extubated 72 hours after reintubation.

Clinical Pearls

1. NPPE is an event that every anesthesia provider is likely to encounter sometime in practice. The underlying event is relief of either acute or chronic upper airway obstruction. Acutely, laryngospasm is the most common precipitating event.

2. The period of airway obstruction necessary to cause NPPE may be surprisingly brief. NPPE may occur quickly or evolve over many hours. The severity may be variable and, because of this, therapy must be individualized.

3. The initial physical processes involve alteration in intrathoracic pressure and hemodynamic relationships, causing an increase in interstitial, then alveolar fluid. Alveolar injury also may occur and is suggested by pink, frothy or frankly bloody pulmonary fluid.

4. Therapy may be simply supplemental oxygen. Alternatively the patient may require intubation with continuous positive airway pressure or PEEP applied. Aggressive hemodynamic support is required on rare occasions.

5. Outpatients developing pulmonary edema after relief of airway obstruction require at least extended observation; admission may be the most prudent strategy.

REFERENCES

1. Kollef MH, Pluss J: Noncardiogenic pulmonary edema following upper airway obstruction. Medicine 70:91–98, 1991.
2. Guffin TN, Har-El G, Sanders A, et al: Acute post-obstructive pulmonary edema. Otolaryngol Head Neck Surg 112:235–237, 1995.
3. Devys JM, Balleau C, Jayr C, Bourgain JL: Biting the laryngeal mask: An unusual cause of negative pressure pulmonary edema. Can J Anesth 47:176–178, 2000.
4. Dolinkski SY, MacGregor DA, Scudceri PE: Pulmonary hemorrhage associated with negative-pressure pulmonary edema. Anesthesiology 93:282–284, 2000.
5. Mandal NG: Negative-pressure pulmonary edema in a child with hiccups during induction. Anesthesiology 94:378–379, 2001.
6. Broccard AF, Liaudet L, Aubert JD, et al: Negative pressure post-tracheal extubation alveolar-hemorrhage. Anesth Analg 92:273–275, 2001.

Marc A. Rozner, PhD, MD

PATIENT 46

An 82-year-old woman with pacemaker complications

An 82-year-old woman is scheduled for an excisional biopsy of a mass in her right breast. She had a pacemaker previously implanted in the right pectoral position. The patient had been seen by her cardiologist a few days before the case. The note from the cardiologist states: "This patient has a dual-chamber pacemaker set to 60 beats/min in the DDDR mode. It was placed for sinus bradycardia 3 years ago, and recent evaluation shows it to be working correctly. She is cleared for surgery."

The patient was not seen by her cardiologist on the day of surgery. She received a balanced general anesthetic. Monopolar electrosurgery was used intraoperatively, and the anesthesiologist noted no intraoperative difficulties. After emergence and extubation, she is taken to the postanesthesia care unit (PACU). The patient is placed on the PACU monitor (Datex AS-3; Datex-Ohmeda, Madison, WI), at which time she is noted to have a heart rate of 135 beats/minute. Although she notes "palpitations," her blood pressure is stable, and she is not in any distress. A 12-lead ECG is ordered (see Figure).

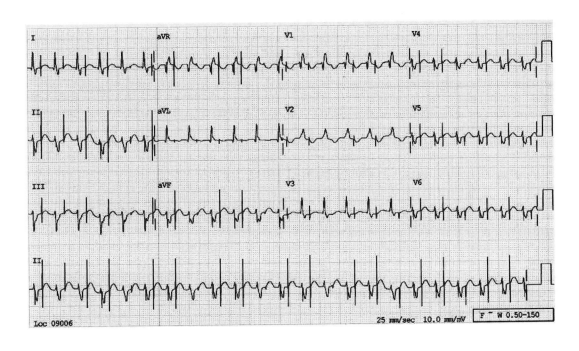

Questions: Interpret the 12-lead ECG.

What is a DDDR pacemaker?

What is the utility of bioimpedance cardiac pacing?

What devices commonly used in the operative and perioperative environment may complicate use of bioimpedance pacemakers?

How should electrosurgical units be used when the patient has a pacemaker?

How should patients with bioimpedance pacemakers be managed perioperatively?

Review the issue of magnets placed near pacemakers.

Interpret the 12-lead ECG. The ECG shows an atrioventricular (A-V) sequentially paced rhythm at 135 beats/min. The A-V delay appears to be 300 msec. The cause of this tachycardia is inappropriate pacemaker response secondary to interference from the PACU respiratory rate monitor. The apparent unusual relationship between the atrial and ventricular artifacts is caused by (1) lack of intrinsic A-V conduction in this patient, (2) an unnaturally long A-V delay of 300 msec, and (3) the short cardiac cycle that results from a rate of 135 beats/min.

What is a DDDR pacemaker? The usual manner to report pacing mode includes at least three characters: the first character indicates the chamber(s) paced, the second character indicates chamber(s) sensed, and the third character identifies the behavior of the pacemaker when an appropriate event is sensed. In DDD mode, the pacemaker ensures that any atrial event (whether intrinsic or paced) will be followed by a ventricular event (whether intrinsic or paced). Additionally, after any quiescent period of appropriate length following any ventricular event, an atrial event is paced. There are caveats for premature atrial contractions, premature ventricular contractions, and high rate behaviors that are specific to devices and can be modified by programming. In modern-day pacemakers, a fourth character (generally *R*) is present to indicate that the generator will detect some form of "exercise" and increase the pacing rate in response to this exercise.

What is the utility of bioimpedance cardiac pacing? Many patients who need artificial cardiac pacing have chronotropic incompetence; that is, they fail to increase their heart rate with increasing oxygen demand, such as during exercise. As a result, modern-day pacing devices attempt to *quantify* exercise and provide increased cardiac output via an increased rate. Many mechanisms exist for determining *exercise,* but the most commonly used (in the United States) include accelerometers, motion sensors, and bioimpedance minute ventilation sensors.

Bioimpedance minute ventilation sensors were introduced in the late 1980s, and these sensors provide one of the earliest indications of the need to increase cardiac output. Minute ventilation sensors are useful in poorly conditioned, physically impaired patients (e.g., a wheelchair-bound patient).

To detect changes in minute ventilation, these devices measure the electrical current required to inject a small signal into the chest. This current changes with chest wall expansion and contraction, and algorithms can be created to *infer* a res-

piratory rate. As this *respiratory rate* increases, the pacemaker increases its lower rate set-point. As this set-point exceeds the patient's intrinsic rhythm, the patient is paced. The following Table lists currently available pacemakers with minute ventilation (bioimpedance) sensing.

Pacemakers With Minute Ventilation
(Bioimpedance) Sensing

ELA Medical
   Brio Series 212, 220, 222
   Talent Series 130, 213, 223
   Opus RM Series 4534
   Chorus RM Series 7034, 7134
CPI-Guidant Pulsar and Pulsar_Max Families
   1170, 1171, 1172, 1270, 1272
Medtronic Kappa 400
Telectronics / St Jude
   Meta Series 1202, 1204, 1206, 1230, 1250, 1254, 1256
   Tempo Series 1102, 1902, 2102, 2902

What devices commonly used in the operative and perioperative environment may complicate use of bioimpedance pacemakers? Many patient monitoring devices *inject* electricity into a patient, and these other injected signals can confuse the pacemaker. Devices that measure respiratory rate via a bioimpedance algorithm are an example. Some ECG instruments also use this type of system to detect lead disconnection. The strong, violent electromagnetic interference from monopolar electrosurgery also induces electrical currents on the body surface.

The injection of electrical signals onto the chest wall can confuse a bioimpedance pacemaker because the signal injected by the nonpacemaker device can interfere with the signal injected by the pacemaker. This confusion often leads to a pacemaker-driven tachycardia.

Pacemakers that use bioimpedance measurements for their activity sensor can produce a pacemaker-driven tachycardia under a variety of settings. Reports have been published detailing inappropriate heart rates in the setting of ventilator-driven hyperventilation, use of noninvasive cardiac output devices, connection to ECG monitors, and use of monopolar electrosurgery (the *Bovie*). Some PACU and intraoperative monitors use a similar bioimpedance detection method for monitoring respiratory rate. The electrical signal from the respiratory rate monitor can fool a bioimpedance pacemaker into believing that the patient is performing maximal exercise. In the setting of maximal exercise, the pacemaker generates the maximum sensor rate (a programmed setting).

Some pacemakers that use bioimpedance sensors now incorporate an additional activity sensor, and these devices can be programmed to *cross-check* the two sensors before driving the patient's heart rate to the maximum rate for exercise. Although these devices are less likely to cause inappropriately fast heart rates than single-sensor models, they still can create short periods of high rate pacing.

How should electrosurgical units be used when the patient has a pacemaker? Monopolar electrosurgery should be avoided whenever possible. In its place, bipolar (two-tip) electrosurgery should be used. Manufacturer guidelines should be followed for placement of electrosurgical current return pads (often, although inappropriately, called the *grounding plate*); these pads should be placed so as to prevent any electrosurgical current from crossing the pacemaker/leads/heart. Thus, in a head and neck or intracranial case, the current return pad should be placed on the posterior-superior aspect of the shoulder contralateral to the implanted pulse generator. In cases in which monopolar electrosurgery is required in multiple sites (e.g., head and neck reconstructive cases with abdominal or lower extremity free flaps), two electrosurgical devices should be used with two pads placed appropriately. For arm procedures, pads can be placed distally on the arm to exclude the generator from the electrosurgical current path.

How should patients with bioimpedance pacemakers be managed perioperatively? Because of the potential for signal misinterpretation and patient injury, many authors now recommend disabling any form of pacemaker rate responsiveness before surgery. The U.S. Food and Drug Administration published an alert about this issue in 1998 (URL, available at http://www.fda.gov/cdrh/safety/minutevent.html). The American College of Cardiologists recommended the disabling of all rate responsiveness to avoid confusion in the operating room.

Review the issue of magnets placed near pacemakers. In general, the routine use of magnets is not recommended because not every device responds to magnet placement with continuous asynchronous pacing. In some devices from CPI-Guidant, Pacesetter, and Vitatron, the magnet mode can be programmed to *OFF*. In many devices from Intermedics and Biotronik, asynchronous pacing is limited to <64 events, after which the device returns to the programmed settings even though the magnet is in place. In many devices from CPI-Guidant, Pacesetter, and others, magnet application provides asynchronous pacing at the lower rate, which might be lower than the patient's intrinsic rate. Such pacing below the patient's intrinsic rate can produce competition and inappropriate R-on-T pacing.

If the anesthetic plan includes magnet application, the magnet behavior must be identified before the start of the case. With some pacemakers (most Medtronic, newer CPI-Guidant, newer Pacesetter), application of a magnet converts the mode to asynchronous pacing with a rate between 85 and 100 beats/min, preventing *Bovie oversensing* and the intermittent inhibition of output. The manufacturers can provide specific information regarding any device.

The Present Patient

The patient has a Telectronics Tempo model No. 2102 pacemaker with a bioimpedance sensing device. She is experiencing a pacemaker-driven tachycardia at the maximum sensor rate, programmed at 135 beats/min. When the respiratory rate monitor was disabled, the patient's heart rate gradually returned to her sinus rate. Had no intrinsic sinus activity been detected, atrial pacing would have begun at the programmed lower rate (in this case, 60 beats/min). Also, in this pacemaker, placement of a magnet would have converted this pacemaker to DOO pacing, with the rate dependent on remaining battery voltage. (In DOO pacing, atrium and ventricle are paced in AV sequential mode with no sensing and no rate responsiveness. This is the definition of asynchronous, non–rate-responsive mode.)

In this case, the injection of electrical signals by the respiratory rate monitor led this pacemaker to *believe* that the patient was exercising, increasing the pacing rate. When these interactions take place, pacemakers with a single, minute ventilation sensor tend to increase their pacing rate up to the *maximum sensor rate* (also called *upper activity rate*). This increase in rate takes place within one to three cardiac cycles. In this patient, the same behavior was observed on enabling respiratory rate monitoring on a Marquette 8010 (GE Medical Systems, Milwaukee, WI).

Concerning the displayed ECG, because this patient's pacemaker had an unusually long programmed interval (300 msec) for the A-V delay, the ECG appears to suggest that the atrial pacing artifact produces the QRS and the ventricular pacing event falls on the T wave. Interrogation of this device showed that it was working correctly. With a rate of 135 beats/min, however, the interval between the QRS complexes would be ≤444 msec. In this setting, with an A-V delay of 300 msec, there would be only 144 msec from a ventricular event until the next paced atrial event. This patient's unusual pacemaker settings, combined with an interaction between the pacemaker and the respiratory rate monitor, produced a pacemaker pseudomalfunction (the belief that a pacemaker is malfunctioning when it is working properly according to programmed instructions).

Clinical Pearls

1. The manufacturer and type of pacing device should be determined before administering an elective anesthetic. The clinician should call the manufacturer and ask if any intraoperative issues are known. Monopolar electrosurgery should be avoided whenever possible; bipolar (two-tip) electrosurgery should be used whenever possible. Manufacturer guidelines should be followed for placement of electrosurgical current return pads.

2. The pacemaker should be interrogated preoperatively and postoperatively to comply with the guidelines for perioperative care from the American College of Cardiologists. The person providing the interrogation should program any rate responsiveness and all rate enhancements (e.g., dynamic A-V delay, rate search hysteresis, atrial fibrillation suppression) to *OFF*, which reduces possible confusion during the case. Despite these recommendations, devices with minute ventilation sensors continue to produce untoward behavior that has the potential to injure a patient.

3. In general, the routine use of magnets is not recommended because not every device responds to magnet placement with continuous asynchronous pacing. If the anesthetic plan includes magnet application, the magnet behavior must be identified before the start of the case. The manufacturers can provide specific information regarding any device.

4. Any device with minute ventilation sensing *must* have the minute ventilation sensor disabled.

REFERENCES

1. Madsen GM, Anderson C: Pacemaker-induced tachycardia during general anaesthesia: A case report. Br J Anaesth 63:360–361, 1989.
2. Van Hemel NM, Hamerlijnck RP, Pronk KJ, et al: Upper limit ventricular stimulation in respiratory rate responsive pacing due to electrocautery. Pacing Clin Electrophysiol 12:1720–1723, 1989.
3. Anderson C, Masden GM: Rate responsive pacemakers and anaesthesia: A consideration of possible implications. Anaesthesia 45:472–476, 1990.
4. Aldrete JA, Brown C, Daily J, et al: Pacemaker malfunction due to microcurrent injection from a bioimpedance noninvasive cardiac output monitor. J Clin Monit 11:131–133, 1995.
5. von Knobelsdorff G, Goerig M, Nagele H, et al: Interaction of frequency-adaptive pacemakers and anesthetic management: Discussion of current literature and two case reports. Anaesthetist 45:856–860, 1996.
6. Levine PA: Response to rate-adaptive cardiac pacing: Implications of environmental noise during craniotomy. Anesthesiology 87:1261, 1997.
7. Wallden J, Gupta A, Carlsen HO: Supraventricular tachycardia induced by Datex patient monitoring system. Anesth Analg 86:1339, 1998.
8. Rozner MA, Nishman RJ: Pacemaker tachycardia revisited. Anesth Analg 88:965, 1999.
9. Wong DT, Middleton W: Electrocautery-induced tachycardia in a rate-responsive pacemaker. Anesthesiology 94:710–711, 2001.
10. Rozner MA, Nishman RJ: Electrocautery-induced pacemaker tachycardia—why does this error continue? Anesthesiology 96:773–774, 2002.
11. Eagle KA, et al: ACC/AHA Guideline update on perioperative cardiovascular evaluation for noncardiac surgery. Anesth Analg 94:1052–1064, 2002.

Kristin Woodward, MD

PATIENT 47

A 3-year-old trauma patient with impaired upper extremity function

A 3-year-old boy is brought to the trauma center. He was ejected from the rear seat of a car, where he was secured by a seat belt but not in a child car seat. The paramedics state that the child was crying on their arrival at the scene. He was placed in a rigid cervical collar and positioned on a pediatric spine board. He had an obvious open humerus fracture and multiple lacerations. He was alert and crying appropriately during transfer and was accompanied by his mother, who was uninjured. Paramedics note that he is tachycardic and tachypneic with satisfactory oxygen saturation. The child is previously healthy and takes no medications. He ate lunch 30 minutes before the accident.

Physical Examination: General appearance: pale and listless. Paramedics comment he was much more active on transport. Weight 15 kg. Temperature 36.2°C; pulse 142, respirations 22; blood pressure 83/37; oxygen saturation 97% in room air. Glasgow Coma Scale score: 12; eyes open, appears confused, and withdraws to pain. Cardiac examination: tachycardic with a nonradiating systolic ejection murmur heard at the left sternal border. Pulmonary examination: lungs clear, although respirations are shallow. Abdominal and extremities: abdomen is tense and nonfocally tender to palpation; multiple lower extremity lacerations and an open left humerus fracture. Neurologic examination: listless, withdraws to pain; pupils equal and reactive; reflexes symmetric, although left upper extremity could not be rigorously tested secondary to the injury. The child has his right hand clinched, and the left hand appears flaccid.

The patient becomes more listless during the primary survey. His heart rate increases to 160 beats/min, and his systolic blood pressure falls to 60 mmHg. He becomes cyanotic, and his respiratory pattern becomes irregular. The laboratory calls and states his hematocrit is 21.7%.

Laboratory Findings: Sodium 148 mEq/L, potassium 3.4 mEq/L, creatinine 1.0 mg/dL, hematocrit 22%. Cervical spine radiographs: normal.

Questions: What is the clinical suspicion?

At what age and weight should children ride in car seats?

What immediate action should be taken in this child's care?

How should the child's spine be stabilized and intubation managed?

Compare cervical spinal cord injuries in a 3-year-old with that in an 8-year-old.

Describe the physical properties of the pediatric cervical spine that predisposes the spine to higher cervical injuries. Are children more or less predisposed to develop cervical spine injuries compared with adults?

What is SCIWORA?

What is the best way to diagnose a cervical spine injury in the pediatric patient? What physical examination features suggest cord injury?

What is the clinical suspicion? Spinal cord injury without radiologic abnormality (SCIWORA).

At what age and weight should children ride in car seats? Pediatric trauma is the number one cause of death in pediatric patients >1 year old. It accounts for 15,000 deaths per year in the United States. The use of child car restraints has reduced the number of fatalities by 71%. Infants < 20 lb should ride in a convertible infant-toddler child restraint device facing backward. Older toddlers can be placed in a similar device facing forward. Older children weighing ≤40 kg need to ride in a booster seat.

What immediate action should be taken in this child's care? Respiratory compromise is always a concern in pediatric trauma patients, and an essential first step includes establishing a definitive airway. Many causes lead to airway compromise in this patient population. Upper airway obstruction by the tongue is the most common cause and should be expected anytime there is an altered level of consciousness. Brainstem or cervical spinal cord injury can lead to hypoventilation. Hypoxemia and hypotension are often attendant to these injuries. Regardless of the cause, the child should have airway patency established (using jaw thrust and oral airway), be assist ventilated if necessary, and administered 100% oxygen. Pediatric self-inflating bags with a reservoir connected to oxygen at 10 to 15 L/min reach a fraction of inspired oxygen (FIO_2) of 60% to 95%. Oxygen saturation should be monitored continuously.

When the child is oxygenating and ventilating, measures should be taken to improve circulation. Hypotension is a sign of uncompensated shock in the pediatric patient. Adequate IV access should be established, including intraosseous access if necessary. Fluid resuscitation should include normal saline boluses at 10 to 20 mL/kg, although after initial resuscitative efforts it may be wise to change to lactated Ringer's solution. If type-specific blood is available, it can be given in 10-mL/kg boluses. Failure to improve hemodynamic stability after initial fluid challenges should prompt one to consider an emergent trip to the operating room.

How should the child's spine be stabilized and intubation managed? Craniospinal trauma always should be considered in a child who has sustained a fall from significant height or been a victim of a major mechanism motor vehicle accident. Spine immobilization begins at the scene by using a rigid cervical collar, securing on a rigid backboard with strapping and further neck immobiliza-

tion, and using log-roll precautions while maintaining the head and neck in a neutral position. Pediatric spine boards have a shallow indentation for the head to rest in; this may aid intubation because it aligns the mouth and trachea. A soft collar does not stabilize a pediatric cervical spine.

The patient is shocky, manifests a declining level of consciousness, and has an orthopedic injury that requires irrigation, débridement, and operative fixation, all suggesting the need for endotracheal intubation. When preparing to intubate, one must presume the patient has a cervical spine injury, and all airway manipulation should be made with the head and neck stabilized in a neutral position. Because all trauma patients should be assumed to have full stomachs, cricoid pressure must be applied until endotracheal intubation is established definitively. Awake fiberoptic intubation is an unlikely option in a pediatric patient without the cooperation of the patient and extensive experience performing this procedure in pediatric patients.

Compare cervical spinal cord injuries in a 3-year-old with those in an 8-year-old. Acute spinal cord injury is uncommon in infants and children but becomes increasingly common in adolescence. Spinal cord damage is more frequent in the upper cervical cord (C1–3) in children <8 years old. In older children, the location of spinal cord injury is similar to adults (C5–7).

Describe the physical properties of the pediatric cervical spine that predispose the spine to higher cervical lesions. Are children more or less predisposed to develop cervical spine injury compared with adults? Young children have more cervical spinous elasticity, the musculature supporting the neck is underdeveloped, and the occiput is large in comparison with the rest of the body, predisposing them to high cervical injuries. Interspinous ligaments are lax, and vertebral bodies are softer. This elasticity is of benefit, however, in comparison with adults because forces are distributed better and vertebral fractures are less common.

What is SCIWORA? SCIWORA is an acronym for *spinal cord injury without radiographic abnormality*. SCIORWA occurs in 5% to 55% of all pediatric spinal cord injuries, is due to the ligamentous cervical spine laxity found in children, and now is considered a major component of pediatric spinal injury. Children <8 years old are at particularly high risk for this type of injury. Although relatively infrequent when compared with older children, cervical spine injuries can be difficult to detect; a history of a major mechanism injury, close neurologic examination, and a high index of suspicion are necessary to identify such injuries. Several prehospital deaths have been attributed to mistreated cervical injuries that previously were thought to be due to head trauma. Spinal cord infarction after SCIWORA has been reported as a major cause of morbidity in this population.

What is the best way to diagnose a cervical spine injury in the pediatric patient? What physical examination features suggest cord injury? The mechanism of injury and physical examination may be the best clues to the possibility of a spinal cord injury in a pediatric patient. A thorough peripheral neurologic examination includes assessing motor, sensory, proprioception, light touch and pinprick, hot and cold, tendon reflexes, and anal tone. However, the extent of the examination varies, depending on the age of the child and the child's ability to participate in the examination. In the awake, verbal patient, complaints of numbness, tingling, or weakness may be sought. In the unconscious patient, evaluation of respiratory effort, vital signs, and reflexes may aid in the diagnosis. The positioning of the upper extremities may establish a level of spinal cord injury. Flexion at the elbows suggests that the C5 root (supplying the biceps) is intact, whereas the C6 level (supplying the triceps) is not. Intact elbow extension, impaired elbow extension (loss of triceps), and impaired motor function at the wrist suggest an injury at the C7 level. Partial cord injuries may present with flaccid paralysis, absent reflexes, and autonomic dysfunction but with sensation intact. Complete cord injuries have loss of sensation as well. Absent upper extremity tone and normal lower extremity function suggest a central-cord syndrome secondary to an extension injury. Flexion injuries cause an anterior-cord syndrome characterized by complete loss of motor, pain, and temperature function but with position and vibratory sensation maintained. Priapism also is a feature of cord injuries.

It currently is not clear what is the best radiologic study to obtain in pediatric patients when you suspect cervical spine injury. CT scans are the best way to look at the bony anatomy. MRI is the best study to evaluate the intraspinal canal or intramedullary hematomas. MRI also is best to study spinal cord tissue, ligaments, intervertebral disks, and other soft tissue structures.

The Present Patient

Because of the left upper extremity finding, this patient was treated as if there were a cervical spine injury. His airway was secured with the head and neck in the neutral position with rapid-sequence intubation with cricoid pressure. He was taken to the operating room, where he was found to have a splenic laceration. His humeral fracture was irrigated, débrided, and externally fixed. Entrapment of the radial nerve was noted at surgery, and the nerve was released. He was taken to the pediatric intensive care unit with stable vital signs. The following day he was alert with a nonfocal neurologic examination. After cervical CT and MRI scans were interpreted as normal, he was extubated.

Clinical Pearls

1. Pediatric patients have an immature and elastic spine that can lead to spinal cord injuries without injury to the bony structures. In approximately 50% to 65% of pediatric cervical spine injuries, no abnormalities are detected on plain films.

2. Patients <8 years old are more susceptible to injury at the upper cervical region (C1–3) because of the greater elasticity of supporting structures, underdeveloped neck musculature, and a disproportionately large head and occiput.

3. A careful neurologic examination in the context of a concerning mechanism of injury is essential in detecting cervical spine injuries. The inability of small children to cooperate fully renders examination difficult. Cervical spine injury should be assumed in the presence of normal radiographs until further evaluation can be undertaken. CT and MRI are useful in characterizing anatomic defects.

4. Neurologic examination should precede pharmacologic paralysis and intubation. When the child is paralyzed and sedated, examination is impossible, and the best opportunity to detect neurologic abnormalities has been lost.

REFERENCES

1. Bruce DA: Head trauma. In Fleisher GR (ed): Textbook of Pediatric Emergency Medicine, 3rd ed. Baltimore, Williams & Wilkins, 1993, pp 1102–1112.
2. Loder RT: The cervical spine. In Morrisey RT, Weinstein SL (eds): Lovell and Winter's Pediatric Orthopedics, 4th ed. Philadelphia, Lippincott-Raven, 1996, pp 763–767.
3. Rasmusen GE, Fiscus MD, Tobias JD: Perioperative anesthetic management of pediatric trauma. Anesthesiol Clin North Am 17:251–262, 1999.
4. Ross AK: Pediatric emergencies. Anesthesiol Clin North Am 19:309–337, 2001.

John D. Lockrem, MD

PATIENT 48

A 55-year-old man with "a simple case of resuscitation"

A 55-year-old man was an unrestrained vehicle driver hit broadside on the passenger side by another vehicle traveling at 25 miles per hour. Paramedics found the patient alert and complaining of abdominal and left leg pain. Pulse rate was 90 beats/min and regular, blood pressure was 100/80 mmHg, and respirations were 20/min. A rigid cervical collar was positioned, and an IV line was started. Pressure was applied to a scalp laceration. A 1-L infusion of lactated Ringer's solution was given during the 20-minute transfer to a trauma center.

Physical Examination: General appearance: Patient alert and in pain. Pulse 105; blood pressure 90/65. Initial survey revealed no airway compromise. Cardiac and pulmonary examination: heart sounds normal; lungs clear to auscultation. Abdominal examination: abdomen distended and tender, particularly in the right upper quadrant; pelvis unstable to vigorous palpation; abdominal ultrasound revealed free fluid.

Laboratory Findings: Hematocrit 34. Arterial blood gases: pH 7.15, PO_2 185, PCO_2 30, base deficit 16. Serum lactate 10 mg/dL. Two large-bore IV catheters are placed in the antecubital fossae, type O-positive blood is obtained from the blood bank, and a urethral catheter is inserted. The patient is transferred rapidly to the operating room for exploratory laparotomy. On arrival in the operating room, the patient's vital signs are unchanged, the abdomen is rigid, and the patient's skin is cool to touch. During a brief preoperative interview, the patient revealed a history of coronary artery disease with a percutaneous transluminal angioplasty performed 18 months earlier. Medications included atenolol and enalapril.

After monitors are placed and the patient is preoxygenated, a rapid-sequence induction and tracheal intubation are performed with inline cervical stabilization and cricoid pressure. Induction medications include etomidate 12 mg and succinylcholine 140 mg.

At laparotomy, a large liver laceration is bleeding profusely, and a retroperitoneal hematoma is identified in the pelvis. As per the pelvic fracture protocol, packed RBCs and fresh frozen plasma infusions are started immediately. After 6 U of packed RBCs, 4 U of fresh frozen plasma, and 6 L of lactated Ringer's solution are administered, the hematocrit is 27, lactate is 9 mg/dL, prothrombin international normalized ratio (INR) is 1.5, and platelets are 80,000. Pulse is 90 beats/min, and blood pressure is 110/85 mmHg. A pulmonary artery catheter is inserted, and the cardiac index is 3.2 L/min/m²; the oxygen consumption index is 125 mL O_2/m². Hemostasis is accomplished with an argon beam coagulator and right upper quadrant packing. The skin layer only is closed, and the patient is sent to interventional radiology for embolization of the bleeding pelvic vessels.

Questions: Define shock.
Can physiologically *driving* patients improve survival?
Are vital signs and physical examination useful to diagnose shock and guide therapy?
What is the utility of acidosis in the diagnosis of shock?
How might the state of individual organs be monitored for shock?

Define shock. Shock is not defined by blood pressure. It is a state of perfusion inadequate to support the body's oxygen needs. Oxygen metabolism is useful to describe the shock state because of the following: (1) oxygen is not stored effectively in the body and must be supplied continuously. Approximately 30% of the available oxygen is metabolized routinely during each circulation time (the oxygen extraction ratio). (2) Oxygen metabolism correlates with survival from shock. (3) Oxygen debt incurred in periods of shock continues to exist even after normalization of vital signs.

Can physiologically *driving* patients improve survival? There is a correlation between the ability to maintain oxygen delivery during consumption at stress response levels (approximately 30% above resting levels) and survival of the shock episode. Metabolic activity is increased during shock. It takes energy to mobilize white cells, to generate fibroblasts, to manufacture acute-phase reactants (including fibrinogen), and to repay oxygen debt. Patients who can generate increased metabolic activity have a survival advantage. Patients (who are often young or athletic) who independently generate a cardiac index of 4.5 $L/min/m^2$, oxygen delivery of 600 mL $O_2/min/m^2$, and an oxygen consumption index of 170 ml $O_2/min/m^2$ have been shown to have improved survival. For patients unable to respond spontaneously to this level, does it improve their survival to achieve these goals pharmacologically? Studies testing this hypothesis are inconclusive. In a prospective randomized trial of a heterogeneous group of severely injured patients, Velmahos et al failed to show an improvement in survival by using fluid resuscitation and inotropes to achieve these hemodynamic goals. Young patients tended to fare well and elderly patients fared poorly; arbitrary group standards were not shown to increase survival. Is there a middle group with limited physiologic reserve who, with vigorous fluid resuscitation, inotropic support, and enhancement of oxygen-carrying capacity, might have their survival enhanced? Using current measures of global oxygen delivery and consumption, this subgroup has yet to be identified. Until tissue metabolic needs can be quantified, clinicians are left with a basic approach to resuscitation, and the ability to respond to stress is a marker for survival rather than a specific treatment goal.

Are vital signs and physical examination useful to diagnose shock and guide therapy? As hypovolemia develops, compensatory mechanisms attempt to maintain perfusion to vital organs. Failure to recognize that a patient is in a compensated state may lead to catastrophic physiologic collapse if resuscitation is not undertaken. More so, normalization of vital signs, including urine output, with initial therapy may restore only a certain level of compensation and not address the underlying oxygen deficit.

Cool skin suggests the shock state and indicates redistribution of blood flow but is nonspecific. Tachycardia generally is present in shock, but medications such as β-blockers impair the response, sympathetic reflexes often are blunted in the elderly, and many patients show a vagal response that counteracts the heart rate increase expected. In a group of patients described by Vayer, heart rate was normal in some shock patients. Blood pressure may be well maintained by adrenergic activity until substantial degrees of hypovolemia are encountered. The shock index, the ratio of heart rate to systolic blood pressure, also has been suggested as a measure of shock. A ratio of >0.9 has been shown to be an indicator of acute circulatory failure that later would require intensive volume support. The shock index also is nonspecific, however.

What is the utility of acidosis in the diagnosis of shock? Lack of oxygen delivery to cells results in anaerobic metabolism. This is an inefficient means to produce the adenosine triphosphate and results in the generation of lactic acid. Lactic acidosis is a marker of shock. Abrahamson reported that all patients who corrected the hyperlactacidemia of shock within 24 hours survived, whereas the mortality of the rest increased in proportion to the time required to normalize the value. Lactic acidosis also has been shown to be an independent predictor for the need of blood transfusion. Sequential analysis of serum lactate levels is a valuable marker of the shock state.

Standard base deficit (BD) is the calculated amount of strong base necessary to titrate a sample of whole blood to a pH of 7.4 with a PCO_2 of 40 mmHg and a hemoglobin of 5 g/dL. This value has been shown to correlate with survival such that patients with a normal Glasgow Coma Scale score and an initial BD of ≥20 have a predicted 50% mortality. Patients with a BD of >15 have been shown to require twice the fluid and 6 times the amount of blood transfusion compared with patients with mild acidosis. Failure to correct acidosis with resuscitation is often an indication of ongoing hemorrhage.

How might the state of individual organs be monitored for shock? The concept of measuring specific organ metabolism has great appeal and likely will guide treatment in the future. Gastric tonometry is a method of assessing perfusion of the stomach and presumably the intestines. The principle is that it is possible to estimate the mucosal PCO_2 by its equilibration with the carbon dioxide in a saline-filled balloon within a hollow viscus. Using the Henderson-Hasselbalch equation, the pHi, or intramucosal pH, can be calculated. The results of studies using pHi to guide therapy are inconclusive. Similar to oxygen consumption variables, the failure to correct pHi over 24 hours predicts higher mortality, but a difference in mortality based on randomized intention to treat, using pHi as a goal of therapy, was not shown. Additionally, there are several assumptions involved that may not be valid in an individual case, and intragastric carbon dioxide may change with nasogastric suctioning and antacid therapy. As the equipment improves in reliability and ease of use, this method promises to be a useful tool. Finally, tissue oximetry has been correlated in the laboratory with perfusion, but at this stage of development, the technique is fraught with clinical problems.

Subsequently, resuscitation of the patient continued in the intensive care unit. When stabilized hemodynamically, CT scans of the head, thorax, abdomen, and pelvis were completed, and an external fixator was applied to the bony pelvis. Over the course of resuscitation, lactate levels decreased to 2 mg/dL, cardiac index increased to 4.0 L/min/m², and oxygen consumption index increased to 1.6. The abdominal packs were removed the next day; the pelvic fracture was fixed internally the next week.

The Present Patient

Despite the efforts of many and the tremendous advances in understanding, the actual tools in the hands of clinicians treating shock essentially have not changed in 20 years. It remains paramount to recognize shock at the earliest phase so that treatment can begin before perfusion is compromised. A high index of suspicion combined with clinical experience is invaluable. In the present case, members of the trauma team recognized the constellation and progression of findings associated with unstable pelvic fractures. A protocol to aggressively resuscitate such patients early in the evolution of the disease process, including early use of blood products, was developed in response to clinical observations in a specific trauma setting.

Clinical Pearls

1. There is currently no one best way to assess perfusion in the traumatically injured patient.

2. Nonetheless, important parameters to measure and trend include basic vital signs, urine output, blood gases, serum lactate, hematocrit, electrolytes, and coagulation tests.

3. Measurement of cardiac output is important in the critically injured patient. Conventionally, this requires placement of a pulmonary artery catheter, but less invasive methods, such as esophageal Doppler, thoracic impedance, transthoracic echocardiography, and sophisticated carbon dioxide monitoring, are clinically available and will be in widespread use in the near future.

4. Patients who can mount on their own a supraphysiologic response after injury seem to have a survival advantage. It is not clear as yet which patients, when driven through volume resuscitation and inotropic support to supraphysiologic parameters, are conferred a survival benefit. The state-of-the-art is insufficient to determine conclusively what individual responses should be.

5. Definitive and specific end points of resuscitation remain elusive, but substantially improved monitors are well on their way to clinical availability.

REFERENCES

1. Mullins RJ: Management of shock. In Mattox KL, Feliciano DV, Moore EE (eds): Trauma, 4th ed. New York, Mc-Graw-Hill, 2000, pp 195–232.
2. Stene JK, Grande CM: Anesthesia for trauma. In Miller RD (ed): Anesthesia, 5th ed. New York, Churchill Livingstone, 2000, pp 2157–2172.
3. Velmahos GC, Demetriades D, Shoemaker WC, et al: Endpoints of resuscitation of critically injured patients: Normal or supranormal. Ann Surg 232:409–418, 2000.
4. Dabrowski GP, Steinberg SM, Ferrara JJ, et al: A critical assessment of endpoints of shock resuscitation. Surg Clin North Am 80:825–844, 2000.
5. Orlinsky M, Shoemaker W, Reis ED, et al: Current controversies in shock and resuscitation. Surg Clin North Am 81:1217–1262, 2001.

Willem Nel, MD

PATIENT 49

A 65-year-old woman with a posttraumatic painful wrist

A 65-year-old woman reports that she slipped and fell 6 weeks ago. Radiographs of the right wrist revealed a nondisplaced distal radioulnar fracture. She was treated with a forearm cast; pain was managed with opioid analgesics and nonsteroidal antiinflammatory drugs. The pain diminished after 36 to 48 hours, but then increased substantially over the subsequent 6 to 7 weeks. Follow-up radiograph at 4 weeks showed satisfactory healing without evidence of nonunion or infection, and the cast was removed. Other causes for persisting pain, such as cervical spine pathology, nerve damage, and systemic disease were ruled out, and she was referred to a chronic pain clinic for further evaluation.

Besides complaints of burning pain, the patient states her right hand is chronically swollen, she has difficulty moving her fingers and wrist, and her hand and forearm intermittently turns cold and blue. Her skin is also extremely sensitive to light touch.

Physical Examination: Targeted examination of right upper extremity compared with left upper extremity: edema, pallor, and hyperhydrosis of the right hand and wrist area. Right distal forearm was cooler than left by 0.8°C when measured using an infrared thermometer.

Laboratory Findings: CBC and C-reactive protein: Normal. Radiographs of wrist and forearm, mammogram, and MRI of cervical spine: All normal. Full-body thermogram: decreased heat emission in the right forearm and hand.

Questions: What is the operating diagnosis?
How should a patient presenting with complaints of chronic pain be evaluated?
Describe the current diagnostic criteria for CRPS.
What is the role of the sympathetic nervous system in producing chronic pain states?
Discuss common tests for evaluating complaints of chronic pain.
How should patients with chronic pain syndromes be treated?
How is SMP differentiated from SIP?
What is the benefit of physical therapy?
Besides sympathetic nerve blocks, how else might a patient's pair be treated?
What medications are effective for the treatment of neuropathic pain?
What therapies are available for patients who do not experience substantial benefit from sympathetic nerve blocks or neuropathic pain medications?

What is the operating diagnosis? Chronic regional pain syndrome (CRPS) type 1.

How should a patient presenting with complaints of chronic pain be evaluated? When diagnosis of any chronic pain syndrome is contemplated, a thorough review of symptoms and discussion of past medical history, including psychological and social history, is necessary. Subsequently, careful examination of the objective physical findings and the results of special testing are important to rule out any other condition that might explain the patient's symptoms.

Describe the current diagnostic criteria for CRPS. Chronic pain syndromes have been recognized for >100 years but have suffered from inconsistencies in their definitions. In 1995, the International Association for the Study of Pain redefined and established diagnostic criteria for painful disorders previously known as *reflex sympathetic dystrophy* and *causalgia*. These disorders were renamed *chronic regional pain syndrome type 1* and *type 2*.

CRPS type 1 has a history of trauma to the affected area associated with pain that is disproportionate to the inciting event in duration or intensity or both. Neuropathic pain, defined as pain in the absence of continuous nociceptive input secondary to altered neural structure or function or both, is usually present and can be characterized by a burning sensation, allodynia, dysesthesias, and anesthesia dolorosa. There are also one or more of the following asymmetric findings:

- Motor dysfunction (movement disorder of the affected area, weakness, tremor, exaggerated tendon reflexes, dystonia, or myoclonic jerks)
- Sympathetic dysfunction (temperature differential of >0.5°C between the affected and unaffected extremity, increased pilomotor activity, color changes)
- Edema and sudomotor dysfunction (hyperhydrosis)
- Dystrophic and atrophic changes (increased or decreased hair and nail growth, skin changes and ulcers, contractures, muscle wasting, bone changes)

In addition to the physical syndrome, there is often an associated psychiatric disorder. Psychiatric disturbances may contribute to the pain syndrome or be a consequence of experiencing chronic pain. Depression, sleep disturbances, emotional lability, and strained interpersonal relations necessitate the involvement of a mental health provider.

CRPS type 2 is a chronic pain syndrome characterized by neuropathic pain that is isolated to the distribution of a specific major nerve after injury to that nerve. There also can be associated findings similar to CRPS type 1 but confined to the distribution of the injured nerve. CRPS type 2 can progress to CRPS type 1. If any of the above-mentioned symptoms and signs occur outside the distribution of the injured nerve, the diagnosis of CRPS type 1 should be considered.

What is the role of the sympathetic nervous system in producing chronic pain states? There are several theories that attempt to explain the pathophysiology of chronic pain syndromes. To understand these mechanisms, it is important to review the pertinent neuroanatomy and physiology of pain transmission and modulation.

The pain transmission pathway is in essence a three-neuron system. The first-order neuron transmits pain impulses from the periphery to the second-order neuron cell body located in the dorsal horn of the spinal cord gray matter. The second-order neuron projects to the thalamus, where it in turn synapses with the third-order neuron that ultimately projects to the sensory cortex where pain is perceived. This pathway has numerous connections at different levels, including the sympathetic nervous system (spinal cord and supraspinal levels) and motivational-affective areas of the brain. Pain perception initiates a response that is designed to protect the body, isolate the injured area, and prevent further injury. Nociceptive inputs from A-delta and C fibers are transmitted to the dorsal horn, where these fibers synapse with nociceptive-specific and wide dynamic range (WDR) second-order neurons. WDR neurons respond to nociceptive and nonnociceptive input. This is an important property that plays a central role in the production of neuropathic pain. With continuous afferent nociceptive input, WDR neurons become hyperexcitable (*windup*). This is a normal response that initially facilitates pain transmission, but also activates the pain inhibition system. The inhibitory system consists of descending inhibitory pathways that are facilitated via α_2-adrenergic, serotoninergic, and opioid receptor activation and an intrinsic spinal cord cholinergic inhibitory system. WDR neurons also activate the preganglionic sympathetic cell bodies in the spinal cord leading to increased sympathetic activity. In some patients, the continued hyperactive state of the WDR neurons owing to ongoing nociceptive input leads to failure of the inhibitory pathway. This failure results in continued pain even in the absence of the original noxious stimulus. The sympathetic nervous system can be involved in the maintenance of neuropathic pain by its role in activation of WDR neurons. There is evidence of abnormal interaction between the postganglionic sympathetic nerves and sensory afferents in the periphery. The exact mechanism is unknown, but tonic activity of the sympathetic nerves and adrenoreceptors on the afferent nociceptors might play a role. This continuous interaction between the afferent sensory neurons and the efferent sympathetic nervous system results in a self-propagating reflex arch that activates pain impulses in the absence of a noxious stimulus. This reflex sympathetic hyperactivity explains some of the symptoms and signs present in CRPS.

Discuss common tests for evaluating complaints of chronic pain. Thermography measures body temperature and is normally symmetric. Asymmetry, either hyperthermia or hypothermia, can be an indication of sympathetic dysfunction. Three-phase bone scans detect areas of increased bone turnover that are present with increased sympathetic activity. Radiographs reveal areas of disuse osteoporosis resulting from chronic pain. These tests and their findings are not unique to CRPS and should be interpreted in context. Initiating treatment should not be delayed, however, while awaiting the results of diagnostic batteries when CRPS is suspected because early intervention is an important factor in the successful treatment of chronic pain states.

How should patients with chronic pain syndromes be treated? A multidisciplinary approach is necessary and may involve occupational and physical therapy and psychiatric counseling as has been discussed. The involvement of complementary services should be individualized to the patient's needs. It is important to set realistic expectations before initiating treatment for any chronic painful condition. It is important to determine the role of the sympathetic nervous system in the maintenance of chronic pain syndromes because this information directs the clinician's treatment plan. Sympathetic nerve blocks are done as diagnostic and therapeutic interventions. If blockade of the sympathetic nerves results in pain relief, the pain syndrome is termed *sympathetically maintained pain* (SMP) versus *sympathetically independent pain* (SIP).

How is SMP differentiated from SIP? Care should be taken to perform pure sympathetic blocks to differentiate between SMP and SIP. Detailed knowledge of the anatomy of the sympathetic nervous system and training in performing specific sympathetic blocks are necessary. The use of fluoroscopy greatly enhances accuracy and success in performing these blocks. The most common sympathetic blocks include stellate ganglion blocks for upper extremity sympathetic blockade and lumbar sympathetic blocks for lower extremity sympathetic blockade. Because the sympathetic chains are in close proximity to somatic nerves, these nerves sometimes can be inadvertently blocked; the patient needs to be informed on what to expect from these blocks and instructed to report the exact physical effects after each block. The patient should experience an increase in temperature in the blocked extremity without any sensory or motor blockade, and the degree and duration of pain relief should be noted. The experienced effect has to be reproducible by repeating the block, usually three to six times, each time taking care to ensure pure sympathetic blockade. Only blocks that are devoid of somatic blockade can determine SMP versus SIP. Besides the diagnostic benefit, a series of sympathetic blocks may diminish pain substantially and for maximal effectiveness should be initiated as soon as possible. Some patients have lasting pain relief with a reduction of pain after each block; this leads to the resolution of pain or reduction to an acceptable level, signaling the end point in treatment. A patient who does not respond to sympathetic blocks has SIP, and management is directed to modalities other than sympathetic blockade.

Another group of patients has temporary reduction of pain after each block, but their pain returns to baseline. These patients may be candidates for a sympathectomy, which may be achieved surgically; with radiofrequency ablation; or after injection of neurolytic agents such as absolute alcohol, glycerol, or phenol. It is important to identify placebo responders. These patients typically have great pain relief after the first blocks, but their duration and intensity of pain relief diminish after subsequent blocks. These patients are not candidates for further sympathetic blocks or neurolytic procedures.

What is the benefit of physical therapy? The most important goal in physical therapy is preserving the function of the affected area. Motor dysfunction is a hallmark of CRPS and requires aggressive therapy to prevent loss of range of motion and contracture formation. Therapy can be facilitated with adequate analgesics and often is most tolerable and effective immediately after a sympathetic block. Patients who have significant spasticity or muscle cramping may benefit from antispasmodics and muscle relaxants, including cyclobenzaprine, tizanidine, carisoprodol, and baclofen.

Besides sympathetic nerve blocks, how else might a patient's pain be treated? Neuropathic pain is difficult to control with traditional analgesics. Nonetheless, combinations of acetaminophen, nonsteroidal antiinflammatory drugs, tramadol, and opioid analgesics should be used to provide pain relief. Care should be exercised when prescribing opioid analgesics because these medications are not effective for neuropathic pain, and doses can escalate quickly, creating opioid dependency. The patient should be informed of the side effects of all medications prescribed.

What medications are effective for the treatment of neuropathic pain? Medications with proven clinical efficacy in the management of neuropathic pain include tricyclic antidepressants, such as amitriptyline and nortriptyline, and anticonvulsants, such as gabapentin and topiramate. Tricyclic antidepressants modulate pain through augmentation of the descending inhibitory pain pathway neurotransmitters and through antidepressant effects. The anticonvulsants suppress abnormal and ectopic electrical activity of injured nerves. The end points of dosing these drugs are relief of pain, development of side effects, or reaching the maximal dose. Before prescribing these drugs, the clinician should be familiar with their effects and side effects.

What therapies are available for patients who do not experience substantial benefit from sympathetic nerve blocks or neuropathic pain medications? Patients who fail relatively conservative management modalities might be candidates for dorsal column stimulation, or in rare cases, a select group of patients might benefit from intrathecal opioid delivery systems. Dorsal column stimulation inhibits dorsal horn cells, including the nociceptive and sympathetic cells; activates A-beta fibers, inhibiting pain transmission (gate control theory); and evokes a neurohumoral response that elevates endorphin and serotonin levels, augmenting descending inhibitory pathways. Intrathecal opioid delivery provides profound analgesia, and this form of opioid delivery is especially beneficial to patients who are taking large doses of oral opioids. The side-effect profile is significantly better because only a fraction of opioid is used in relation to oral therapy. Tolerance develops and care needs to be taken to escalate dosing over months and years. This form of opioid delivery also can be abused, and careful patient selection is important.

The Present Patient

Aggressive therapy was instituted in the patient, beginning with a series of stellate ganglion blocks, followed immediately by physical therapy. Analgesia was provided with oxycodone 20 mg twice daily, ibuprofen 800 mg 3 times daily, and gabapentin titrated over a 2-week period to 900 mg 3 times daily. Her symptoms improved dramatically over 3 weeks until she had only minor residual pain. Oxycodone and ibuprofen were withdrawn over 10 days and replaced by tramadol 50 mg 3 times daily. Gabapentin was continued for another 3 months and stopped. The patient continues to have minor pain that is controlled with tramadol 50 mg twice daily. She continues with motion therapy of her wrist and hand to maintain function and has had a good outcome with only minor residual disability.

Clinical Pearls

1. CRPS should be considered when the degree of pain is unusual for the injury and is associated with one or more asymmetric findings, such as motion abnormalities, sympathetic dysfunction, sudomotor dysfunction, swelling, and dystrophic or atrophic changes.

2. Early diagnosis and prompt, aggressive treatment are imperative. This disease responds favorably to early treatment and is significantly resistant to improvement when well established.

3. A multimodal approach to treatment should be considered that includes sympathetic blockade and motion therapy complemented by analgesics and neuropathic pain medication.

4. CRPS often is associated with significant depression and psychosocial disorders. This necessitates the involvement of mental health providers with specific experience in the management of chronic pain patients.

5. Realistic goals need to be set as end points to treatment. The patient must understand that some degree of permanent disability is possible, and a 50% reduction in baseline pain would be considered a good outcome.

REFERENCES

1. Monti DA, Herring CL, Schwartzman RJ, et al: Personality assessment of patients with complex regional pain syndrome type I. Clin J Pain 14:295–302, 1998.
2. Oerlemans HM, Oostendorp RA, de Boo T, et al: Signs and symptoms in complex regional pain syndrome type I/reflex sympathetic dystrophy: Judgment of the physician versus objective measurement. Clin J Pain 15:224–232, 1999.
3. Wilson PR: Complex regional pain syndrome–reflex sympathetic dystrophy. Curr Treat Options Neurol 1:466–472, 1999.
4. Heaver JE, Willis WD: Pain pathways: Anatomy and physiology. In Raj PP (ed): Practical Management of Pain, 3rd ed. 2000, pp 107–116.
5. Johnson BW: Pain mechanisms: Anatomy, physiology and neurochemistry. In Raj PP (ed): Practical Management of Pain, 3rd ed. 2000, pp 117–144.
6. Kirkpatrick AF (ed): Reflex Sympathetic Dystrophy Syndrome Association of America (RSDSA), Clinical Practice Guidelines, 2nd ed. 2000.
7. Klein F, Riedl B, Sieweke N, et al: Neurological findings in complex regional pain syndromes — analysis of 145 cases. Acta Neurol Scand 101:262–269, 2000.
8. Harden RN: A clinical approach to complex regional pain syndrome. Clin J Pain 16(2 suppl):S26–32, 2000.
9. Stanton-Hicks M: Complex regional pain syndrome (type I, RSD; type II, causalgia): Controversies. Clin J Pain 16(2 suppl):S33–40, 2000.

Howard J. Miller, MD

PATIENT 50

A 46-year-old woman fails to awaken after general anesthesia

Preoperative Evaluation: A 46-year old, 75 kg woman, with a septic left knee joint underwent emergency surgical irrigation and debridement under general anesthesia. She had a long history of smoking, but was otherwise healthy. She last ate food 3 hours prior to arriving in the operating room. She did not regularly take any medications and she had no known drug allergies. She had one previous operation, emergent exploratory laparotomy for a ruptured ectopic pregnancy. Records from her previous operation described that she had received a transfusion of two units of packed red blood cells prior to her surgery and that she underwent general anesthesia, with a rapid sequence induction, without intraoperative or postoperative incident.

Intraoperative Events: The patient underwent a general anesthetic. A rapid sequence induction was performed, uneventfully, with sodium thiopental 300 mg and succinylcholine 100 mg. She was intubated with a 7.0 I.D. endotracheal tube. Maintenance was with oxygen, isoflurane, and fentanyl (total dose of 200 micrograms). No further relaxants were administered. The operation lasted 90 minutes.

At the conclusion of surgery, the patient failed to breathe spontaneously despite an arterial saturation of 100%, end-tidal carbon dioxide of 50 mm Hg, and end-tidal isoflurane concentration of 0.1%. Peripheral stimulation of the ulnar nerve revealed fade with train of four.

Questions: What does peripheral nerve suggest as to the mechanism for failure to arouse?
Discuss the laboratory tests available to confirm the diagnosis.
What is the treatment?
Why was this event not observed during the patient's prior surgery?

What does peripheral nerve suggest as to the mechanism for failure to arouse? Atypical plasma cholinesterase

Succinylcholine (Sch) is a depolarizing muscle relaxant that mimics acetylcholine (Ach) at the motor end-plate, binding to the Ach receptor, resulting in depolarization. Unlike Ach, Sch does not readily dissociate from the receptor, possibly causing a desensitization of the receptor and a flaccid paralysis. Succinylcholine is hydrolyzed to choline and succinylmonocholine by pseudocholinesterase, an enzyme manufactured in the liver and usually abundant in the plasma. Pseudocholinesterase may be deficient quantitatively or qualitatively. Quantitiative deficiencies (decreased amounts of *normal* enzyme) may be noted in severe liver disease, malnutrition, catabolic states, malignancies, burns, during pregnancy, or with administration of oral contraceptives. More difficult to characterize are qualitative deficiencies of plasma cholinesterase (*abnormal* enzyme).

Discuss the laboratory tests available to confirm the diagnosis. Two alleles are associated with production of pseudocholinesterase. An individual may be homozygous normal (N/N), homozygous atypical (A/A), or heterozygous (N/A). Several atypical enzymatic forms are described by the laboratory analysis necessary to characterize them, and they include dibucaine-resistant, fluoride-resistant, and silent (meaning there are no satisfactory laboratory tests) qualitative pseudocholinesterase deficiencies.

The dibucaine-resistant assay for plasma cholinesterase is the most common qualitative test used. The incidence of the heterozygote form (N/A) is 1/25. The homozygous atypical incidence (A/A) is 1/2500. Kalow and Genest, in 1957, described the "**dibucaine number**" assay to characterize and differentiate this enzymatic form from the natural allelic state. Described simplistically, serum from the patient under study is combined with dibucaine and benzoylcholine and the degree of hydrolysis determined. It should be noted that in the absence of dibucaine, serum from all allelic states would result in total hydrolysis of benzoylcholine. However, the addition of dibucaine will impair hydrolysis to different extents, depending upon the allelic state as described below:

Serum from N/N genotype + benzoylcholine + dibucaine → 20% hydrolysis or **80% inhibition.**
Serum from N/A genotype + benzoylcholine + dibucaine → 40–60% hydrolysis or **40–60% inhibition.**
Serum from A/A + benzoylcholine + dibucaine → 80% hydrolysis or **20%inhibibition.**

The percentage that dibucaine inhibits the hydrolysis of benzoylcholine by pseudocholinesterase is the dibucaine number. Therefore, the dibucaine numbers for the various genotypes are as follows: N/N = 80, A/N = 40–60, and A/A = 20.

While normal pseudocholinesterase will result in a termination of Sch effect in 5–10 minutes, the heterozygous atypical form will likely have a prolongation of Sch effect of about 25 minutes, often clinically insignificant. However, the homozygous-atypical individual may have a duration of Sch action of 3–4 hours or more, certainly significant.

Under normal circumstances, train-of-four stimulation of a peripheral nerve in the presence of succinylcholine results in equal declines in each component of the train of four and no tetanic fade. This has been termed a "Phase I" blockade. However, with excessive doses of Sch, typically 7–10 mg/kg, or during prolonged Sch infusions not guided by peripheral nerve stimulation, a different pattern of electrical stimulation is observed. Fade on train-of-four stimulation (progressive declines in successive twitches) and tetanic fade associated with administration of Sch is termed "Phase II" blockade, and the exact etiology of this phenomenon is unknown. Besides excessive dosing and prolonged infusions, this pattern of stimulation could be observed if usual doses of Sch were not being metabolized normally (usually 90–95% of a normal Sch dose is quickly metabolized after administration, leaving only a small quantity to reach the neuromuscular junction). This situation is consistent with pseudocholinesterase deficiency and was observed in this patient. The patient's pseudocholinesterse deficiency was not recognized during previous Sch administering because packed red blood cells were administered prior to that procedure. Banked blood maintains substantial pseudocholinesterase activity for at least four weeks.

What is the treatment? The treatment of Phase II blockade is controversial. Though some have attempted to reverse a Phase II block with anticholinesterases, e.g.. edrophonium or neostigmine, reversal is not always reliable. Another solution is to transfuse blood products, but this is not an appropriate use of these products due to the risks associated with transfusion, i.e. transmission of infectious disease and transfusion reactions. Perhaps the best alternative is to sedate and ventilate the patient until the patient's full strength returns and the patient can adequately maintain their own oxygenation and ventilation once extubated.

The patient was ventilated until normal peripheral nerve stimulation was observed. Sedation was discontinued, and she was extubated when she met the usual criteria; further recovery was unremarkable. A sample of the patient's blood was sent for determination of dibucaine number, which was found to be 35. The patient was diagnosed as being homozygous for dibucaine-resistant atypical pseudocholinesterase and was counseled to inform all future anesthesiologists and health care providers of this finding.

Clinical Pearls

1. It is prudent for the practitioner to establish the return of train-of-four, using a peripheral nerve stimulator, after giving succinylcholine and before the administration of additional muscle relaxants. Failure to observe return of normal twitches suggests the presence of atypical plasma cholinesterase.

2. Substantial pseudocholinesterase activity persists in stored blood products for over 4 weeks and can obscure the presence of atypical cholinesterase forms. Blood products are not normally considered appropriate treatment for atypical plasma cholinesterase.

3. A key management strategy for prolonged paralysis of any nature is to maintain a controlled airway, mechanically ventilate the patient with supplemental oxygen, and provide appropriate sedation until the diagnosis has been determined and appropriate treatment instituted, or until spontaneous return of full muscular activity is achieved.

4. While administration of anticholinesterases in the setting of Phase II blockade had been suggested, supporting the patient as in 3 above is highly recommended.

5. While not discussed, the nondepolarizing muscle relaxant mivacurium, also metabolized by pseudocholinesterase, might lead to a similar clinical picture in the presence of atypical plasma cholinesterase. Reversal with anticholinesterases should be undertaken with the greatest care, as overcoming the competitive antagonism may be difficult when mivacurium is not being metabolized.

REFERENCES

1. Pantuck EJ: Plasma cholinesterase: gene and variations. Anesth Analg 77:380–386, 1993.
2. Lovely MJ, Patteson SK, Beuerlein FJ, Chesney JT: Perioperative blood transfusion may conceal atypical pseudocholinesterase. Anesth Analg 70:326, 1990.
3. Donati F, Bevan DR: Long-term succinylcholine infusion during isoflurane anesthesia. Anesthesiology 58:6, 1983.
4. Viby-Mogensen J: Succinylcholine neuromuscular blockade in subjects heterozygous for abnormal plasma cholinesterase. Anesthesiology 55:231, 1981.
6. Viby-Mogensen J: Succinylcholine neuromuscular blockade in subjects homozygous for atypical plasma cholinesterase. Anesthesiology 55:429, 1981.
7. Kalow W, Genest K: A method for the detection of atypical forms of human serum cholinesterase: Determination of dibucaine numbers. Can J Biochem Physiol 35:339–346, 1957.

INDEX